Intelligent Systems Reference Library

Volume 233

Series Editors

Janusz Kacprzyk, Polish Academy of Sciences, Warsaw, Poland

Lakhmi C. Jain, KES International, Shoreham-by-Sea, UK

The aim of this series is to publish a Reference Library, including novel advances and developments in all aspects of Intelligent Systems in an easily accessible and well structured form. The series includes reference works, handbooks, compendia, textbooks, well-structured monographs, dictionaries, and encyclopedias. It contains well integrated knowledge and current information in the field of Intelligent Systems. The series covers the theory, applications, and design methods of Intelligent Systems. Virtually all disciplines such as engineering, computer science, avionics, business, e-commerce, environment, healthcare, physics and life science are included. The list of topics spans all the areas of modern intelligent systems such as: Ambient intelligence, Computational intelligence, Social intelligence, Computational neuroscience, Artificial life, Virtual society, Cognitive systems, DNA and immunity-based systems, e-Learning and teaching, Human-centred computing and Machine ethics, Intelligent control, Intelligent data analysis, Knowledge-based paradigms, Knowledge management, Intelligent agents, Intelligent decision making, Intelligent network security, Interactive entertainment, Learning paradigms, Recommender systems, Robotics and Mechatronics including human-machine teaming, Self-organizing and adaptive systems, Soft computing including Neural systems, Fuzzy systems, Evolutionary computing and the Fusion of these paradigms, Perception and Vision, Web intelligence and Multimedia.

Indexed by SCOPUS, DBLP, zbMATH, SCImago.

All books published in the series are submitted for consideration in Web of Science.

Janmenjoy Nayak · Asit Kumar Das ·
Bighnaraj Naik · Saroj K. Meher · Sheryl Brahnam
Editors

Nature-Inspired Optimization Methodologies in Biomedical and Healthcare

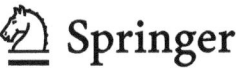

Editors
Janmenjoy Nayak
P.G. Department of Computer Science
Maharaja Sriram Chandra Bhanja Deo
(MSCB) University
Baripada, Odisha, India

Bighnaraj Naik
Department of Computer Applications
Veer Surendra Sai University of Technology
Sambalpur, Odisha, India

Sheryl Brahnam
Department of Information Technology
and Cybersecurity
Missouri State University
Springfield, MO, USA

Asit Kumar Das
Department of Computer Science
and Technology
Indian Institute of Engineering Science
and Technology
Howrah, West Bengal, India

Saroj K. Meher
Systems Science and Informatics Unit
Indian Statistical Institute (ISI)
Bangalore, India

ISSN 1868-4394　　　　　　ISSN 1868-4408　(electronic)
Intelligent Systems Reference Library
ISBN 978-3-031-17546-6　　ISBN 978-3-031-17544-2　(eBook)
https://doi.org/10.1007/978-3-031-17544-2

© The Editor(s) (if applicable) and The Author(s), under exclusive license to Springer Nature Switzerland AG 2023

This work is subject to copyright. All rights are solely and exclusively licensed by the Publisher, whether the whole or part of the material is concerned, specifically the rights of translation, reprinting, reuse of illustrations, recitation, broadcasting, reproduction on microfilms or in any other physical way, and transmission or information storage and retrieval, electronic adaptation, computer software, or by similar or dissimilar methodology now known or hereafter developed.

The use of general descriptive names, registered names, trademarks, service marks, etc. in this publication does not imply, even in the absence of a specific statement, that such names are exempt from the relevant protective laws and regulations and therefore free for general use.

The publisher, the authors, and the editors are safe to assume that the advice and information in this book are believed to be true and accurate at the date of publication. Neither the publisher nor the authors or the editors give a warranty, expressed or implied, with respect to the material contained herein or for any errors or omissions that may have been made. The publisher remains neutral with regard to jurisdictional claims in published maps and institutional affiliations.

This Springer imprint is published by the registered company Springer Nature Switzerland AG
The registered company address is: Gewerbestrasse 11, 6330 Cham, Switzerland

Foreword

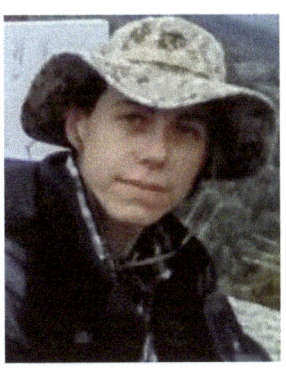

Today's healthcare industries yield critical and massive amounts of data from various sources such as biomedical research, hospital records, clinical records of patients, clinical examination results, and different health IoT devices. These data require proper management and analysis to produce meaningful information. Managing and analyzing this vast data resource with conventional methods is time-consuming and expensive. Therefore, by providing relevant solutions for improving healthcare services, industries are hunting for lower costs, better outcomes, and value-based solutions to generate and systematically analyze the vast data resources now available.

Emerging technologies based on optimization methodologies are vital in handling this vast amount of data. Having focused my research the last couple of years on new optimization methods for generating ensembles, I find the chapters in this book, *Nature-Inspired Optimization Methodologies in Biomedical and Healthcare*, highly suggestive. The bulk of the chapters offers many new algorithms and practical tips that researchers and practitioners should find beneficial. Different types of medical data are addressed, and various methods for combining nature-inspired optimizations with deep learning and other neural networks are presented. This volume also provides a literature review covering the complete history of nature-inspired optimization, an overview of the state-of-art, and many valuable references.

Prof. Loris Nanni
Dipartimento di Ingegneria
dell'Informazione
University of Padova
Padua, Italy

Preface

Healthcare always provides a wider scope of research among the researchers because of the drastic increase in healthcare technology from the last few decades. In the current decade, intelligent healthcare is providing many advances in the diagnosis and other medical treatments. Generally, healthcare is described as the mechanism of diagnosing illness and other intellectual and physical downturn to enhance the quality of human health. Therefore, healthcare systems have been established to reach the requirements of the indigent people. The healthcare systems require precise information and adequately managed health facilities to provide services to the needy people. Several intelligent healthcare systems are able to provide reliable solution for many complex medical problems. Proper measurement of results plays an important role in the healthcare and biomedical fields as it forms the base for medical evaluation, diagnosis, and prognosis process. In addition, the present healthcare system is also facing many difficulties such as time delay in diagnosis process, lack of important information of patient, exploration of voluminous patient data, and so on. Therefore, proper measurement of results and delivering quality service to patients are considered as the significant goals of healthcare system. Moreover, the increasing amount of patient and other medical data with the convergence of related healthcare domains is leading the medical research into a different direction. The current trends and techniques give unique opportunity for solving different trivial tasks of medical and healthcare. But such techniques are on a real need of extracting the convenient patterns for the characterization of target problems and developing intelligent mechanism underlying the noisy and fabricated data, which may ultimately transform such knowledge into real-life solutions. In recent decades, nature-inspired optimization algorithms have gained rising popularity in solving complex problems of different domains because of the knowledge discovery and evolution of natural computing. The ability to resolve the non-deterministic polynomial problems is considered as the fundamental cause for the popularity of nature-inspired optimization approaches. As nature-inspired optimization algorithms offer robust computational tools for complex optimization problem, numerous algorithms have been developed by the researchers. Currently, nature-inspired optimization approaches have been utilized in biomedical and healthcare system to solve the key issues of healthcare sector such as providing quality service at low cost and to enhance quality of healthcare services.

The problems in the healthcare industry, such as predicting, planning, scheduling, have not been effectively formulated, and many nature-inspired optimization algorithms are not well known to the healthcare sector. Therefore, the primary purpose of this book is to provide a detailed perception of the application of nature-inspired optimization algorithms in the healthcare sector to provide effective computer-aided diagnosis and prediction for preventing disease at the early stages. With this reasoning, the proposed book starts with the fundamentals of nature-inspired optimization techniques, implementations, and mechanisms allied with them. It is a pile of various recently developed nature-inspired optimizations and other amalgamated approaches utilized for the field of healthcare and bioengineering. Besides, the book is an ample collection of the latest and advanced intelligent methods integrated with nature-inspired optimization approaches. It will head for the challenges encountered by the hospitals and healthcare organizations for practical investigation, depository, and analysis of data. Further, the book will assist in focusing on future research challenges and guide the practitioners and researchers. Also, a particular prominence will be on the accumulation of applicable advanced mechanisms, automated tools, and possible approaches for resolving sophisticated biomedical problems to data scientists, experts, and research scholars in a broader sense. In addition, many researchers and students would benefit from this book as it provides in-depth knowledge of the theory and application of nature-inspired optimization approaches and allied hybrid technologies in the healthcare sector. Moreover, researchers can also have the scope to find a lot of unexplored areas to carry out novel research in the future. This volume comprises 12 chapters and is organized as follows:

Chapter 1 provides a brief description of the most significant nature-inspired optimization algorithms that have been developed from the past to the present and their role in solving computationally complex problems in real-life applications of various domains. In addition, Mohammed Aarif K. O. et al. have also provided an overview of the performance of different nature-inspired optimization algorithms along with their challenges and further research directions.

In Chap. 2, an inferring classic model has been proposed by R. Jayashree for the efficient prediction of spreading patterns of coronavirus infection using swarm learning approach known as the Recursive Particle Swarm Optimization algorithm. In the proposed model, author makes use of recursive particle swarm optimization algorithm for finding the optimal hyperparameters. Moreover, the recursive particle swarm optimization algorithm automatically updates the features whenever infected person transfers from the state of symptomatic to recovery/death or asymptomatic to symptomatic/recovery because of its dynamic nature. The suggested model has been evaluated using data provided by the official coronavirus website, and the results indicate that the suggested model attains better accuracy in predicting patterns of coronavirus infection in comparison to the Bayesian Monte Carlo version.

Chapter 3 is about developing an optimized ensemble learning machine-based framework for the accurate prediction of obesity levels from physical conditions and eating habits. The system developed by Geetanjali Bhoi et al. makes use of gradient boosting decision tree approach for handling noisy and high variance data. Moreover, the suggested approach also makes use of artificial particle optimization approach for finding optimal hyperparameters of the model. The authors have identified 16 distinct factors relevant to obesity and determined age, gender, height, weight, and family history with overweight as the most significant factors of predicting obesity levels. The developed system has been evaluated, and results indicate that the developed system efficiently predicts distinct obesity level of patients when compared with other similar approaches.

In Chap. 4, Natalia Obukhova et al. suggested an approach for color correction with minimum error using the perceptual metric CIEDE2000. In this approach, a separate target function is used to represent each color of the palette. The approach also makes use of third-order polynomial with 11 coefficients to represent each color channel as the algorithm matches with the palette. Basically, the algorithm used to estimate transformation function coefficients based on multi-objective optimization involves three steps. In the first step, the starting point is determined by the least square method. Next, Broyden–Fletcher–Goldfarb–Shanno algorithm is used for performing line search. Finally, in the last step, Nelder-Mead Algorithm has been used in the solution refinement. The developed approach has been validated, and results indicate that for all colors from palette, error rate is less than 1. After matching, if the error is more than 1 then the difference between colors will be visible to observer.

Chapter 5 developed a data-driven heart failure detection model using extreme gradient boosting an ensemble learning technique. The system developed by Etuari Oram et al. uses of dataset consisting of clinical and lifestyle information of 299 heart failure patients, including 105 women and 194 men. 13 features are captured to represent the clinical and lifestyle information of heart failure patients. Then the optimal parameters of extreme gradient boosting ensemble learning technique such as subsample, L2 regularization, L1 regularization, learning rate, max depth, and max delta step have been determined using Gravitational search algorithm. Finally, the model has been evaluated, and empirical results indicate developed system obtains better performance when compared with other similar approaches.

Chapter 6 introduces an approach that combines the capability of various nature-inspired optimization algorithms along with a learning model of artificial neural networks for generating more rationalized and precise output of the neural network. Initially, the functionality of various nature-inspired optimization algorithms, such as genetic algorithm, particle swarm optimization algorithm, differential evolution, colony optimization algorithm, bat algorithm and black hole algorithm along with their advantages and disadvantages, has been explained by Soumen Kumar Pati et al. Then, the nature-inspired optimization algorithms have been integrated with artificial neural networks to solve complex optimization problems. From the experimental results, it is concluded that hybrid models have produced better performance in terms of accuracy, precision, and convergence on global optima.

Chapter 7 is about extracting relevant information from medical reports using fuzzy theory and nature-inspired optimization algorithms. Initially, sentence tokenization has been applied by Chirantana Mallick and Asit Kumar Das to pre-process the extracted data. Then, BioBERT model has been applied to perform removal of stopwords, stemming operations and vectorization. Therefore, a structured data is produced in feature extraction for processing each report and then similar sentences are clustered using Fuzzy C-means clustering. Next, clusters are defuzzified and base summaries are constructed using multiple similarity clustering measures and a bi-objective strength measure. Finally, report summary has been produced by using an ensemble summarising approach, which makes use of Pareto evolutionary algorithm. Generally, the method has two objective functions. The method has been evaluated using PubMED MEDLINE dataset that contains publicly available biomedical reports and outcomes reveal that the recommended method obtained better performance in comparison with related state-of-the-art methods.

Chapter 8 aims in developing an efficient prediction model for the early detection of polycystic ovarian syndrome using extreme learning machine and Bayesian optimization approaches. Initially, Swapnarekha et al., have applied random oversampling technique to overcome the class imbalance problem. Then the optimal hyperparameters of the Extreme learning machine were chosen using the Bayesian optimization algorithm. The developed system has been validated using PCOS dataset consisting of 541 instances of women with 42 attributes and the outcomes reveal that developed model outperformed other similar approaches in terms of accuracy, precision, recall, and F1 score.

In Chap. 9, Diviya Prabha and Rathipriya have focused on classifying diabetes tweets using a capsule network and Gravitational Search Algorithm. At first, Twitter API is used to retrieve the diabetes tweets from Twitter and classified into five different classes. Then the developed system was applied to classify tweets as positive, strong positive, negative, strong negative, and neutral and the results concluded that recommended approach attained better classification results compared to existing methods.

Chapter 10 examines and finds the appropriate technique for developing heart failure prediction models. In the developed model, Dukka Karun Kumar Reddy et al. have applied various nature-inspired optimization algorithms to identify and predict cardiovascular diseases. The authors have also analyzed the performance metrics of Tree-based machine learning classification tasks by extracting the relevant features using hyperparameter tuning. The empirical results reveal that hyperparameter tuning with optimization techniques can substantially enhance the overall performance of the proposed system in predicting cardiovascular disease.

In Chap. 11, Suresh Kumar et al. have developed a hybrid deep learning model based on a Long Short Term Memory Network and Firefly algorithm for detecting Chronic Obstructive Pulmonary Disease at its early stages. The recommended model also assessed the relative effectiveness of various modeling paradigms to identify the best model for detecting chronic obstructive pulmonary disease on the dataset of 563 hospital or emergency ward visits in China–Japan Friendship Hospital performed between February 2011 and March 2017. Further, the authors have used random search, hyperband, and firefly algorithms to acquire the appropriate hyperparameters for the suggested LSTM model. The experimental results show that LSTM with Firefly algorithm has obtained superior results than the LSTM-Random Search and LSTM-Hyperband in the detection of chronic obstructive pulmonary disease.

Chapter 12 proposes a novel evolutionary algorithm-based feature selection approach to determine the most relevant attributes for the efficient diagnosis of breast cancer at an early stage. In the suggested model, Satyajit Panigrahi et al. have combined the Genetic Algorithm with Ant Colony Optimization to enhance the search operation in the global search space. Then the nature of breast tumors has been determined from the reduced attribute subset using Random Forest classifier. Finally, the recommended system is evaluated on the Wisconsin Diagnostic Breast Cancer dataset, and the empirical outcomes demonstrate the efficacy of the developed approach over other popular single algorithms and ensemble learners.

Baripada, India	Janmenjoy Nayak
Howrah, India	Asit Kumar Das
Sambalpur, India	Bighnaraj Naik
Bangalore, India	Saroj K. Meher
Springfield, USA	Sheryl Brahnam

Contents

1	**Nature-Inspired Optimization Algorithms: Past to Present**		1
	K. O. Mohammed Aarif, P. Sivakumar,		
	Mohamed Yousuff Caffiyar, B. A. Mohammed Hashim,		
	C. Mohamed Hashim, and C. Abdul Rahman		
	1.1	Introduction	2
		1.1.1 Why Do We Need Nature-Inspired Optimization Algorithms?	4
		1.1.2 Classification of Optimization Algorithms	4
	1.2	Background	6
		1.2.1 Natural Computing	6
		1.2.2 Algorithm	7
		1.2.3 Optimization	8
		1.2.4 Metaheuristic	9
	1.3	Broad Review on Nature-Inspired Optimization Algorithms	12
		1.3.1 Genetic Algorithms	12
		1.3.2 Ant Colony Optimization	13
		1.3.3 Swarm Intelligence	16
		1.3.4 Artificial Bee Colony (ABC)	21
		1.3.5 ACO-Ant Colony Optimization	23
		1.3.6 BAT Algorithm	23
	1.4	Theoretical Analysis and Applications	24
		1.4.1 Applications	25
	1.5	Discussions, Challenges, Open Issues and Future Recommendations	26
	1.6	Conclusion	28
	References		30
2	**Preventing the Early Spread of Infectious Diseases Using Particle Swarm Optimization**		33
	R. Jayashree		
	2.1	Introduction	33

xiii

	2.2	Literature Review of the Status of Research and Development in the Subject	35
	2.3	Methodology	37
		2.3.1 Pattern Prediction with Prior Knowledge	39
	2.4	Experiments and Results	40
		2.4.1 Running Environment	40
		2.4.2 Performance Metric	42
	2.5	Conclusion and Future Enhancement	45
	References		45
3	**Optimized Gradient Boosting Tree-Based Model for Obesity Level Prediction from patient's Physical Condition and Eating Habits**		49
	Geetanjali Bhoi, Etuari Oram, Bighnaraj Naik, and Danilo Pelusi		
	3.1	Introduction	50
	3.2	Literature Study	54
	3.3	Understanding Factors Associated with Obesity	55
	3.4	Proposed Approach	59
		3.4.1 Artificial Physics Optimization	59
		3.4.2 APO Based GBT for Obesity Prediction	60
	3.5	Experimental Result and Analysis	65
	3.6	Conclusion	66
	References		67
4	**Multi-Objective Optimization Algorithms in Medical Image Analysis**		71
	Natalia Obukhova, Alexandr Motyko, and Alexandr A. Pozdeev		
	4.1	Introduction	71
	4.2	Perceptual Method of Color Correction Based on Multi-Objective Optimization	77
		4.2.1 Loss-Function for Perceptual Color Correction	77
		4.2.2 Multi-Objective Optimization	78
		4.2.3 Color Correction Method	81
	4.3	Experimental Results	90
	4.4	Conclusion	93
	References		95
5	**Heart Failure Detection from Clinical and Lifestyle Information using Optimized XGBoost with Gravitational Search Algorithm**		97
	Etuari Oram, Bighnaraj Naik, Geetanjali Bhoi, and Danilo Pelusi		
	5.1	Introduction	98
	5.2	Literature Survey	99
	5.3	Exploratory Data Analysis of Heart Failure Data	101
	5.4	Proposed Method	104
		5.4.1 Gravitation Search Algorithm	104

	5.4.2	GSA-Based XGB for Heart Failure Detection	105
5.5		Results and Analysis	109
5.6		Conclusion	111
References			111

6 NIANN: Integration of ANN with Nature-Inspired Optimization Algorithms ... 113
Soumen Kumar Pati, Ayan Banerjee, Manan Kumar Gupta, and Rinita Shai

6.1	Introduction		114
6.2	Literature Review		115
6.3	Integration of Artificial Neural Network and Optimization Algorithm		120
	6.3.1	Artificial Neural Network (ANN)	120
	6.3.2	Optimization Algorithm	123
	6.3.3	Integration of ANN and OA	130
6.4	Experimental Results and Discussion		131
	6.4.1	Experimental Setup	133
	6.4.2	Discussion on ANN	133
6.5	Conclusion		140
References			142

7 Hybridization of Fuzzy Theory and Nature-Inspired Optimization for Medical Report Summarization ... 147
Chirantana Mallick and Asit Kumar Das

7.1	Introduction		148
7.2	Literature Survey		150
7.3	Proposed Methodology		152
	7.3.1	Preprocessing	153
	7.3.2	Fuzzy C-Means Clustering	155
	7.3.3	Defuzzification X-Cut	156
	7.3.4	Generate the Base Summaries	156
	7.3.5	Nature Inspired Optimization	157
7.4	Experimental Results		161
	7.4.1	Experimental Setup	163
	7.4.2	Performance Evaluation W.r.t ROUGE	164
	7.4.3	Compare Performance with Different Summarising Approaches W.r.t ROUGE	166
7.5	Conclusion and Future Direction		167
References			171

8 An Optimistic Bayesian Optimization Based Extreme Learning Machine for Polycystic Ovary Syndrome Diagnosis ... 175
H. Swapnarekha, Pandit Byomakesha Dash, Janmenjoy Nayak, and Ashanta Ranjan Routray

8.1	Introduction	176

	8.2	Related Work	178
	8.3	Proposed Work	181
		8.3.1 Extreme Learning Machine	181
		8.3.2 Bayesian Optimization (BO)	182
		8.3.3 Proposed ELM + BO Method	184
	8.4	Discussion of Result Analysis and Simulation Setup	185
		8.4.1 Dataset Overview and Environmental Setup	185
		8.4.2 Result Analysis	186
	8.5	Conclusion	187
	References		191
9	**Diabetes Twitter Classification Using Hybrid GSA**		195
	V. Diviya Prabha and R. Rathipriya		
	9.1	Introduction	195
	9.2	Related Works	197
	9.3	Tweets Extraction	198
	9.4	Methodology	198
		9.4.1 GSA	198
		9.4.2 CNN	202
		9.4.3 GRU	203
		9.4.4 LSTM	203
		9.4.5 Embedding Layer	204
		9.4.6 Dropout Layer	204
		9.4.7 Maxpooling	205
		9.4.8 Output Layer	205
	9.5	Data Collection	205
	9.6	Data Pre-processing	205
		9.6.1 Conversion and Correction	206
		9.6.2 Tokenization	206
		9.6.3 Stop Words	206
		9.6.4 Lemmatization	207
		9.6.5 Word Stemming	207
		9.6.6 Word Representation	207
		9.6.7 Bag of Word	207
		9.6.8 TF-IDF	208
		9.6.9 Word2Vec	208
	9.7	Proposed Capsule Network with GSA	208
		9.7.1 Capsule Network	209
		9.7.2 Capsule Network with GSA Algorithm	210
	9.8	Conclusion	216
	References		217

10 Advance Machine Learning and Nature-Inspired Optimization in Heart Failure Clinical Records Dataset ... 221
Dukka Karun Kumar Reddy, H. S. Behera, and Weiping Ding
- 10.1 Introduction ... 222
  - 10.1.1 Cardiovascular Disease (CVD) ... 223
- 10.2 Related Works ... 225
- 10.3 Tree Based Algorithms ... 226
- 10.4 Natured Inspired Optimization (NIO) ... 226
- 10.5 Basic Preliminaries of Optimization Techniques ... 229
  - 10.5.1 Bat Algorithm ... 229
  - 10.5.2 Hybrid Bat Algorithm ... 230
  - 10.5.3 Hybrid Self Adaptive Bat Algorithm ... 231
  - 10.5.4 Firefly Algorithm ... 233
  - 10.5.5 Grey Wolf Algorithm ... 234
- 10.6 Experiment Setup and Datasets Descriptions ... 235
  - 10.6.1 System Environment ... 235
  - 10.6.2 Heart Failure Clinical Records Data Set ... 236
- 10.7 Results ... 236
- 10.8 Conclusion and Future Work ... 238
- References ... 245

11 Early Detection of Chronic Obstructive Pulmonary Disease Using LSTM-Firefly Based Deep Learning Model ... 247
P. Suresh Kumar, Pandit Byomakesha Dash, B. Kameswara Rao, S. Vimal, and Khan Muhammad
- 11.1 Introduction ... 248
- 11.2 Literature Study ... 251
- 11.3 Proposed Method ... 251
  - 11.3.1 Firefly Optimization Algorithm ... 251
  - 11.3.2 Long Short-Term Memory (LSTM) ... 254
  - 11.3.3 LSTM + Firefly Methodology ... 256
- 11.4 Experimental Setup ... 257
  - 11.4.1 Dataset ... 257
  - 11.4.2 Simulation Environment ... 259
  - 11.4.3 Performance Measures ... 259
- 11.5 Result Analysis ... 260
- 11.6 Critical Discussion ... 265
- 11.7 Conclusion ... 265
- References ... 266

12 GACO: A Genetic Algorithm with Ant Colony Optimization—Based Feature Selection for Breast Cancer Diagnosis ... 269
Satyajit Panigrahi, H. Swapnarekha, and Sharmila Subudhi
- 12.1 Introduction ... 269
- 12.2 Related Work ... 273

12.3	Preliminaries		274
	12.3.1	Data Normalization	274
	12.3.2	Principal Component Analysis (PCA)	276
	12.3.3	Genetic Algorithm (GA)	276
	12.3.4	Ant Colony Optimization (ACO)	277
	12.3.5	Random Forest Algorithm (RF)	279
12.4	Proposed System		279
	12.4.1	Data Preprocessing Component (DPC)	280
	12.4.2	Evolutionary Algorithm-Based Feature Selection Component (EAFSC)	280
	12.4.3	Proposed GACO_RF Component (GRC)	282
12.5	Results and Discussions		284
	12.5.1	Dataset Description	284
	12.5.2	Data Preprocessing	284
	12.5.3	GA Parameters Estimation	284
	12.5.4	GACO Parameter Estimation	285
	12.5.5	Performance Comparison of Evolutionary Feature Selection Methods	287
	12.5.6	Performance Metric	289
	12.5.7	Performance Comparison of Proposed GACO_RF Model	289
12.6	Conclusion		290
References			291

Chapter 1
Nature-Inspired Optimization Algorithms: Past to Present

K. O. Mohammed Aarif, P. Sivakumar, Mohamed Yousuff Caffiyar,
B. A. Mohammed Hashim, C. Mohamed Hashim, and C. Abdul Rahman

Abstract Nature-inspired algorithms are class of novel methods and processes for computing, analyzing, and solving various optimization problems. Nature-Inspired Optimization Algorithms (NIOAs) are bio inspired computational intelligence techniques gives an enormous drive for solving many complex problem as it exploits an exceptionally unique, strong, convincing and engaging behavior which is competent to give ideal outcomes. In the past few decades, several Nature-Inspired Optimization Algorithms has been proposed. However, very limited efforts have been made to provide a comprehensive investigation of NIOAs. In this chapter we present an overview of most significant NIOAs established from past to present days and their role in resolving complex computationally hard problems in various field of application. This overview endeavors to give a more extensive point of view and significant illumination to comprehend NIOAs. This also features the achievement, challenges and future research direction concerning recent NIOAs.

Keywords Nature-inspired optimization algorithms · Swarm intelligence (SI) · Artificial intelligence · Particle swarm optimization · Bat algorithm (BA) · Artificial bee colony · Cuckoo

---

K. O. Mohammed Aarif (✉) · M. Y. Caffiyar · B. A. M. Hashim · C. M. Hashim · C. A. Rahman
C.Abdul Hakeem College of Engineering and Technology, Melvisharam, Tamil Nadu, India
e-mail: aarifko.ece@cahcet.edu.in

M. Y. Caffiyar
e-mail: yousuff.ece@cahcet.edu.in

B. A. M. Hashim
e-mail: hashimba.ece@cahcet.edu.in

C. M. Hashim
e-mail: hashim.ece@cahcet.edu.in

C. A. Rahman
e-mail: cabdulrahman.ece@cahcet.edu.in

P. Sivakumar
Dr. N.G.P. Institute of Technology, Coimbatore, Tamil Nadu, India

© The Author(s), under exclusive license to Springer Nature Switzerland AG 2023
J. Nayak et al. (eds.), *Nature-Inspired Optimization Methodologies in Biomedical and Healthcare*, Intelligent Systems Reference Library 233,
https://doi.org/10.1007/978-3-031-17544-2_1

1.1 Introduction

Optimization is principal in numerous applications, like designing, business exercises, and modern plans. Clearly, the points of enhancement can be anything-to limit the energy utilization and expenses, to expand the benefit, result, execution, and productivity. It is no embellishment to say that enhancement is required all over the place, from designing plan to business arranging and from Internet directing to occasion arranging. Since assets, time, and cash are constantly restricted in real world applications, we need to track down answers for ideally utilize these important assets under different requirements. Numerical improvement or writing computer programs is the investigation of such preparation and plan issues utilizing numerical apparatuses. Since generally genuine world applications are frequently exceptionally nonlinear, they require refined Optimization instruments to handle. These days, virtual experiences become a fundamental apparatus for settling such enhancement issues with different proficient pursuit algorithms.

Behind any virtual experience and computational techniques, a common underlying theme is that the model must be simulated using a computational model that takes inputs to produce the desired results. The fundamental parts and the manners in which they cooperate decide how an algorithm works and the proficiency and execution of the algorithm. Optimization issues as a rule start with the definition of the issue, for example, minimization of cost, energy, resource utilized, or augmentation of profit and quality.

From this problem explanation the true capacity is formed, either as an expansion or minimization work. The following stage is to recognize the limitations related with the problem, which could be either uniformity or imbalance imperatives. The boundaries related with the genuine capacity and the imperatives must be identified and their limits obviously expressed. The ideal answer for the problem must found via search, for which the inquiry or arrangement space should be defined. The provisional area of the arrangement in the inquiry space or the nearby district where the arrangement might actually be found too must be at first known, on the grounds that that is the place where the quest for the ideal needs to start. Assuming the data about the nearby area where the arrangement is probably going to be found isn't accessible, then, at that point, the quest for the ideal needs to begin from an irregular area in the pursuit space. Assuming that the space is very huge and multi-faceted, it is neither common sense nor achievable to do a comprehensive pursuit of the arrangement space. Assuming there are no targets in the issue yet just imperatives, then, at that point, it is an achievability issue. If the true capacity furthermore requirements are divisible in the plan factors, it is a distinct Optimization issue. Given any numerical capacity of plan factors and imperatives, assuming it is feasible to separate them as far as the factors then it is a detachable issue. The optimization issues and procedures are sorted into a few classes based on the qualities of the function, the related variables, and imperatives.

- Continuous and Discrete Optimization
- Deterministic and Stochastic Optimization

- Constrained and Unconstrained Optimization
- Linear and Non-linear Optimization
- Single and Multi Objective Optimization

NIAs are universal metaheuristic algorithms which has become the standard for assessing the likelihood of various conditions. One of the primary notes of attention is zeroing in on encrypting plans or the strategy in which the arrangements address privileged nature propelled local area discovery algorithms. This should be possible through arbitrarily inspecting the inquiry space of the issue as different up-and-comer arrangements. Thusly, these arrangements are upgraded as far as single target or multi-objective capacities. Other than this important part, arrangement portrayal, there are additionally two vital parts for any metaheuristic algorithm, these are increase and broadening which are likewise alluded to as Exploitation and investigation. Both of these thoughts insinuate how the chase is accomplished. While Optimization centers on a global space to produce different arrangements, the strengthening would zero in on a neighborhood space also taking advantage of the data accessible around here, rather than a global one. Strengthening points on fostering the great arrangements found, for which it needs to go through a choice stage to distinguish the ideal or best arrangement, while expansion, then again, points on expanding the variety of the arrangements through randomization, which points on forestalling the answer for be caught in the neighborhood ideal locale. Joining the two systems considers the arrangement to arrive at a proficiency top which is distinguished and chosen from a comprehensive space [1].

Optimization algorithms are a wide- range of algorithms that are designed to be efficient in with a numerical establishment that have been intended to track down the ideal arrangement under limitations. On the off chance that they start at similar beginning point they show up at similar last arrangement since the conventional algorithms are deterministic. The old style, subsidiary based algorithms are issue subordinate and depend on the true capacity scene, so they won't be reasonable for issues with discontinuities. Besides, they won't be reasonable for complex, non-straight, multi-modal issues [2]. Any issue which seems, by all accounts, to be incredibly intricate or difficult to tackle utilizing conventional strategies can be addressed by removing a leaf from nature. Inspiration can be acquired by concentrating on nature and how such issues are managed in organic species. Nature-inspired algorithms do not need algorithm of subsidiaries; henceforth they are without slope and are not issue explicit. Regardless of whether the algorithm begins at similar beginning point for rehashed runs, it will not end up with a similar arrangement. There is some in-fabricated stochasticity in the algorithm, with demands and arbitrary strolls. Since nature-inspired algorithms have begun to create what's more show promising outcomes, there has been a boom in their applications in different fields. These incorporate designing, industry, financial matters, correspondence, software engineering, networks, business the board, etc.

1.1.1 Why Do We Need Nature-Inspired Optimization Algorithms?

These algorithms are profoundly effective in tracking down streamlined answers for complex and multi-modular issues. The customary improvement approach in math observing the primary request subsidiary of the true capacity and comparing it to zero to get the basic focuses. These basic focuses then give the greatest or least worth according to the goal work. The computation of inclinations or considerably higher request subordinates needs additional figuring assets and is more blunder inclined than different techniques.

Further, one can imagine that it is so multifaceted to find reply for an enhancement issue with more number of elements like global merger, locality convergence, role of the core optimization strategy, role of the multi-grid recursion, and properties of the streamlining models. Nonetheless, by utilizing these nature inspired algorithms, the issue can be settled with less computational endeavors and time intricacy. These algorithms utilize a stochastic way to deal with observe the best arrangement in the enormous pursuit space of the issue.

1.1.2 Classification of Optimization Algorithms

Nature-inspired optimization algorithms are broadly classified in light of the source of inspiration as:

- Classical Methods
- Natural Evolutionary Algorithms
- Swarm Intelligence Algorithms
- Biological Based Algorithms
- Science Based Algorithms
- Other Algorithms

NIOAs are metaheuristic algorithms and an arising field of exploration since most recent twenty years. These algorithms reenact the aggregate conduct of normal multitudes like echolocation conduct of bats, blazing conduct of bees, searching conduct of bumble bees, and so on to tackle perplexing issues of different spaces. Swarm knowledge based algorithms, a subset of nature-inspired algorithm, deals with numerous specialists (groups) that are enduring and effort as one to accomplish the ideal result. These algorithms are grouped in light of their regular wellspring of motivations, for example, physical based, science based, bio-enlivened and etc. A large portion of this present reality optimization issues, applied in designing disciplines, are rigid, and the retort for these issues doesn't exists in polynomial time. Furthermore, these enhancement issues are too difficult to even consider demonstrating numerically. Nature-propelled algorithms give close to ideal answers for such issues involving meta heuristic strategies for streamlining complex capacities.

In light of the nature and attributes of the goal work, imperatives, design, and some other boundaries related with the issue, the methods for tackling the NIOAs can be categories as follows:

- Linear programming
- Simplex strategy
- Re-examined simplex strategy
- Kamarkar's strategy
- Deterioration guideline
- Duality hypothesis
- Transportation issue
- Non-straight programming
- Quadratic programming
- Mathematical programming
- Kuhn-Tucker conditions
- Dynamic programming
- Whole number programming
- Stochastic programming
- Lagrange multiplier strategy

These conventional strategies have been examined in the accompanying segments with basic models where appropriate.

NIOAs are motivated by normal peculiarities, including swarm insight, natural frameworks, physical and compound frameworks and, and so on [3]. NIOAs incorporate bio-enlivened algorithms and physical science and science based algorithms; the bio-enlivened algorithms further incorporate swarm knowledge based and developmental algorithms [3]. NIOAs are a significant branch of man-made consciousness (AI), and NIOAs have gained critical headway over the most recent 30 years. Up to this point, countless normal NIOAs and their variations have been proposed. Thus far, a large number of common NIOAs and their variants have been proposed, such as genetic algorithm (GA) [4], particle swarm optimization (PSO) algorithm [5], differential evolution (DE) algorithm [6], artificial bee colony (ABC) algorithm [7], ant colony optimization (ACO) algorithm [8], cuckoo search (CS) algorithm [9], bat algorithm (BA) [10], firefly algorithm (FA) [11], immune algorithm (IA) [12], grey wolf optimization (GWO) [13], gravitational search algorithm (GSA) [14] and harmony search (HS) algorithm [15–17]. The primary desire of this chapter is to give an outline of the historical backdrop of the nature-inspired algorithm and analyze a portion of the new nature-inspired algorithms for optimization. In this manner, the section is coordinated as follows. Section 1.2 sketch the elementary design of Natural computation, Algorithm, Optimization, and Metaheurisrics. Section 1.3 describes the broad review on past significant NIOAs with their variants and applications, followed by brief discussions on present dominant NIOAs in Sect. 1.4. Section 1.5 present some tuning and control parameters of future NIOAs. Section 1.6 presents the conclusion and future research directions.

1.2 Background

The background information is elaborately discussed in this section.

1.2.1 Natural Computing

Natural Computing demonstrates a multidisciplinary field of examination zeroed in on the investigation of new standards of algorithm inside regular cycles [2]. The convergence of normal and transformative computation with regards to AI and natural computation is shown in Fig. 1.1. A few applications in engineering can be planned as enhancement issues.

Natural Computing is the study of computationally efficient algorithmsin most common way of separating thoughts from nature to foster imputation frameworks, or utilizing normal materials (e.g., atoms) to perform algorithm. It very well classified into three principle branches.

(1) Computing motivated naturally: it utilizes nature as motivation for the optimization of critical thinking methods. The primary thought of this division is to foster commutation apparatuses (algorithms) by captivating motivation from nature for the arrangement of intricate issues.
(2) The reenactment and copying of nature through registering: it is fundamentally an engineered cycle pointed toward making designs, structures, practices, and life forms that (don't really) look like 'life-as far as we-might be concerned'. Its items can be utilized to copy different regular peculiarities, in this manner expanding how we might interpret nature and experiences about PC models.

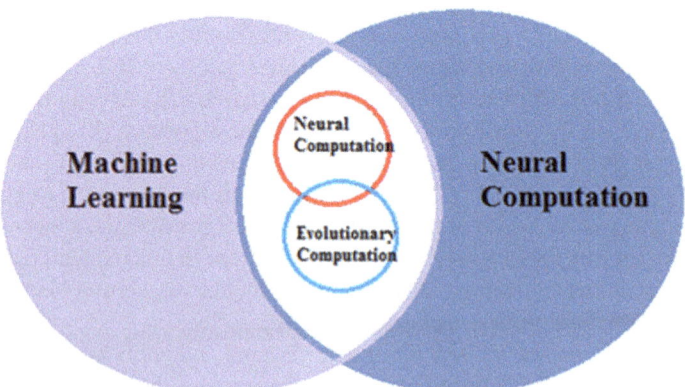

Fig. 1.1 Convergence of normal and transformative computation with regards to AI and natural computation

1 Nature-Inspired Optimization Algorithms: Past to Present

(3) Computing with normal materials: it compares to the utilization of novel regular materials to perform algorithm, consequently establishing a genuine novel figuring worldview that comes to substitute or enhance the current silicon-based PCs.

1.2.2 Algorithm

The graphical representation of genetic algorithm is shown in Fig. 1.2. Numerous normal processes have inspired streamlining algorithms. Notwithstanding, a large portion of them share a typical hidden model, which uncovers how they work. We start with a straightforward model that catches the primary elements. The provocation for putting together algorithms with respect to nature is that the normal cycles concerned are known to create beneficial outcomes, for example, tracking down an ideal worth of some feature. This perception has encouraged many algorithms in view of nature. Regardless of their reasonability, processes showed on nature have consis-

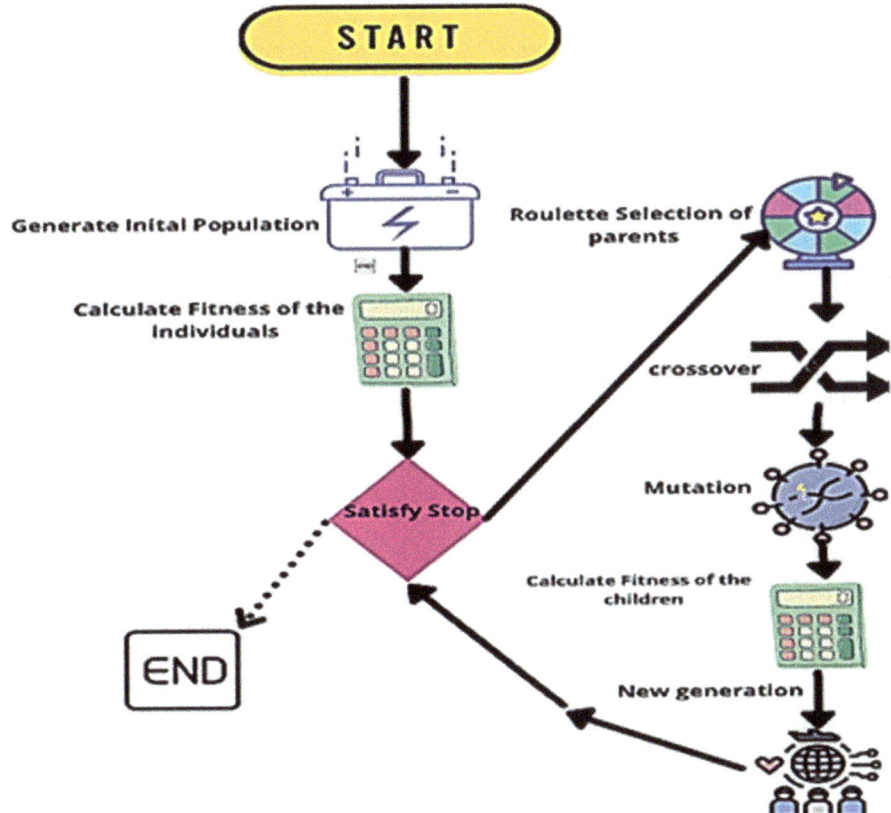

Fig. 1.2 Graphical representation of Genetic Algorithm

tently been taken with uncertainty. Standard numerical strategies, similar to straight composing computer programs, rest on outstanding speculative foundations. So their comprehension, and their cutoff points, can be attempted scientifically. Conversely, nature- centered methods are extraordinarily delegated heuristics considering peculiarities whose properties are not seen, even all of the time by science. Basically, an algorithm is a bit by bit system of giving computations or directions. Numerous algorithms are iterative. i.e.allows algorithms to be shortened by uttering that convinced stages will recurrence till mentioned to halt. The real advances and systems rely upon the algorithm utilized and the setting of interest. For instance, a basic algorithm of tracking down the square foundation of any certain number $k > 0$ or x, can be composed in Eq. (1.1) as beginning from a conjecture arrangement $x_0 = 0$, say, $x_0 = 1$.

$$xt + 1 = (1/2)(xt + (k/xt)) \qquad (1.1)$$

Here, t is the emphasis counter or list, likewise called the pseudo-time or age counter.

This iterative condition comes from the adjustment of $x_2 = k$. We can see that x_5 after only five cycles (or ages) is extremely near the valid esteem.

The explanation that this iterative cycle works is that the series $x_1, x_2, \ldots, x_t$ combines to the genuine worth $sqrtk$ because of the way that.

Nevertheless, a decent decision of the underlying worth x_0 will accelerate the combination. An off-base decision of x_0 could make the emphasis fizzle; for instance, we can't utilize $x_0 = 0$ as the underlying speculation, and we can't utilize $x_0 < 0$ either since $sqrtk > 0$ (for this situation, the cycles will move toward another root: $sqrtk$).So a reasonable decision should be a ballpark estimation. At the underlying advance, if $x_02 < k$, x_0 is the lower bound and k/x_0 is upper bound. On the off chance that $x_02 > k$, x_0 is the upper bound also k/x_0 is the lower bound. For different emphases, the new limits will be x_t and k/x_t. Indeed, the worth x_t+_1 is dependably between these two limits x_t and k/x_t, and the new gauge x_t+_1 is accordingly the mean or normal of the two limits. This ensures that the series merges to the genuine worth of $sqrtk$. This technique is like the notable separation technique.

It merits calling attention to that the end-product, however united perfectly here, may rely upon the beginning (introductory) surmise. This is an extremely normal component and inconvenience of deterministic systems or algorithms.

1.2.3 Optimization

Optimization, otherwise called numerical programming, assortment of numerical standards and strategies utilized for taking care of quantitative issues in many disciplines, including material science, science, designing, financial matters, and business. The subject developed from an acknowledgment that quantitative issues in clearly various disciplines share significant numerical components practically speaking. As a result of this shared trait, numerous issues can be planned and tackled by utilizing the brought together arrangement of thoughts and strategies that make up the field of improvement.

Quickly developing biomedical and medical services information have incorporated numerous scales going from atoms,people, to populaces and have associated different elements in medical services frameworks (suppliers, pharma, payers) with expanding data transfer capacity, profundity, and goal. Those information are turning into an empowering asset for speeding up essential science revelations and working with proof based clinical arrangements. Albeit the strategies for removing designs from information have been around for hundreds of years, it is still very hard to change enormous information into important information by these conventional method for examination. This spurs the improvement of current investigation techniques, which are planned to find significant portrayals or designs of information utilizing streamlining and AI strategies.From an expansive perspective, there are two sorts of uses in biomedical information where streamlining and AI techniques are generally utilized. One spotlights on the information disclosure by investigating verifiable information to give bits of knowledge on what occurred and why it occurred. Strategies like information measurable demonstrating,pattern detailing and perception as an affiliation and connection examination have been regularly utilized in this sort of uses. One more kind of use, on the other hand, center around forecast and dynamic applications that utilization a known dataset (also known as the preparation dataset), and which incorporates input information elements and reaction values, to fabricate a prescient model and scale it to make forecasts utilizing concealed information (otherwise known as the test dataset).

On a general note, biomedical information frequently include huge volumes, high aspects, imbalanced classes, heterogeneous sources,boisterous information, deficiency, and rich settings. Such requesting highlights are additionally driving the optimization of mathematical optimization calculations couple with AI calculations. For instance, it has been a challenge to manage road obstructions in the biomedical information region given the pervasive presence of information difficulties, for example, imbalanced datasets, feebly organized or unstructured information, loud and equivocal naming. Additionally, the streamlining calculations ought to increase to the intricacy of biomedical information that is typically large scale, high-layered, heterogeneous, and uproarious. It is additionally of much interest to study and return to customary AI points like grouping, order,relapse, and aspect decrease and transform them into strong modified approaches for the recently arising biomedical information issues, for example, electronic clinical records investigation and heterogeneous information combination.

1.2.4 Metaheuristic

Metaheuristic is the best strategy for achieving long-term optimization and are deterministic. For instance, the simplex technique in direct writing computer programs is deterministic. Some deterministic enhancement algorithms allow for an additional benefit of being able to run them under different configuration. For instance, the notable Newton-Raphson algorithm is inclination based, as it utilizes the capacity values and their subsidiaries, and it functions admirably for smooth unimodal issues. In any case, assuming there is some intermittence in the goal work, it doesn't work-well. For this situation, a non-slope algorithm is adored. Non-inclination based or slope free algorithms don't utilize any subordinate, however just the capacity values. Hooke-Jeeves design search and Nelder-Mead downhill simplex are instances of slope free algorithms.

For stochastic algorithms, overall we have two sorts: heuristic and metaheuristic, however their distinction is diminutive. In general, heuristic signifies 'to find' or 'to find by experimentation'. Excellence answers for an extreme improvement issue can be initiate in a sensible measure of time,however, no assurance that ideal arrangements are obtained. It trusts that these algorithms work more often than not, however not constantly. This is great when we don't really need the best arrangements but instead great arrangements which are effectively reachable.

Further improvement over the heuristic algorithms is the supposed metaheuristic algorithms. Here meta-signifies 'past' or 'more elevated level', and they by and large perform better compared to basic heuristics. What's more, all metaheuristic algorithms utilize specific trade off of randomization and neighborhood search.

Consequently, nearly all metaheuristic algorithms plan to be reasonable for global improvement. Heuristics is a set of algorithms for solving complex numerical problems, especially for tasks where the goal is to minimize the amount of computation required for a given input or problem. The intricacy of the issue of interest makes it difficult to look through each conceivable arrangement or blend, the point is to track down great attainable arrangement in a good timescale. There is no assurance that all that arrangements can be found. Indeed, there is no assurance that all that arrangements can be found and it may be a combination of the many difficulties and delays would make the process all but impossible. The thought is to have a productive however reasonable algorithm that works well for all inputs, including those that do not have any meaningful outputs and will-work most the time and can create great quality arrangements. Among the observed quality arrangements, it is normal some of them are almost ideal, however there is no assurance for such optimality.

Two significant parts of any metaheuristic algorithms are: increase and expansion, or abuse and investigation. Broadening means to produce assorted arrangements to investigate the inquiry space on the worldwide scale, while escalation means to zero in on the pursuit in a neighborhood locale by taking advantage of the data that a current decent arrangement is found around here. This is in blend with the determination of the best arrangements. The determination of the best guarantees that the arrangements will combine to the optimality, while the expansion by means of randomization maintains a strategic distance from the arrangements being caught at neighborhood optima and, simultaneously, increments the variety of the arrangements. The great blend of these two significant parts will as a rule guarantee that the worldwide optimality is reachable. Metaheuristic algorithms can be grouped in numerous ways. One way is to characterize them as: populace based and direction based. For instance, hereditary algorithms are populace based as they utilize a bunch of strings, so is the particle swarm optimization (PSO) which utilizes various specialists or particles. Then again, reenacted toughening utilizes a solitary specialist or arrangement which travels over the plan space or search space in a piecewise style. A superior transfer or arrangement is acknowledged 100% of the time, while a not-very great change can be acknowledged using a specific likelihood. The means or changes follow a direction in the inquiry space, with a non-zero likelihood that this direction can arrive at the global ideal.

Metaheuristic algorithms, particularly those in light of multitude knowledge, structure a significant piece of contemporary worldwide improvement algorithms [18, 19]. Genuine models are simulated annealing [22], molecule swarm improvement [20, 21] and firefly algorithm [22]. They work astoundingly effectively and enjoy numerous upper hands over conventional, deterministic techniques and algorithms, and in this manner they have been applied in practically all area of science, designing and industry [23]. Notwithstanding such a gigantic accomplishment in applications, numerical examination of algorithms stays restricted and many open issues are as yet unsettled. There are three testing regions for algorithm investigation: intricacy, assembly and without no lunch hypothesis. Intricacy investigation of conventional algorithms, for example, speedy sort and framework reverse are grounded, as these algorithms are deterministic. Interestingly, intricacy investigation of metaheuristic stays a difficult undertaking, somewhat due to the stochastic nature of these algorithms. Notwithstanding, great outcomes do exist, concerning randomization search procedures [2].

Assembly investigation is another difficult region. One of the principle hardships concerning the assembly investigation of metaheuristic algorithms is that no conventional structure exists, however significant examinations have been completed utilizing dynamic frameworks and Markov processes. Notwithstanding, intermingling investigation actually stays one of the dynamic exploration regions with many empowering results [24].Along the numerical investigation of advancement algorithms, another similarly testing, but productive region is the hypothesis on algorithm execution and correlation, prompting a wide scope of without no lunch (NFL) hypotheses [25]. While in very much presented instances of enhancement where it's useful space structures limited areas, NFL hypotheses do hold [26].

In the field of evolutionary calculation, it is normal to look at reformed calculations utilizing a huge test set, particularly at the point when the test set includes work streamlining. If we compare several examining algorithms with all conceivable functions, the efficiency of one of the algorithms will be, on regular.. This is because of the way that, when a calculation is assessed, we should search for the sort of issues where its exhibition is great, to portray the kind of issues for which the calculation is reasonable.

1.3 Broad Review on Nature-Inspired Optimization Algorithms

Since the mid 1990s there was a piece of AI that zeroed in on the insight of computational frameworks and on how they can embrace an approach to "thinking" like the human mind does; with rules and choices. This class of examination, named Computational Intelligence (CI), was conceived due to the primary hereditary algorithm that caused researchers to inquire as to whether nature peculiarities and different kinds of practices could likewise propose techniques for tackling genuine issues. So CI essentially engaged on (1) AI, (2) fluffy rule based frameworks, (3) neural organizations and (4) developmental algorithms.

There are numerous nature-Inspired algorithms, around 100 distinct algorithms and their variations are available in the recent research [27]. Clearly, it is unimaginable to incorporate even a decent part of these algorithms. In this manner, our accentuation is on the algorithms that can be considered as representatives from the past to present research. Likewise, our accentuation here is on giving detailed description and background about every algorithm, the closeness and contrasts of various algorithms and the techniques utilized for producing novel results, choice of the finest solution and further significant features.

1.3.1 Genetic Algorithms

Genetic Algorithm (GA) is an evolutionary algorithm developed by Holland [Holland] in 1975, based on Darwinian development of natural organizations. Its principle qualities are the three genetic administrators: crossover, mutation and selection [16, 37]. A bunch of solutions from a populace that are encrypted as dualistic or genuine strings, called chromosomes. Another populace of resolutions are produced utilizing such genetic administrators. By crossover the two child solutions can be created from two parent solutions by crossover, which basically trades one portion or various sections of one parent solution with its partners. Then again, another solution can be created by transforming the slightest bit or numerous pieces of one solution. Transformation can just flip between 0 and 1 for twofold strings at least one areas. The nature of a still up in the air by its wellness that is a standardized worth related with the capacity values of the target. If there should arise an occurrence of expansion issues, the wellness can be corresponding to the goal. Choice is finished by picking the most fittest solution as per their wellness.

It is a definite technique, however some numerical examination should be possible utilizing binomial dispersions and different instruments [29, 30].

There are numerous benefits of GA over customary optimization algorithms. Two of the most outstanding are the capacity to manage composite issues and parallelism. GA can manage different kinds of optimization, regardless of whether the goal (wellness) work is fixed or non-stationary, direct or nonlinear, ceaseless or irregular, or

1 Nature-Inspired Optimization Algorithms: Past to Present

with arbitrary commotion. Since numerous off-springs in a populace behave like free specialists, the populace (or any subgroup) can investigate the inquiry space in numerous bearings at the same time. This component marks it perfect to correspond the algorithms for execution. Various boundaries and even various gatherings of encoded strings can be controlled simultaneously. Be that as it may, genetic algorithms additionally have a few weaknesses. The plan of a wellness work, the utilization of populace size, the decision of significant boundaries such as the pace of mutation and hybrid, and the choice rules of the new populace ought to be done cautiously. Any improper decision will make it troublesome for the algorithm to join or it will essentially deliver useless outcomes. In spite of these downsides, GA stay one of the best generally utilized improvement algorithms in present day nonlinear optimization.

1.3.1.1 GA Variation

There are a few dozen GA variations which aggregately can be called genetic algorithms. Various variations depend on the different mutations in essential genetic administrators. For the crossover operators, the multi-site or N-site hybrid and uniform cross, rearranged hybrid uses the random permutations for two guardians at N-focuses, and afterward rearranged off springs are changed back by means of an opposite stage. Essentially, transformation can be accomplished by flipping arbitrarily picked bits; by bitwise reversal, which modifies the entire string; or by irregular mutation, where the string is supplanted by a new (irregular) one with likelihood.

Genetic algorithms are crossbred and integrated to solve problems like mapping language to DNA, creating artificial genomes, or using artificial intelligence to solve real world problems. For instance, gradient based techniques can be utilized to improve the presentation of genetic algorithms. The global inquiry capacity of genetic algorithms is utilized to guarantee a high likelihood of tracking down global optimality, while the subordinates or nearby data can be utilized to accelerate neighborhood search. For this methodology, genetic algorithms can be used to detect variants of specific traits. The algorithms will look for genetic signals that can be used to predict whether or not a trait will be passed on.

1.3.2 Ant Colony Optimization

The working procedure of the ant colony optimization (ACO)is shown in Fig. 1.3. The ant colony optimization (ACO) was created by Marco Dorigo in 1992 [6], what's more ACO endeavors to mirror the scrounging conduct of social ants in a colony. All subterranean ants/specialists utilize a compound courier, called track, to speak with other subterranean ants, their communications are neighborhood, in view of nearby data. Track is saved by every specialist, and such synthetic will likewise dissipate. The model for track affidavit and dissipation might shift marginally, rely upon the

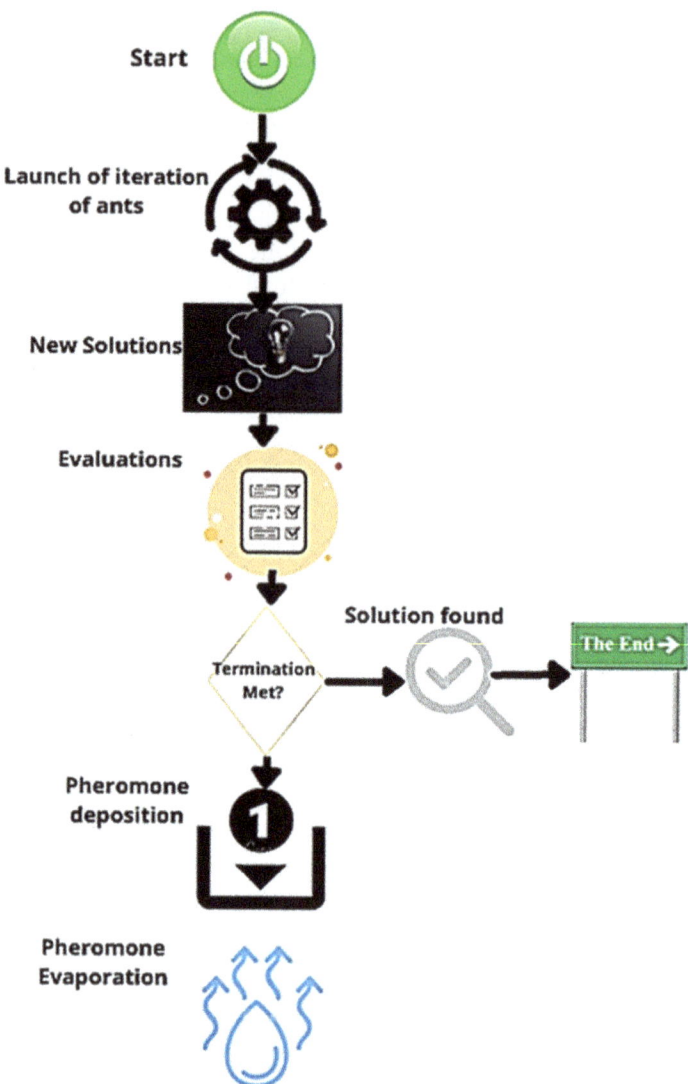

Fig. 1.3 Working procedure of ACO algorithm

variations of ACO. Nonetheless, by and large, steady statement and outstanding rot are utilized in the writing. According to the execution perspective, for instance, an answer in an organization optimization issue can be a way or course. Every specialist will investigate the organization ways furthermore store track when it moves. The nature of this arrangement is connected with the track focus on the way. Simultaneously, track will dissipate as time. At an intersection with various courses, the likelihood of picking a specific still up in the air by a choice model, contingent upon the standardized convergence of the course, the allure of the course (for instance, the distance of the in general way), and relative wellness of this course, contrasting and all others. It merits bringing up that ACO is a blended of methodology and a few straightforward conditions like track testimony and vanishing as well as the way determination probability.

A few types of bugs are equipped for responding to critical optimizations, which are indications that activate responses that are hereditarily encrypted, a sort of aberrant correspondence in light of their exhibition measure. A specific term for this peculiarity is "stigmergy" [27, 28]. Numerous subterranean ant species show stigmergy. Throughout food exploration, ants store track on their way that is distinguished by different ants what's more impacts their way. Consequently, a more grounded grouping of tracks recommends a more noteworthy possibility of disclosure of food, and that implies ants will trail that way and waive their own, subsequent in the old track disappearing. This cycle results in a track trail, assisting different ants with arriving at the food source effectively, as different subterranean ants have recently recognized it. Ant province enhancement (ACO) is firmly connected with its organic motivation. Fake subterranean ants are free, non concurrent substances coordinating to see as a decent answer for the front and center concern. Their fundamental objective is to track down a decent answer for a given optimization issue. They update the upsides of fake tracks by navigating the way, each state in turn.

1.3.2.1 Application

Subterranean ant state advancement is a strong metaheuristic algorithm. It very well may be utilized to track down the briefest way among a bunch of ways for a specific hub. This property can be applied to the mobile sales rep issue [33] and work task issue [31]. ACO can be utilized incorporate the issues of dynamic enhancements, multi-objective optimization [33] and cross breed procedures planned utilizing different enhancement methods [34].

The algorithm of ant state enhancement was worked from motivation by the rummaging conduct of ants. At the point when ants look for food, they at first investigate the region around their home in an irregular manner. Whenever a food source is found, the subterranean ants convey it back to the home, simultaneously storing a synthetic pheromone trail on the ground. This trail is planned to direct different subterranean ants to the food source, which will additionally store more pheromone in the path. As time passes by, a portion of the pheromone is dissipated, and the path might vanish on the off chance that it isn't refreshed with more pheromone. This roundabout correspondence between subterranean ants has been displayed to empower the subterranean ant colony to lay out the most limited way to the food source [35, 36]. The regular peculiarity of strengthening of short (top notch) ways, and dissipation (failing to remember ways that are not great), has enlivened a bunch of strategies known as subterranean ant state advancement.

1.3.3 Swarm Intelligence

The investigation of oneself getting self-organizing [9] aggregate keen conduct of swarms has been a subject of broad examination since the mid-1990s. The SI algorithms are extremely strong since they have inborn parallelism and are versatile. The swarm insight algorithms are very viable in addressing complex, non-straight streamlining issues with diminished time, space, and computational intricacy. SI algorithms are portrayed by numerous hunt specialists that quest for the ideal arrangement in equal, accordingly being productive. They share data among the individuals from the swarm, utilize their aggregate insight, and are self-coordinated and transformative in nature [37]. These algorithms have been intended to tackle issues that have been shown to be NP-hard for the old style algorithms. Noticing the conduct of a flock of birds flying in nature shows that there is no restriction to the number of birds in the flock. The arrangement of an enormous flock includes countless individuals looking over a huge region for quality food and watching themselves against hunters.

The swarm insight algorithms fuse the searching systems of natural life forms like creatures, birds, and bugs. The specialist with the best scavenging procedure gets by in the climate since food is fundamental for endurance. This includes a hunt process, and the specialists with the more efficient search methodology succeed immediately thought about to others in the serious climate. There are a few variables associated with such scavenging exercises - the attributes and size of the specialist, its intelligence, social conduct, area of food and amount, and the work expected to find the food. The presence of hunters and different risks sneaking in the climate and the capacity of the specialists to avoid such powers and break from them or safeguard themselves against such hunters likewise assume an imperative part in endurance. Additionally, since the climate is dynamic, the quality, amount, and area of food continue to change with time because of utilization and other changes that happen throughout some stretch of time. This requires the organic entity to be versatile furthermore flexible to the evolving conditions. The input of the past achievements of the flock, also dividing of data between the flock individuals with respect to food quality and area make it simpler to find food. A few animal varieties display social scavenging which upgrades their odds of coming out on top in finding food and henceforth eventually prompts better possibilities of endurance. This likewise requires great relational abilities among individuals from the populace and a sharing procedure. To deal with this, ordinarily there is an ordered progression in the gathering of life forms with a such pioneer exercises. Correspondence of the find (quality and amount of food) is done in more ways than one relying upon the animal varieties and type of organic entity. A portion of the individuals return to a focal place where every one of the individuals from the gathering are available and spread the data about the quality, area, and distance of the food source. Some of the time, the individuals are driven back to the area of food by the part which has found the food source. In different species, the correspondence is done through communicating of data which could be heard by individuals from their own bunch as well as by hunters, expanding the risk of being assaulted. The benefits also drawbacks of the various kinds of correspondence about food revelation among the various species shift.

The SI algorithms are here and there inefficient when the dimensionality of the inquiry space is enormous. Except if the algorithms have been planned specifically, the pursuit could consume a large chunk of the day over high-layered spaces. The pursuit spaces could be organized or on the other hand unstructured. Utilizing populaces of search specialists joined with heuristics has a significant impact on the arrangement of perplexing designing plan issues. The nature inspired algorithms are novel in accomplishing compelling arrangements effectively with the most un-computational assets. Neighborhood search alludes to looking for the ideal arrangement in the neighborhood of the current arrangements. This will prompt investigation of the variations of the arrangement. A grouping of steps where the means are steered in a specific bearing (rising or drop) is comparable to slope climbing. A few stages could be in the inverse heading to empower the algorithm to emerge from nearby optima. In any case the search could be begun from a few different places in the arrangement space. The historical backdrop of past triumphs could be used in the flow search. In practically all of the developmental algorithms, there is a populace of search specialists that search the arrangement space, searching for the ideal arrangement. They are fundamentally iterative in nature, attempting to make do upon the current arrangements with each succeeding cycle. This ad lib is in the type of another populace which incorporates the fittest individuals from the past age as well as new individuals made by some instrument that is specific to an algorithm. In this cycle, the more fragile individuals from the populace get disposed of. The benefit of populace based search is that it happens in equal and it very well may be coordinated to investigate potential locales of the space that were already neglected where the ideal arrangement could be found.

1.3.3.1 Particle Swarm Optimization

The working procedure of PSO algorithm is shown in Fig. 1.4. Particle swarm optimization (PSO) pulled in an enormous number of scientists to resolve the CD issue. PSO structures an invigorating, consistently growing exploration subject, called swarm intelligence that implies employed with a populace of particles, which in this situation are known as a swarm of particles. These elements transfer and pursuit in the state space of potential arrangements to recognize the ideal arrangement.

Particle swarm optimization also increases your performance, by minimizing the time spent on particle system state changes, allowing for more complex effects that are not possible with state changes. The new particle system also provides a better simulation of particle systems that are created using dynamic systems. Additionally, the particle system includes an integrated, scalable performance tracking system that can make sure that the particle system performs at the maximum level possible. The system enables particle systems to dynamically scale based on the current performance, and even dynamically change their behavior.

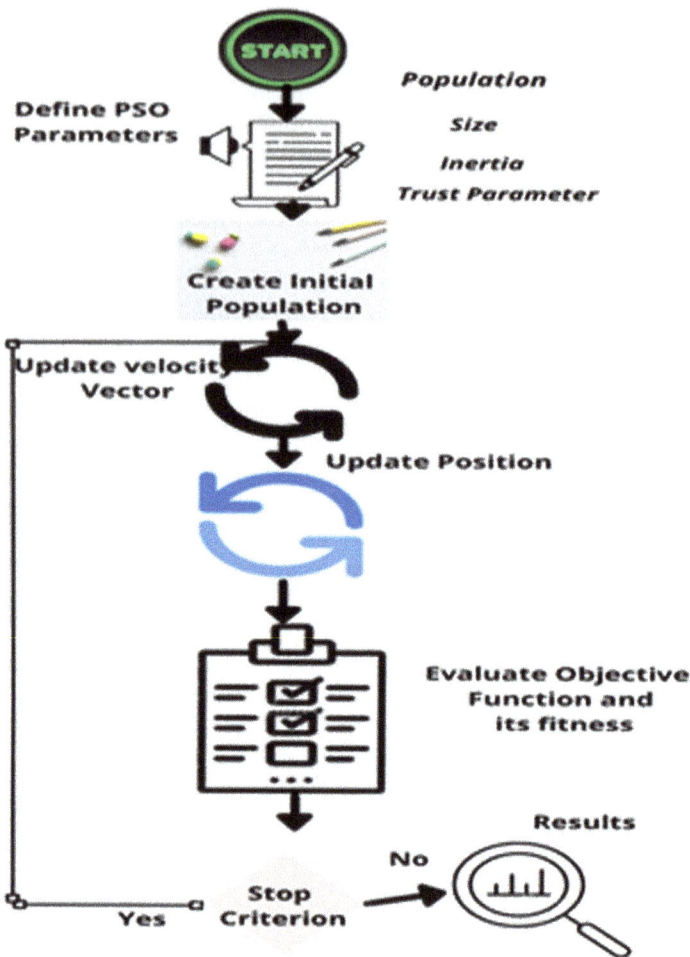

Fig. 1.4 Working procedure of PSO algorithm

PSO involves particles as a bundle called a swarm (Fig. 1.4). The subdivisions are permitted toinvestigate the hunt space and directed by their dormancy, distance from the person Particle's most popular position and distance from the swarm's most popular position.The elements speak with one another to combine in a solitary space quicker. Another explanation that PSO is appealing is that there are not many boundaries to change. One rendition, with slight varieties, workswell in a wide assortment of uses. Particle Swarm Optimization has been utilized for approaches that can be utilized across awide scope of uses, as well concerning explicit applications zeroed in on a particular necessity [39].

1 Nature-Inspired Optimization Algorithms: Past to Present

1.3.3.2 Application of Particle Swarm Optimization

PSO was first used to prepare neural networks, From that point forward, numerous areas of utilization have been found, for example, broadcast communications, information mining, combinatorial optimization power frameworks and sign handling. This algorithm has been utilized primarily to address unconstrained, single-objective improvement issues, obliged issues, multi objective enhancement issues and issues with powerfully evolving scenes. Furthermore, half breeds of PSO have been created utilizing a few advancement algorithms, which further improve the algorithm [40].

1.3.3.3 Firefly

] The operational procedure of fireflies algorithm is shown in Fig. 1.5. Firefly algorithms were acquainted with manages muddled issues having all things considered equity or imbalance based rules. Firefly algorithms treat multi-modular capacities with better effectiveness when contrasted with other swarm algorithms. Like the insect based what's more honey bee based algorithms, firefly algorithm additionally embraces an essential arbitrary population based search, in this way advancing savvy gaining from a gathering of shifted arrangements furthermore bringing about most extreme intermingling and mistake free result. The algorithm uses the normal conduct of fireflies by which bio luminescence or blazing signs to different fireflies to track down prey, tracking down mates or just common correspondence. These fireflies show attributes like that of swarm insight due to their self-association and decentralized choice taking capacity. The power of blazing is viewed as a mark of readiness for the male firefly. Be that as it may, in the regular algorithm, all fireflies are viewed as gender neutral, and consequently, all fireflies are known to be commonly drawn in along these lines. The appeal of the firefly is straightforwardly relative to the light force (or blazing), which thus further goes about as a sign of qualification for a potential "up-and-comer arrangement".

There are a few variations of firefly-based algorithms which have numerous application regions in practically all areas of science and correspondence. Well known among the rundown of variations are Adaptive Firefly Algorithm (AFA), Discrete Firefly Algorithm (DFA), Multi-Objective FA (MOFA), Lagrangian FA (LFA), Chaotic FA (CFA), Mixture FA (HFA) and FA-based Memetic Algorithm (FAMA), to give some examples. DFA is utilized to take care of NP-hard planning issues, and in picture division, MOFA is utilized for taking care of multi-objective burden dispatch issues and LFA finds utility in power framework improvement unit responsibility issues, though FAMA is applied for electrical burden determining.

1.3.3.4 Applications

Firefly-based algorithms are acknowledged to have a large group of uses, some of which indicated under. Obliged [41] and multi-modular capacity optimization [42]

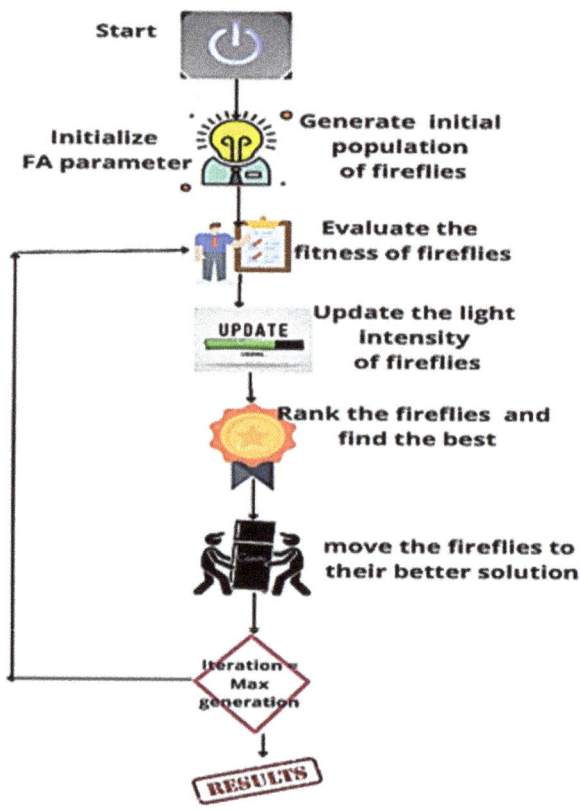

Fig. 1.5 Operational procedure of fireflies algorithm

in stochastic processes and stochastic optimization [62] are proficiently managed by firefly based algorithms. Such algorithms additionally find utilization in falcon based Levyflight frameworks [43], in blended variable underlying optimization [4] and for tackling nonconvex monetary dispatch issues [44]. The survey by [45] additionally supports giving better intelligence in regards to the algorithm, [46] in 2014 for precise present moment weight anticipating, [47] for greyscale picture watermarking, [48] for capacitated office area issue, and [49, 50] for coronary illness expectation and the presentation of oppositional and layered based firefly algorithms. Firefly algorithms may likewise be utilized for taking care of NP-difficult issues, with balance and additionally imbalance driven requirements, exceptionally difficult arrangement issues, consistent and discrete hunt space areas, combinational improvement spaces, equal computational areas and multi-objective hunt difficulties. The firefly algorithm can be utilized related to different strategies, for example, multi-esteemed rationale (for example harsh set hypothesis), cell learning automata and fake brain organizations to foster mixture draws near. Firefly-based algorithms are additionally utilized to tackle load dispatch issues [51], financial exchange cost determining [52], picture pressure [53], fabricating cell arrangement [54], work shop booking [55] and energy protection [56].

1.3.3.5 Differential Evolution

Differential evolution (DE) is a mathematical description that describes how a change in fitness can lead to an evolutionary change that affects a particular individual. There are numerous DE variations, and they have been applied in a wide scope of fields. This part gives a short prologue to the fundamental DE and its fundamental execution subtleties and variations. Crucial combination properties as far as populace change are likewise talked about.

Differential evolution (DE), created by Storn and Price [46], involves a change administrator as far as the distinction of two unique arrangement vectors. DE is comparability to design search and genetic algorithms because of its utilization of hybrid what's more change. Indeed, DE can be reflected as an additional optimization to genetic algorithms with express refreshing conditions, which brand it conceivable to do some hypothetical investigation. DE is a stochastic pursuit algorithm with self-putting together propensity and does not utilize the data of subsidiaries. Hence, it is a populace based, subordinate free strategy. Also, DE involves genuine numbers as arrangement strings, so no encoding and deciphering is required.

Differential evolution comprises of three principle steps: change, hybrid, and choice. Transformation is completed by the change plot. For every vector x_i at anytime, or generation t, we first arbitrarily pick three particular vectors x_p, x_q, and x_r at t.

Differential evolution (DE) showed a few benefits in the optimization of the local area recognition issue. DE starts the hunt with a populace, like the past algorithms. A solitary substance from the populace, which is involved people, is chosen and utilized as the objective vector, and it is utilized to create the freak vector by the freak activity. Fundamentally, this kind of algorithm identifies the upgraded arrangement paying little heed to introductory boundary values; it has a quick combination, as well as requiring a couple of control boundaries. The exhibition of this method is vigorously dependent on the change conspire, and the control boundaries. Despite the fact that there are different transformations conspires, the accompanying techniques are the most frequently utilized [46]: While the boundaries are basically qualities expected for the technique to work, like the populace size, hybrid size, and the scale factor.

1.3.4 *Artificial Bee Colony (ABC)*

The working principle of ABC algorithm is shown in Fig. 1.6. Artificial Bee Colony is a revolutionary, free-form, non-linear optimization [17] depends on the conduct of bumble bees living in a province while attempting to look for food sources to support themselves. An artificial settlement has bees as specialists, while the food

Fig. 1.6 Working principle of ABC algorithm

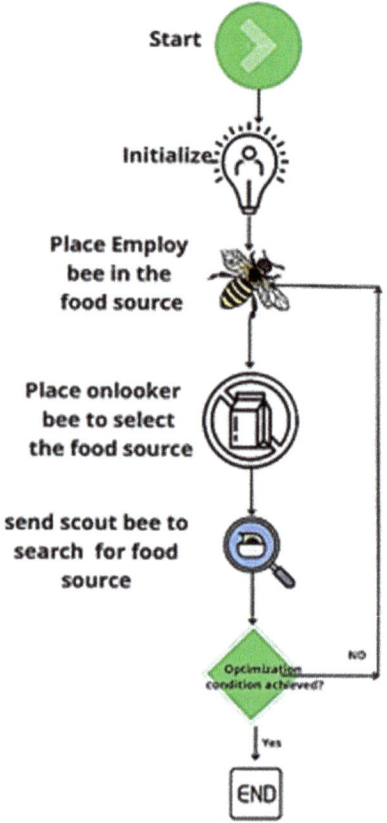

is the arrangement that should be painstakingly extricated by them, to get by and save their assets too. Karaboga introduced the ABC algorithm, and there are three sorts of bees: utilized foragers, scouts and spectators. A utilized forager partners with one food source and offers it with different bees by specific likelihood; scouts are responsible for looking through new food sources and spectators observe food sources through imparting data to utilized foragers.

1.3.4.1 Application

Artificial Bee Colony is utilized in a small scale of the operation. The first colony of artificial bee colonies was established in a small farm [36]. In this instance the bee colonies is being operated in a controlled manner and it's being maintained and monitored through remote monitoring system. Cross breeds of the ABC algorithm, which are utilized in numerous extraordinary areas of gadgets have additionally been proposed and created [26].

1.3.5 ACO-Ant Colony Optimization

ACO metaheuristic comprises of a state of artificial insects developing arrangements iteratively by emulating the rummaging conduct of social subterranean insects. ACO involves pheromone as a synthetic courier and the pheromone focus as the sign of quality answers for an issue of interest. According to an execution perspective, arrangements are connected with the pheromone focus, prompting courses and ways set apart by the higher pheromone fixations as better answers for inquiries of the issue. Subsequently, the two central matters in ACO algorithms are the likelihood of picking a course and the focus pace of pheromone, where the likelihood of picking a course from hub I to hub J.

The hunt cycle of Bee Colony Optimization (BCO) is coordinated by participation and transformation of the bee province, the objective is to find the biggest food source [47, 48]. As such, the BCO optimization calculation begins with the representative bees that save a dietspring to them when they left from the store to stake the dietcradle data with spectators on different region. Then, at that point, spectators decide the food source by watching worker bees' moves and attempting to work on this source. A worker bee turns into a scout in instance of leaving the food source to investigate new food sources haphazardly. The level of scout, worker also experienced worker are generally resolved physically [47]. Both ACO and BCO need to hybrid activity that makes them moderately sluggish with regards to combination, however, they are effective with regards to look through space investigation. In any case, as far as possible the subspace abuse, indeed, absence of hybrid activity is a typical event in some metaheuristic algorithms.

1.3.6 BAT Algorithm

To find their direction even in a total obscurity, bats utilize modern echolocation to plan their general climate. By transmitting a short beat of sound waves and afterward paying attention to their reverberations, they might distingue at any point prey from objects and hazardous hunters. In light of this way of behaving, Xin-She Yang et al. fostered a new enhancement calculation, called the BA. BA falls into something very similar class of calculations, called swarm knowledge, for example, PSO, and ACO. BA utilizes a populace of bats for the inquiry of the worldwide ideal. Not long after its appearance in the writing, BA begins to draw in the consideration of a few scientists all over the planet because of its two significant qualities. The first, BA is profoundly proficient and solid in the pursuit of the worldwide ideal for low layered issues. The second is its simple design. BA is so natural to carry out that it tends to modified utilize any scripting languages under two or three dozen lines of codes. The bat calculation has been utilized to tackle a few designing issues. It was utilized to enhance the brushless DC wheel engine, measuring battery for energy capacity [6], power framework stabilizer and power dispatch. Besides, specialists likewise found different uses of BA in many teaches, for example, the way arranging of uninhabited combat air vehicle (UCAV), underlying harm location, shortcoming analysis, picture handling, and others, for example, stream shop booking or just arranging sports instructional courses. Be that as it may, as the issues' intricacy expands, the calculation's presentation might show some untimely assembly. This untimely assembly of the calculation might be because of the need the investigation capacity. To conquer this inadequacy, some scientists have proposed a few upgrades with the plan to improve the standard BA's presentation for general advancement use, while others altered BA to fit for specific explicit undertakings like the mobile sales rep issue, huge scope support structures, primary dependability, coronary failure discovery, miniature lattice the executives and others. The recently proposed calculation was tried on a few complex benchmarks and the outcomes were contrasted and those of 20 other norm and refined calculations including 6 gotten to the next level variations of BA. The non-parametric measurable tests showed the prevalence of the directional bat calculation. This calculation was effectively applied to tackle 190 A. Chakri et al.probabilistic obliged issues, run of the mill to underlying dependability based plan enhancement field.

1.4 Theoretical Analysis and Applications

As discussed in Sect. 1.2, albeit the NIOAs reenact different populace practices, every one of them are the iterative strategies and have a few normal attributes which fulfill the Reynolds model [54] and this model depicts the essential guidelines for the conglomeration movement of the mimicked herd made by a conveyed conduct model.

1. Randomicity: Randomicity is the vulnerability of an occasion with a specific likelihood what's more can improve the worldwide pursuit capacity of people. All the NIOAs in state people randomly, which can cover the space as extensive as could be expected, a few different systems have been taken on in them which can improve the investigation and abuse capacities

2. Data Interactivity: The people in the NIOAs should trade data straightforwardly or in a roundabout way, which can build the likelihood of acquiring the worldwide ideal. For example, GA, IA and DE embrace the hybrid administrator.

3. Optimality: The individuals in the NIOAs push toward the worldwide best arrangement through various systems of data trade.

In expansion to the previously mentioned normal attributes of hypothetical execution, these normal NIOAs are fluctuated to various renditions to deal with various issues, including combinational improvement issues (COPs) and multi-objective enhancement issues (MOOPs). Comparable variation strategies are embraced to work on the enhancement execution of NIOAs, for instance, versatile innovation, fluffy hypothesis, disarray hypothesis, quantum hypothesis and hybridization innovation.

A vital yet in addition exceptionally commonsense inquiry is the means by which to pick a algorithm for a given issue. This might be certainly connected to another inquiry: what sort of issues would an algorithm be able to address most actually. In numerous applications, the issue viable appears to be fixed; we need to utilize the right instrument or techniques to address in the best manner. Consequently, there are two sorts of decisions and accordingly two important inquiries:

- For a given kind of issues, what is the best algorithm from use's point of view?
- For a given algorithm, what sorts of issues would it be able to tackle?

The principal question is more enthusiastically than the subsequent inquiry; however the last option isn't not difficult to answer all things considered. For a given kind of issues, there might be a bunch of productive algorithms to take care of such issues. Be that as it may, much of the time, we may not know how effective an algorithm can be before we really attempt it. Maybe at times, such algorithms in any case ought to be created. In any event, for existing algorithms, the decision generally relies upon the aptitude of the chief, the assets and the sort of issues. Preferably, the best accessible algorithms and devices ought to be utilized to take care of a given issue; nonetheless, the appropriate utilization of these instruments might in any case rely upon the experience of the client. Likewise, the assets like computational expenses and programming accessibility what's more time permitted to deliver the arrangement will likewise be significant variables in choosing what algorithms and techniques to utilize.

In any case, for new algorithms, as in the instances of most nature-inspired algorithms, we need to do broad investigations to approve and test their presentation. Clearly, any explicit information about a specific issue is useful 100% of the time for the proper decision of the best and most productive strategies for the enhancement From the algorithm advancement perspective, how to best consolidate issue explicit information is still a continuous testing question.

1.4.1 Applications

The applications of nature-motivated algorithms in designing are exceptionally assorted and to cover a decent part of these applications might take a major volume. In the present book, probably the furthest down the line advancements will be assessed and presented. Consequently, in the remainder of this part, we will momentarily feature a couple of applications to show the variety and adequacy of nature-motivated advancement algorithms.

- Underlying improvement: Design enhancement in structural designing is basically underlying improvement on the grounds that the principle errands to configuration structures to expand the exhibition record and to limit the expenses, dependent upon complex rigid configuration codes. Regular models are pressure vessel configuration, speed minimizer plan, vault and pinnacle plans, as well as blend of advancement with limited component reenactment and different plans.

- Booking and Routing: Scheduling issues, for example, aircraft planning and vehicle directing can have significant true applications. The notable model is the alleged mobile sales rep issue that expects to visit every city precisely once so the in general voyaged distance should be limited. Nature-inspired algorithms have been utilized to take care of such extreme issues with promising outcomes.
- Picture handling: Image handling is a major region with a tremendous writing. Picture division and element determination can frequently be formed as an enhancement issue, and consequently can be handled by improvement strategies in blend with customary picture handling procedures [54]. Picture programmed enlistment and grouping can be addressed utilizing nature-motivated algorithms with great execution.
- Information mining: Data mining is a functioning exploration region with different applications. Order and bunching can be firmly connected with streamlining and numerous half breed procedures have as of late been created by brushing customary information mining strategies, for example, k-mean bunching with nature-inspired advancement algorithms, for example, the firefly algorithm, and cuckoo search and bat algorithm. Later concentrates by Fong et al. showed that such half and half techniques can acquire excellent results [55]. For instance, Senthilnath et al. looked at more than twelve different bunching algorithms, they reasoned that the methodology based the firefly algorithm would be able to get the best outcomes with minimal measure of computational endeavors.Clearly, there are numerous different applications and contextual investigations, intrigued readers can allude to more specific writing and the later parts of this section.

1.5 Discussions, Challenges, Open Issues and Future Recommendations

Regardless of the viability of nature-enlivened systems and their notoriety, there are as yet many testing matters regarding such algorithms,particularly according to hypothetical points of view. However analysts know the essential components of how such algorithms can function practically speaking, it isn't exactly clear why they work and under precisely what circumstances. Moreover, all nature-motivated algorithms have procedure subordinate boundaries, and the upsides of these boundaries can influence the presentation of the process viable. In any case, it isn't clear what the best qualities or sets are and how to tune these boundaries to accomplish the best presentation.

Moreover, there are a few hypothetical examinations of some nature-inspired algorithms [56, 57], it actually misses the mark on bound together numerical system to break down all algorithms to get inside and out comprehension of their dependability, combination, paces of union and power. Each of these algorithms is different as far as both the hunt techniques included and the pursuit control. Every one of them, in any case, has a nearby pursuit strategy consolidated into their design, which is utilized to strengthen the pursuit and merge to a nearby ideal. This neighborhood search methodology is at the center of reenacted strengthening, only way in which we could hope to preserve and expand. Higher values might lead the algorithm to investigate various bowls of fascination, while lower values permit the technique to move toward the neighborhood ideal. In GAs, it is the change administrator that acts like a neighborhood search technique. The distinction, in any case, is that transformation isn't a 'slope climber' and stops after one neighborhood search. The number of inhabitants in arrangements is developed in equal, permitting the investigations of numerous bowls of fascination.

As we have seen from the above comprehensive investigation, appropriate variation and variety are critical to guarantee the great exhibition of an algorithm. Variation can be done in various parts (of an algorithm), like the age of the populace, choice of arrangements, elitism, substitution of arrangements, change of boundaries also by and large equilibrium between investigation and abuse. Variety can likewise show up in many places, for example, the ways of creating new arrangements, choice and substitution of existing arrangements, exploratory moves, randomization, and above all to keep a decent equilibrium in investigation and double-dealing. In spite of the achievement of nature-inspired algorithms, there are still some trying, open issues that should be tended to. These open issues incorporate the equilibrium of investigation and double-dealing, determination instruments, perfect proportion of randomization, also boundary tuning as well as boundary control.

As referenced in the fundamental text, quite possibly the most difficult issue is the way to balance investigation and double-dealing in a algorithm so it can manage a huge scope of issues effectively. In all actuality, how much investigation and abuse may rely upon the sort of issue, and hence, somewhere in the range of deduced information on the issue to be tackled can assist with deciding such equilibrium. In any case, it isn't known instructions to consolidate such information successfully. For instance, angle/subordinate data got from the goal capacity can be exceptionally helpful for abuse, yet, assuming such double-dealing is excessively solid, it can make the framework be caught in a neighborhood ideal, subsequently forfeiting the chance of tracking down the genuine worldwide optimality.

To adjust investigation and double-dealing, a perfect proportion of arbitrariness is required. In any case, nobody realizes what sum is the perfect sum. At one limit, assuming there is no haphazardness, an algorithm turns into a deterministic algorithm, and in this manner loses the capacity to investigate. At the other limit, on the off chance that the inquiry is overwhelmed by a high level of irregularity, the algorithm turns into an arbitrary hunt, and in this manner altogether lessens its capacity to take advantage of the scene data. Truth be told, it isn't known how to control arbitrariness appropriately in order to adjust investigation and double-dealing most successfully.

Another significant issue is the choice system and it isn't known what choice is best. An appropriate choice strain is critical to keep a solid populace. For instance, when numerous arrangements have comparative wellness, mathematically talking, their wellness values may nearly be something very similar, in this way how to choose specific arrangements becomes interesting. Run of the mill approaches incorporate re-scaled wellness values, positioning of arrangements, and versatile elitism [2].

Nonetheless, it isn't clear assuming they can work for all algorithms and on the off chance that there is other better ways of dealing with choice. Then again, as the presentation of practically any procedure will rely upon its boundary settings, how to tune these boundaries to accomplish the best exhibition is a more significant level optimization issue. Indeed, this is the optimization of an enhancement algorithm. It is as yet an open inquiry. Likewise, how to control the boundaries by differing their qualities to accomplish the best generally speaking presentation is additionally a key testing issue. It is trusted that productive devices can be created to settle a wide reach of enormous scope issues in true applications. Future exploration headings ought to zero in on such main points of contention and difficulties.

1.6 Conclusion

In this book chapter, we have attempted to investigate most significant nature-inspired optimization algorithms and their role in resolving complex computationally hard problems in various field of application. As we have seen from the above essential investigation, appropriate variation and variety are critical to guarantee the great exhibition of a algorithm. Variation can be completed in various parts (of a algorithm), like the age of the populace, determination of arrangements, elitism, substitution of arrangements, change of boundaries furthermore generally speaking harmony between investigation and abuse. Variety can likewise show up in many places, for example, the ways of producing new arrangements, choice and substitution of existing arrangements, exploratory moves, randomization, and above all to keep a decent equilibrium in investigation and abuse. Notwithstanding the accomplishment of nature-inspired algorithms, there are still some trying, open issues that should be tended to. These open issues incorporate the equilibrium of investigation and double-dealing, determination components, perfect proportion of randomization, also boundary tuning as well as boundary control.

Unfortunately, it isn't practical to investigate each nature-propelled algorithm in detail. The activity would be both monotonous and unnecessarily dreary; thus, our zero in is on nonetheless, we have likewise examined momentarily a few other nature-inspired algorithms to show that the models and standards in all actuality do reach out to numerous different algorithms. The models that we have depicted show how NIAs work, yet in addition give experiences regarding processes in numerous regular frameworks. Notwithstanding, we should close by taking note of that the strategies we acquire from nature don't copy regular cycles; they are just models. Similarly as with all models, they exclude many subtleties, and some of the time, the distinctions can be pivotal. Additionally, it is essential to understand that nature can give a larger number of examples than ways of planning algorithms. It is additionally informative to concentrate on the ways they are utilized in nature. These give a few significant examples. Here and there, a cycle that is imperative in nature is viewed as an issue in registering. For instance, think about hereditary algorithms. Untimely union in GAs alludes to the peculiarity wherein all individuals from the populace get the same hereditary make-up, subsequently halting the hunt before an answer has been reached. In genuine populaces, be that as it may, intermingling assumes a vital part: it fixes alleles in a populace, so empowering it to procure new characters.

Maybe, the greatest contrast between critical thinking in nature and that in PC algorithms is that the algorithms essentially consistently treat issues as one off. That is, they are treated as shut frameworks, secluded from whatever other issues that might be put to them. Regular frameworks, then again, take care of many issues, regularly in equal, so they treat critical thinking in an alternate manner. One outcome of regarding issues as shut frameworks is just computational strategies don't gain for a fact. They for the most part approach every issue again. Indeed, even in AI, algorithms advance just neighborhood information from cases that are introduced to them with regards to a specific issue. They don't hold that information to utilize later on different issues. Normal frameworks, interestingly, ordinarily hold information acquired as a matter of fact. Youthful creatures gain from each insight, developing a collection of 'arrangements' over the long run. Similarly, populaces are molded by their current circumstance, which chooses for qualities the most appropriate to tackle future issues. A remarkable illustration of the above is the different manner by which improvement is taken on in algorithm versus in nature. Numerous human issues are acted like streamlining. Besides, the issues are presented inside a shut setting. Not much is thought of. So the point becomes to track down the very best conceivable arrangement, for example the highest mark of the tallest mountain. Indeed, the greater part of the hypothetical examinations completed in past work are tied in with demonstrating intermingling of NIOAs.

Clearly, there are different issues and open issues also. The above discussion has quite recently centered a couple of central questions. This multitude of difficulties can introduce once in a lifetime kinds of chances for additional exploration in investigating transformation and variety in metaheuristic algorithms. It very well may be normal more hypothetical outcomes will show up from now on, and any hypothetical outcomes will give colossal knowledge into understanding metaheursitic algorithms. It is trusted that effective devices can be created to settle a wide reach of enormous scope issues in genuine applications. Future examination bearings ought to zero in on such main points of interest and difficulties.

Finally, the survey can fill in as a directing point for scholars and researchers of the area inspired by moving toward the issue of local area location with computational models inspired by development in nature by giving a total outline and classification that can acquaint them with the main parts of this space.

References

1. Yang, X.S.: Nature-inspired optimization algorithms: Challenges and open problems. J. Comput. Sci. **46**, 101104 (2020)
2. Yang, X.S.: Metaheuristic optimization: Nature-inspired algorithms and applications. In: Yang, X.S. (eds.) Artificial Intelligence, Evolutionary Computing and Metaheuristics. Studies in Computational Intelligence, vol. 427. Springer, Heidelberg (2013). https://doi.org/10.1007/978-3-642-29694-9-16
3. Fister, I., Yang, X.-S., Fister, I., et al.: A brief review of nature-inspired algorithms for optimization. Elektrotehni Ski Vestnik **80**(3), 1–7 (2013)
4. Soni, V., Sharma, A., Singh, V.: A critical review on nature inspired optimization algorithms. In IOP Conference Series: Materials Science and Engineering, Vol. 1099, No. 1, p. 012055. IOP Publishing (2021)
5. Hayes-Roth, F.: Review of adaptation in natural and artificial systems by John H. Holland, The U. of Michigan Press, 1975. ACM SIGART Bull. **53**, 15 (1975)
6. Kennedy, J., Eberhart, R.: Particle swarm optimization. In: Proceedings of the 1995 IEEE International Conference on Neural Networks, Perth, WA, Australia, 27 November–1 December 1995; pp. 1942–1948
7. Storn, R., Price, K.: Differential evolution-a simple and efficient heuristic for global optimization over continuous space. J. Glob. Opt. **11**, 341–359 (1997)
8. Dervis, K., Bahriye, B.: A powerful and efficient algorithm for numerical function optimization: Artificial bee colony (ABC) algorithm. J. Glob. Optim. **39**, 459–471 (2007)
9. Colorni, A., Dorigo, M., Maniezzo, V.: Distributed optimization by ant colonies. In: Proceedings of the 1st European Conference on Artificial Life, pp. 134–142, New York, UK, 11–13 November 1991
10. Yang, X. S., Deb, S.: Cuckoo Search via Lévy Flights. In: Proceedings of the 2009 World Congress on Nature and Biologically Inspired Computing, pp. 210–214, Coimbatore, India, 9–11 December 2009
11. Yang, X.S., Gandomi, A.H.: Bat algorithm: A novel approach for global engineering optimization. Eng. Comput. **29**, 464–483 (2012)
12. Yang, X.S.: Nature-Inspired Metaheutistic Algorithms, 2nd edn. University of Cambridge Beckington, Luniver Press, UK (2008)
13. Bersini, H., Varela, F.J.: The immune recruitment mechanism: a selective evolutionary strategy. In: Proceedings of the International Conference on Genetic Algorithms, San Diego, CA, USA, vol. 13–16, pp. 520–526 (1991)
14. Mirjalili, S., Mirjalili, S.M., Lewis, A.: Grey Wolf Optimizer. Adv. Eng. Softw. **69**, 46-61 (2014)
15. Esmat, R., Hossein, N.P., Saeid, S.: GSA: A gravitational search algorithm. Inform. Sci. **179**, 2232–2248 (2009)
16. Geem, Z.W., Kim, J.H., Loganathan, G.V.: A new heuristic optimization algorithm: Harmony search. Simulation **76**, 60–68 (2001)
17. Lim, T.Y.: Structured population genetic algorithms: A literature survey. Artif. Intell. Rev. **41**, 385–399 (2014)
18. Chaurasia, G.S., Singh, A.K., Agrawal, S., Sharma, N.K.: A meta-heuristic firefly algorithm based smart control strategy and analysis of a grid connected hybrid photovoltaic/wind distributed generation system. Sol. Energy **150**, 265–274 (2017)
19. Auger, A., Doerr, B.: Theory of Randomized Search Heuristics: Foundations and RecentDevelopments. World Scientific (2010)
20. Kirkpatrick, S., Gellat, C.D., Vecchi, M.P.: Optimisation by simulated annealing. Science **220**, 671–680 (1983)
21. Mareli, M., Twala, B.: An adaptive Cuckoo search algorithm for optimisation. Appl. Comput. Inform. **14**(2), 107–115 (2018)
22. Yang, X.S.: Firefly algorithms for multimodal optimization. In: Watanabe, O., Zeugmann, T. (eds.) SAGA 2009. LNCS, vol. 5792, pp. 169–178. Springer, Heidelberg (2009)

23. Glover, F., Laguna, M.: Tabu search. In: Du, D.Z., Pardalos, P.M. (eds.) Handbook of Combinatorial Optimization. Springer, Boston, MA (1998). https://doi.org/10.1007/978-1-4613-0303-9_33
24. Gutjahr, W.J.: Convergence analysis of metaheuristics. Ann. Inf. Syst. **10**, 159–187 (2010)
25. Igel, C., Toussaint, M.: On classes of functions for which no free lunch results hold. Inform. Process. Lett. **86**, 317–321 (2003)
26. Villalobos-Arias, M., CoelloCoello, C.A., Hernandez-Lerma, O.: Asymptotic convergence of metaheuristics for multiobjective optimization problems. Soft. Comput. **10**, 1001–1005 (2005)
27. Kougianos, E., Mohanty, S.P.: A nature-inspired firefly algorithm based approach for nanoscale leakage optimal RTL structure. Integr. VLSI J. **51**, 46–60 (2015)
28. Holland, J.H., Taylor, C.E.: Adaptation in natural and artificial systems: an introductory analysis with applications to biology, control, and artificial intelligence. Complex adaptive systems. Q Rev Biol. **69**(1), 88–9 (1994)
29. Das P., Jana B., Acharyya S.: A new variant of genetic algorithm for solving gene selection problem. In: Giri, D., Buyya, R., Ponnusamy, S., De, D., Adamatzky, A., Abawajy, J.H. (eds.) Proceedings of the Sixth International Conference on Mathematics and Computing. Advances in Intelligent Systems and Computing, vol. 1262. Springer, Singapore (2021). https://doi.org/10.1007/978-981-15-8061-1-25
30. Bonabeau, E., Dorigo, M., Theraulaz, G.: Swarm Intelligence: From Natural to Artificial Systems. Oxford University Press, Oxford (1999). Print ISBN-13: 9780195131581, https://doi.org/10.1093/oso/9780195131581.001.0001
31. Surowiecki, J.: The Wisdom of Crowds. Anchor Books (2004), ISBN:978-0-385-72170-7
32. Pei, Y., Wang, W., Zhang, S.: Basic ant colony optimization. In: Proceedings of the 2012 International Conference Computing Science Electronics Engineering ICCSEE 2012, vol. 1, pp. 665–667 (2012). https://doi.org/10.1109/ICCSEE.2012.178
33. Reddy, T.N.: Optimization of K-means algorithm: ant colony optimization. In: 1st International Conference Computing Methodology Communication (ICCMC 2017), pp. 530–535 (2017)
34. Zhai, Y., Xu, L., Yang, Y.: Ant colony algorithm research based on pheromone update strategy. In: Proceedings of the 2015 7th International Conference Intelligent Human-Machine Systems Cybernetics IHMSC 2015, vol. 1(2), pp. 38–41 (2012). https://doi.org/10.1109/IHMSC.2015.143
35. Deneubourg, J.-L., Aron, S., Goss, S., Pasteels, J.M.: The self-organizing exploratory pattern of the argentine ant. J. Insect Behav. **3**(2), 159–168 (1990)
36. Blum, C., Roli, A.: Metaheuristics in combinatorial optimization: Overview and conceptual comparison. ACM Comput. Surv. **35**(3), 268–308 (2003)
37. Dorigo, M., Stützle, T.: Ant Colony Optimization. MIT Press (2004), ISBN: 9780262042192
38. Eskandar, H., Sadollah, A., Bahreininejad, A., Hamdi, M.: Water cycle algorithm-A novel metaheuristic optimization method for solving constrained engineering optimization problems. Comput. Struct. **110**, 151–166 (2012)
39. Khamparia, A., Khanna, A., Nguyen, N.G., Le Nguyen, B. (eds.): Nature-Inspired Optimization AlgorithmsRecent Advances in Natural Computing and Biomedical Applications (2021). https://doi.org/10.1515/9783110676112, Published by De Gruyter 2021
40. Jamil, M., Zepernick, H.J.: Multimodal function optimisation with cuckoo search algorithm. Int. J. Bio-Inspired Comput. **5**(2), 73–83 (2013)
41. Yang, X.S., He, X.S.: Why the firefly algorithm works?. In: Yang, X.S. (eds.) Nature-Inspired Algorithms and Applied Optimization. Studies in Computational Intelligence, vol. 744. Springer, Cham (2018). https://doi.org/10.1007/978-3-319-67669-2_11
42. Fisher, L.: The Perfect Swarm: The Science of Complexity in Everyday Life. Basic Books (2009), ISBN-13: 9780465020850
43. Fister, I., Fister, I., Yang, X.S., Brest, J.: A comprehensive review of firefly algorithms. Swarm Evol. Comput. **13**(1), 34–46 (2013)
44. Fister, I., Yang, X.S., Brest, J., Fister, I.: Modified firefly algorithm using quaternion representation. Expert Syst. Appl. **40**(18), 7220–7230 (2013)

45. Fister, I., Perc, M., Kamal, S.M., Fister, I.: A review of chaos-based firefly algorithms: Perspectives and research challenges. Appl. Math. Comput. **252**, 155–165 (2015)
46. Storn, R., Price, K.: Differential evolution—a simple and efficient heuristic for global optimization over continuous spaces. J. Glob. Optim. **11**, 341–359 (1997). https://doi.org/10.1023/A:1008202821328
47. Shunmugapriya, P., Kanmani, S.: A hybrid algorithm using ant and bee colony optimization for feature selection and classification (AC-ABC Hybrid). Swarm Evol. Comput. **36**, 27–36 (2017). ISSN 2210-6502, https://doi.org/10.1016/j.swevo.2017.04.002
48. Yang, X.S., Deb, S.: Engineering Optimisation by Cuckoo Search. Int. J. Math. Model. Numer. Optim. **1**, 330–343 (2010). https://doi.org/10.1504/IJMMNO.2010.035430
49. Levy flight algorithm for optimization problems—a literature review. Appl. Mech. Mater. **421** (2013). https://doi.org/10.4028/www.scientific.net/AMM.421.496
50. Yang, X.S., Deb, S.: Cuckoo Search via Lévy flights. In: 2009 World Congress on Nature & Biologically Inspired Computing (NaBIC), pp. 210–214 (2009). https://doi.org/10.1109/NABIC.2009.5393690
51. Osaba, E., Yang, X.S.: Soccer-inspired metaheuristics: Systematic review of recent research and applications. In: Osaba, E., Yang, XS. (eds.) Applied Optimization and Swarm Intelligence. Springer Tracts in Nature-Inspired Computing. Springer, Singapore (2021). https://doi.org/10.1007/978-981-16-0662-5_5
52. Yang, X.S.: A new metaheuristic bat-inspired algorithm. In: Nature Inspired Cooperative Strategies for Optimisation (NICSO 2010), vol. 284, pp. 65–74. Studies in Computational Intelligence. Springer, Berlin (2010)
53. Walton, S., Hassan, O., Morgan, K., Brown, M.R.: Modified cuckoo search: A new gradient free optimisation algorithm. Chaos Solitons Fractals **44**(9), 710–718 (2011). ISSN 0960-0779, https://doi.org/10.1016/j.chaos.2011.06.004
54. Reynolds, C.: Flocks, herds, and schools: A distributed behavioral model. Comput. Graph. **21**, 25–34 (1987)
55. Fong, S., Deb, S., Yang, X.S., Li, J.Y.: Metaheuristic swarm search for feature selection in life science classification. IEEE IT Prof. **16**(4), 24–29 (2014)
56. Clerc, M., Kennedy, J.: The particle swarm: explosion, stability, and convergence in a multidimensional complex space. IEEE Trans. Evol. Comput. 58–73 (2002)
57. Chen, S., Peng, G.H., He, X.S., Yang, X.S.: Global convergence analysis of the bat algorithm using a markovian framework and dynamic system theory. Expert Syst. Appl. **114**, 173–182 (2018)

Chapter 2
Preventing the Early Spread of Infectious Diseases Using Particle Swarm Optimization

R. Jayashree

Abstract Alpha, beta, delta and gamma are variations of contemporary coronavirus, the extreme acute respiratory syndrome. Community health care organizations are obliged to discover, avert and regulate infections in the populace. Precaution techniques manipulate the unfolding of today's infectious diseases like coronavirus variations to some extent. Identification of modern-day infection in the preliminary stage is very vital to govern its spreading. In this chapter, an easy inferring archetypal is proposed for the forecast of the spreading pattern of today's infectious illnesses using a swarm learning approach in which every particle is benefited from the other particle's experience despite available neighbourhood statistics. An evaluation of the features of the anticipated archetypal is received by the use of a Recursive Particle Swarm Optimization algorithm that calls for repetitively fixing a quadratic programming problem. The version is derived from training data which provides insight into the force of the spread of the latest infectious illnesses. The proposed version performs on par with the advanced Bayesian Monte Carlo version. The anticipated approach empirically assesses authorized data provided by the World Health Organization. The computation takes a look at consequences, and displays a better accuracy of the predicted pattern of infection spreading.

Keywords Particle Swarm optimization · Coronavirus · Recursive particle Swarm optimization · Bayesian Monte Carlo · Machine learning

2.1 Introduction

Swarm learning is the knowledge gained from sharing experiences among members without sharing confidential data. The advantage of this learning over the conventional methods is it protects the privacy of the individuals and boosts collaboration and records trade, especially within the medical subject [1]. Machine learning (ML)

R. Jayashree (✉)
Department of Computer Science, SRM Institute of Science and Technology, Kattankulathur Campus, Chennai, Tamil Nadu 603203, India
e-mail: jayashrr@srmist.edu.in

© The Author(s), under exclusive license to Springer Nature Switzerland AG 2023
J. Nayak et al. (eds.), *Nature-Inspired Optimization Methodologies in Biomedical and Healthcare*, Intelligent Systems Reference Library 233,
https://doi.org/10.1007/978-3-031-17544-2_2

algorithms locate patterns with skilled records, therefore, accumulating the capability to become aware of the found-out styles in other records properly. Agrawal et al. [2] proposed the Particle Swarm Optimization algorithm (PSO) in 1995 to discover the premier answer simplest with goal function, unbiased of gradient or differential objectives. This approach is widely used in a variety of applications, which include photograph and film evaluation, model and restructuring of present-day power systems, electronics, electromagnetic, and so on. The PSO algorithm outperforms the Bayesian Monte Carlo (BMC) approach when the number of iterations in ML is huge [3]. The distributed regulation within the system is the benefit of PSO. As a result, the search system is not affected when failure occurs in any particle. The PSO is clean, easy and simplest wherein few parameters needed to be adjusted [2]. A Recursive Particle Swarm Optimization (RPSO) is proposed to clear up dynamic optimization in which the facts are obtained one after another [4]. The position of the particle is updated recursively based on the primordial and continuous information.

Since 2015, Machine Learning techniques assisted the detection of outbreaks where still improvements are needed. For example, automated outbreak detection systems, Artificial Neural networks, and Logistic Regression methods [5–7]. Quantitative prediction is set in place of simple prevention and control of variances which is the more challenging part. For privacy and computational reasons, epidemiological data are generally reported in huge numbers which can be grouped by weeks/months or by geographical locations. This enables predictions based on a history of data [8]. In general, outbreaks extend over geographical boundaries. Therefore, predictive model includes Interaction, spatial and temporal features. This provides additional insight into the study of infectious disease spreading patterns. Confirmed Infected Persons (IP) provide indirect information which is inadequate in the prediction of future effects of infection spreading on the population. Thus, the expected number of IPs can be expressed as a spatial and temporal function related to the prior information [9].

Testing the entire susceptible is not possible in a region/country with a large population [10]. Particularly, the situation is highly complicated in some infectious diseases (ID) detection, like coronavirus variants, since a noteworthy part of positive IPs remain undetected because of the lack of key characteristics (that is, asymptomatic) of the diseases [11]. Therefore, the logistic function with space, time and interaction factors provides the basic model for the determination of the total number of infected/confirmed IPs [11]. The number of confirmed, active and recovered data with time intervals is important in the estimation of the optimization approach using the PSO technique. Quantitative differences among various coronavirus waves are exposed through Spatio-temporal connectivity in their transmission scales, and patterns [12]. The detection of rapid deviations in the projected count of IPs provides an early warning about the state transition [13]. The anticipated model guides controlling and preventing the disease from spreading in any densely populated geographical location.

The transmission pattern of infectious diseases like coronavirus gives dynamic heterogeneity of the disease and optimization insight which enables us to understand the pharmaceutical and non-pharmaceutical strategies [12]. The DZNE (Deutsches Zentrum fur Neurodegenerative Erkrankungen) is the part of the Helmholtz Association of German Research Centres in which the research members identified perfect data for testing Swarm Learning [1]. They are,

- Non-infectious diseases: acute myeloid and acute lymphoblastic leukaemia.
- Infectious diseases: tuberculosis and corona variants.

The new coronavirus variant, Omicron, spreads 3 times faster than the delta variant of COVID-19 [14]. A large number of spike protein, mutations, on Omicron affect the antibodies' ability to recognize and block virus infection. Compare to the Delta variant, Omicron contains very few symptoms thus early detection and isolation of the susceptible is difficult [14]. To overcome this problem, a model is proposed with 'interaction' features to identify the global maxima with PSO for the determination of the spreading pattern of the coronavirus infection. The results show that the improved model with RPSO outperforms the BCM model in terms of the performance evaluation, Kolmogorov–Smirnov test.

2.2 Literature Review of the Status of Research and Development in the Subject

In late November 2021, a new coronavirus variant was first identified and named Omicron, spreading fast in more than 89 countries [15]. According to 'Times' news [16], the new variant overtakes the delta variant by increasing it six times in 8 days. Reinfection occurs majorly in the people who got infected with one variant and then later a mutated variant [17]. The new coronavirus variant has higher transmissibility, which may result in severe consequences.

The Machine learning algorithm, and calculation, are basic to create sagacious decisions that help trained professionals and radiologists to get more information to shield themselves from misdiagnosing a patient. Many scientists and researchers around the world are actively working on the early prediction of ID and its impact. However, only a few research groups are discussed here.

The machine learning algorithms detect patterns on trained data and gain the ability to find the learned pattern for testing data. Agrawal et al. [2] introduced PSO with Acceleration and in detail explained the Swarm optimization technique which is widely used in medical research because knowledge sharing happens among every node without confidential data sharing between nodes. Thus, swarm learning protects data. The swarm learning approach provides knowledge by exchanging information across nodes in the network with machine learning algorithms. Since its formation in eras in the past, this technique is considerably used for resolving tough continuous Global optimization issues [11]. In report [1], swarm learning-based collaborative studies have been performed to check an innovative approach for studying information saved in a decentralized manner. Many research institutions from various parts of the world like Germany, Netherlands and Greece participated in this research. The swarm learning technique finds out the people vulnerable to getting infected in an optimized manner [18]. The PSO is a swarm aptitude method that is stirred via the cleverness, knowledge sharing, and communal conduct of fish-schooling and bird-flocking [19, 29].

In South Africa, the Omicron is spreading much faster than its previous variants. Health Security Agency of the UK found that two-dose vaccination is not as effective on the new variant as in the delta variant [15]. Researchers in South Africa and Europe found that the omicron symptoms are milder than the delta variant. Researchers in the UK warned that the new variant may cause tens of thousands of additional deaths. At the Health Research Institutes virologist Alex Sigal (Africa), and Sandra Ciesek (Germany) conducted research that concluded that the currently available vaccines are 40% less potent against the new coronavirus variants [14, 20, 21]. Additionally, at the Karolinska Institute, virologists Daniel Sheward and Murrell analysed the effect of virus and vaccination on healthcare workers [20]. Zhan et al. [22] demonstrated the novel particle swarm optimization in forecasting the changing characteristics of ID. Zreiq Rafat et al. [23] investigated four phenomenological epidemic models in addition to the SIR version so that the cumulative number of confirmed IPs of coronavirus and the feasible end-date of the ID are envisaged. The constraints identification for optimized generalized logistic (GL) is a challenging task in the non-linear least-squares problem [11].

A prominent science journal from the US published a study on immense coronavirus epidemiology in Tamil Nadu and Andhra Pradesh (the south Indian states) for 85 thousand patients [24]. The fatality rate is 2.1% in the year 2020 [24]. Nagarajan Karikalan et al. [25] studied publicly available 1959 patients' detail in Karnataka state, India, and identified 68% of epidemiological contacts of influential patients through a social network analysis approach.

Time-series based early detection techniques are studied for ID [7, 9]. Liu Yang et al. [12] described how the organism reacts to a disease using 16,000 transcriptomes which are largely available just like X-ray images. Artificial intelligence and swarm learning are suitable for analysing data like transcriptomes. Swarm Learning generated remarkably better outputs compared to the particles in the network erudite separately. The proposed spatiotemporal evaluation technique chaperon efforts to control and avert the spread of the latest disorder not just in India but additionally in different densely populated global metropolises [12]. In July 2020, randomly tested 28 thousand patients' data along with their other details like ethnicity, age, gender and race in 46 states and 1013 US counties [10]. This study provided evidence that the mobility of the community using geographical data is applied in monitoring the spread of ID. Li Baolei et al. [4] experimented on a network model with a recursive PSO algorithm and provided accurate results for dynamic problems.

2.3 Methodology

A superior feature of the anticipated model is subject to stingy input data. Required inputs are:

(1) Total number of IP.
(2) Daily number of new IP.
(3) Period between infection and recovery.
(4) Period between infection and death.

Consider the following notations:
In Table 2.1 the 'd' is the number of days from 1st day of report to recovery or death reported.
That is, d = 1, 2,..., day.
The cumulative number of deaths is the sum of the number of new deaths from day 1 to d. Similarly, the cumulative number of recoveries computed as shown in Eqs. (2.1) and (2.2),

$$\hat{C}\Omega(d) = \sum_{n=1}^{d} \Omega'(n) \tag{2.1}$$

$$\hat{C}P(d) = \sum_{n=1}^{d} P'(n) \tag{2.2}$$

Table 2.1 Notations and descriptions

Notation	Description
$\Omega'(d)$	Identified number of deaths on day d
$P'(d)$	Identified number of recoveries on day d
$\hat{C}_\Omega(d)$	Overall count of deaths reported on day d
$\hat{C}_P(d)$	Overall count of recoveries reported on day d
r_{min}	Minimum number of days from infection to recovery
r_{max}	Maximum number of days from infection to recovery
τ_{min}	Minimum number of days between infection and death
τ_{max}	Maximum number of days between infection and death
T(d)	Represent total number of IPs on day d
N(d)	Represent number of new IPs on day d
A(d)	Represent number of active IPs on day d
Rd_j	Predicted rate of death, j days infection
Rr_k	Predicted rate of recovery, k days infection

The ĈΩ(d) and

$$\hat{C}\text{Þ}(d)$$

are the lower and upper limit of the 95% acceptance random time interval that elapses between infection and death/healing respectively. Susceptible individuals can be either symptomatic or asymptomatic and can be a part of infected or infective people.

Those parameters are expected through abating the total of the quadratic mistakes among the actual collective range and the forecasted ones. An estimated technique for the optimization trouble received the usage of an RPSO set of guidelines. The T(d) is the overall quantity of IPs that are believed to observe a GL function. Initially, the feature of GL is S-shaped, used for modelling growth curves. Consider into account the subsequent variants [11]:

$$T(d) = \begin{cases} 0, & d < 0 \\ a, & d \geq 0 \end{cases} \quad (2.3)$$

where $a = \frac{w}{(1+xE)^{1/z}}$, $E = e^{-yd}$ and (w, x, y, z) are parameters that represent the quadruplet for the Q (w, x, y, z) quadratic programming with optimal value. From Eq. (2.3), the count of new IP on d is inferred as,

$$N(d) = \begin{cases} 0, & d \leq 0 \\ T(d) - T(d-1), & d > 0 \end{cases} \quad (2.4)$$

Let $\omega 1 = (d - \tau_{max}, d - \tau_{max+1}, \ldots, d - \tau_{min})$, and

$$\omega 2 = (d - r_{max}, d - r_{max+1}, \ldots, d - r_{min})$$

Consequently, from Eq. (2.4) the new death count on d is exhibited as the summation of a linear amalgamation of the count of new IPs of ω1 which is given as,

$$\Omega(d) = \sum_{i=\tau_{min}}^{\tau_{max}} Rd_i N(d-i) \quad (2.5)$$

from Eq. (2.4) the overall count of IPs recovered on d is the total of a linear combination of the count of new IPs of ω2. Thus, we define:

$$\text{Þ}(d) = \sum_{i=r_{min}}^{r_{max}} Rr_i N(d-i) \quad (2.6)$$

From Eqs. (2.3), (2.5) and (2.6), the count of active IPs on d is defined as given in Eq. (2.7),

$$A(d) = \{A(d-1) + T(d)\} - \{\Omega(d) + Þ(d)\} \qquad (2.7)$$

which is the likelihood of an IP death or recovery 'd' days after being infected. Formulating a Global Optimization problem to locate the factors of the GL function is a very difficult and demanding situation [11]. Consequently, derive an approximate solution via the usage of a PSO. In general, PSO finds the global minimum and/or maximum by moving the collection of particles through the search space. The position of particles represents a probable solution and its velocity constitutes the rate of adjustments of the position for the current location [2]. There are two extremes in the solution space they are, local and global. Compute the fitness value and set the contemporary fitness value as the new local best if the computed value is better than the 'Best-Fitness' value. The global best is the 'Best-Fitness' value of all particles.

Now the global best is selected based on the best fitness value of a particle of all particles. The proposed version indicates better accuracy and balance as opposed to BCM models while predicting the quantity of active IPs. The idea is primarily based on the optimization method which is used in the PSO algorithm. As the problem is solved, an IRR (Infection-to-recovery rate) evaluation is calculated as the summation of the likelihood between Infection and recovery:

$$\text{IRR} = \sum_{i=r_{min}}^{r_{max}} Rr_i, \qquad (2.8)$$

where $i = r_{min}, \ldots, r_{max}$.

Similarly, estimate an IDR (Infection-to-death rate) as the summation of the likelihood between infection and death:

$$\text{IDR} = \sum_{j=\tau_{min}}^{\tau_{max}} Rd_j, \qquad (2.9)$$

where $j = \tau_{min}, \ldots, \tau_{max}$.

From Eqs. (2.8) and (2.9) we get, IRR + IDR = 1.

2.3.1 Pattern Prediction with Prior Knowledge

Interaction is an essential factor in the prediction pattern of infectious diseases like typhoid and coronavirus. For simplicity, the interaction effects of IPs are added up linearly. Prediction is carried out through the knowledge gained from the neighbourhood. This enables the analysis of the nearest proximity to the function [8]. Asymptomatic individuals can be recovered or dead. Similarly, asymptomatic individuals can become unregistered recovered individuals which may be unnoticed through the infection [26]. Identifying asymptomatic individuals and unregistered recovered is not an easy task. Estimating the rate of IPs recovery or demise after a period 't' and evaluating the rates at the time 't + Δt', where 'Δt' is small-time duration, from the previous values. The PSOs based on ML is aware of archetypal limitations [26]. The RPSO is a computational approach which is used to minimize the mismatch among predictions and real observations of the IPs through iterative searching [26]. This method enhances particle prediction solution and therefore (2.7) at time € is written as,

$$A(€) = \{A(€ - 1) + T(€)\} - \{\Omega(€) + Þ(€)\} \qquad (2.10)$$

Then at € + Δ€, (2.10) is written as,

$$A(€ + Δ€) = \{A((€ + Δ€) - 1) + T(€ + Δ€)\} - \{\Omega(€ + Δ€) + Þ(€ + Δ€)\} \qquad (2.11)$$

This meta-heuristic gradient-free method transport the particle towards a satisfactory solution. Assemble the transmission networks of the detected IPs at some stage employing the spatiotemporal connectivity of any two IPs [12]. Prediction of transmission patterns of ID helps to govern and prevent the spreading of diseases which is a difficult task in any densely populated location.

2.4 Experiments and Results

Consider the following:

1. Time duration from symptomatic/asymptomatic to recovery is a minimum of 4 days—a maximum of 34 days with the distribution of 22 and to death as a minimum of 5 days—a maximum of 21 days [31].
2. The time duration for confirmed IPs to recover is a minimum of 10 days—a maximum of 40 days with a distribution of 28 days and to die is a minimum of 11 days—a maximum of 27 days [31].
3. The date, d = 1, corresponds to 3rd March 2020. The cumulative rate of infection is shown in Fig. 2.1 [27].

2.4.1 Running Environment

The whole experimentation is performed on Windows 10 operating system with Python 3.8.6 installed on it. Different types of environments and libraries of python for deep learning models are used for supporting the experimental setup. The main libraries and tools of Python that supported the experimentation include Numpy, Scipy, Anaconda, Tensorflow, Spyder IDE, and Pycharm. These all used for different purposes to improve the execution process.

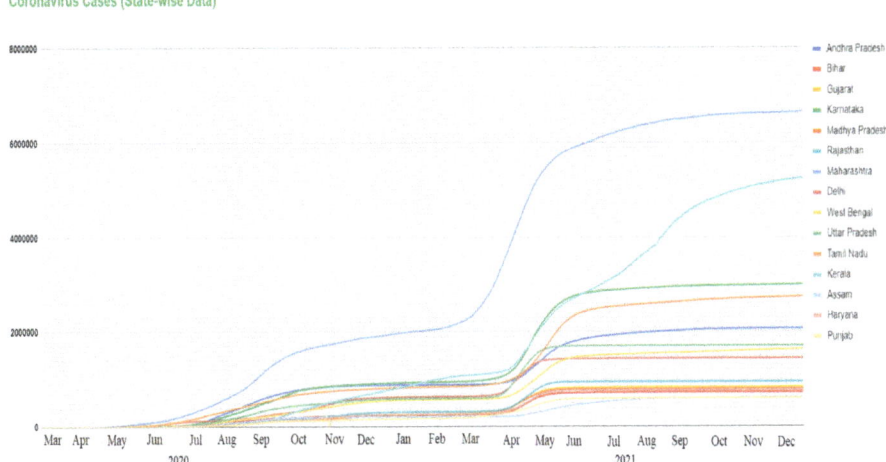

Fig. 2.1 Coronavirus state-wise data sourced from official website

The dataset is sourced from the official Indian website regarding coronavirus cases for 28 states and 7 Union Territories from March 2020 to Jan 2022, a totally of 586 days. Lakshadweep Island is excluded from the dataset because only in Jan 2021 were the first confirmed cases reported in Lakshadweep, which is nearly a year after the pandemic outbreak in India [32–34]. The first 15 states/union territories with the highest registered cases are depicted in Fig. 2.1 [27]. The daily Infected, death, recovered and total cases are sourced from [28]. The subsequent parameter distribution conjectured from the training information is studied, which affords appreciated records of the ailment as well as the aptness of the archetypal. The rate of infection in the case of coronavirus has a high degree of uncertainty inside the fashion as shown in Fig. 2.2.

To evaluate the enactment of the anticipated method, run it on first and second wave datasets considering the count of deaths, recovered, active and unregistered cases throughout the first and second wave of the outbreak, respectively. Acquire the GL curves from (2.7), (2.8) and (2.9). There are possibilities of conversion from asymptomatic to unregistered recovery or symptomatic and from symptomatic to recovered or dead. Thus, estimation of a variety of instances at 'Δt' in RPSO from (2.11) is displayed in Fig. 2.3. The daily rate of IP in the estimated (RPSO) and reference (BMC) model is shown in Fig. 2.4 for 35 Indian states for coronavirus. The equivalent prophecy from the reference BMC version [8] fitted to the equal records. Excessive aberration with actual information examination proves the performance of the RPSO method compared to the reference version.

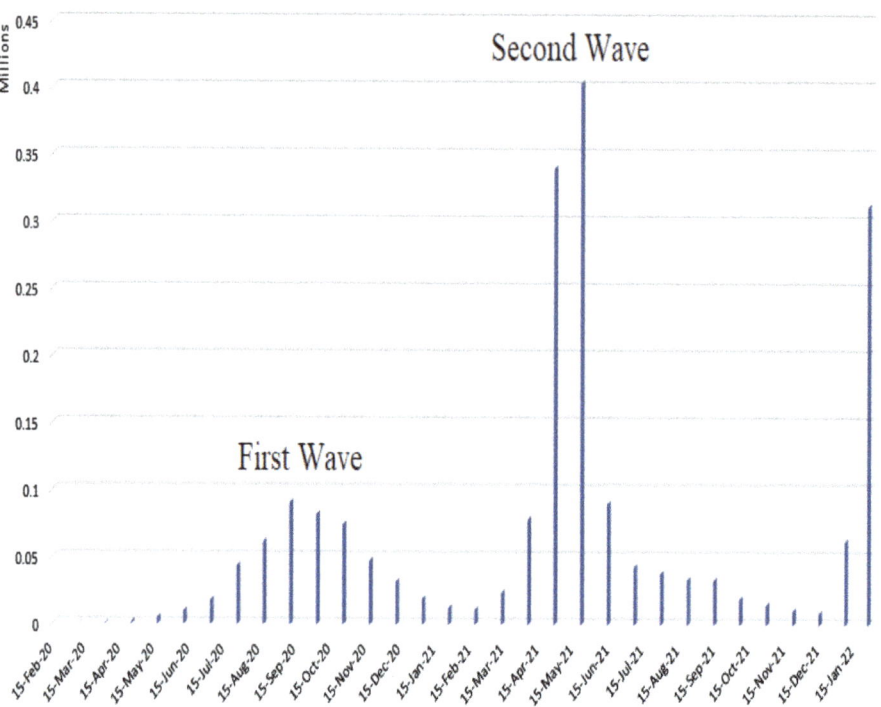

Fig. 2.2 The number of daily new cases from January 2020 to January 2022

2.4.2 Performance Metric

The Kolmogorov–Smirnov (KS) test identifies logistic distribution in the given data. This test defines the Hypothesis as,

- Ho: Distribution is normal.
- Ha: Distribution is not normal.

Critical Value: If the p-value, Asymptotic Significance (2-tailed), is less than 0.05, reject the normality assumption. Otherwise, conclude that there is insufficient evidence to suggest that the distribution is not normal. Carry out a Kolmogorov–Smirnov check for testing the speculation that the prediction errors are typically distributed [30]. The KS test is conducted on days 240 and 580 from the date of the first report at a 95% confidence interval. The consequences are displayed in Table 2.2 and the null hypothesis cannot be rejected at the 5% importance degree.

From (2.8) and (2.9), compute relative deviation prediction for both scenario for $d = day + 1,\ldots, 586$. In both scenarios, the maximum amount of deviation is 9.8% which is 2.5 times better than the reference model.

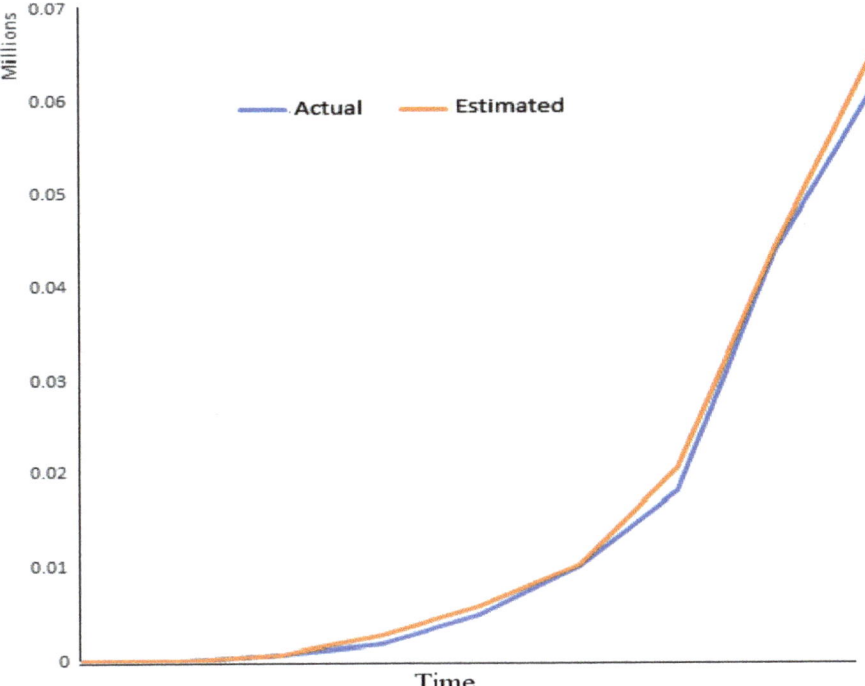

Fig. 2.3 GL curves for estimated and actual data

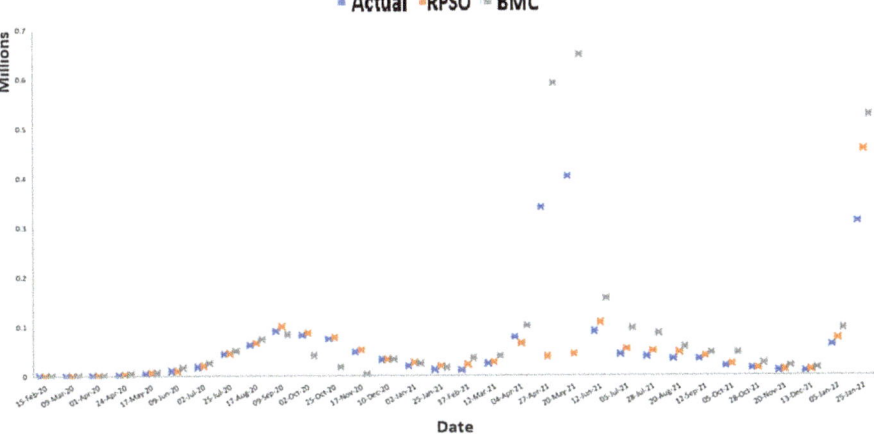

Fig. 2.4 Actual number of daily cases with estimated and reference model

Table 2.2 KS test value for 95% confidence interval

Day	Hypothesis	P-value	KS statistics	CR value
240	H0	0.0752	0.1130	0.1225
580	H0	0.3447	0.0639	0.1003

In Fig. 2.5 blue and red colors represent an increase and decrease in values. Since there is no decreasing value, Fig. 2.5 contains the only blue colour in the waterfall chart.

In Fig. 2.6, the highest range of frequency distribution in BMC is between 25 and 30; the daily number of IP is greater than 0.6 million. Whereas the highest range of frequency distribution in RPSO is between 20 and 25 and the daily number of IP is to the maximum of 0.5 million. Thus, compare to the dataset obtained from WHO which is 0.45 million [28], RPSO provides better prediction than the BMC model as shown in Figs. 2.5 and 2.6.

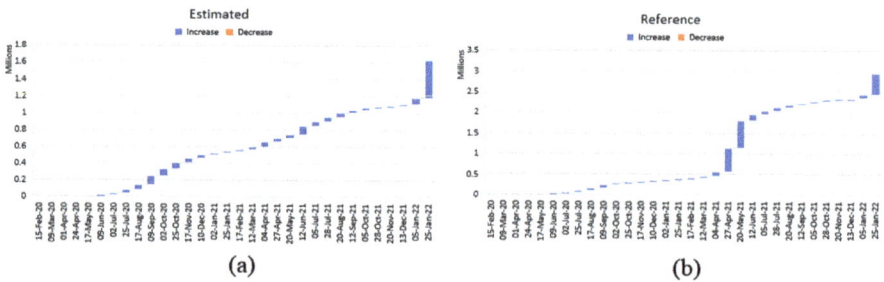

Fig. 2.5 Waterfall chart for daily cases for **a** estimated model **b** reference model

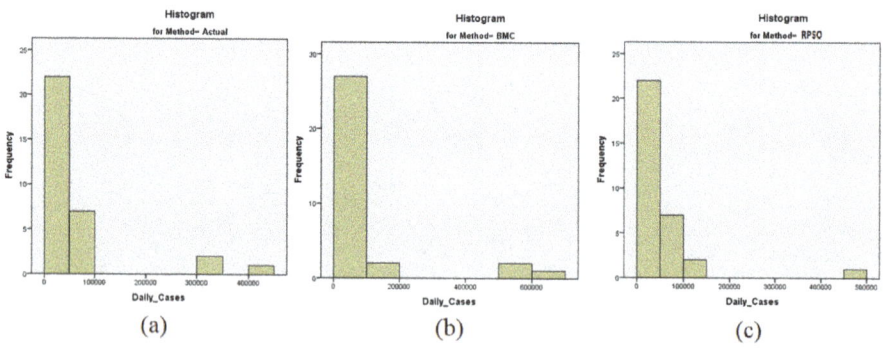

Fig. 2.6 Histograms for frequency of IPs. **a** Daily cases dataset from WHO. **b** Predicted daily cases using BMC. **c** Predicted daily cases using RPSO

2.5 Conclusion and Future Enhancement

The BMC algorithm adds significant computational overhead to the task of finding the optimal hyper-parameter values, while for the PSO algorithm the overhead is insignificant. Instead of static PSO, RPSO is dynamic which updates whenever IP transfers from the set of symptomatic to recovery/death or asymptomatic to symptomatic/recovery. The presented model with interaction factors is sufficient to identify the dynamic nature of coronavirus. The primary intention is to forecast the number of active IPs using RPSO with the help of parameters provided on the official website for coronavirus. The experimental results show that RPSO predicts 90% accurately which is almost 15% greater than the reference model, BMC. It is expected that if the proposed method is run periodically, then provide beneficial for the public fitness government for making knowledgeable choices and for that reason mitigate the impact of the outbreak.

Furthermore, future recommendation of the research trend is to use the recommended approach for location-based interconnection of IPs. Representing IPs as nodes and using edges to connect one another. A network can be built which results in a network of ID spreading patterns in that particular geographical location. This is a tough task since the location of the IP is not static.

References

1. DZNE—German Center for Neurodegenerative Diseases. In: AI with Swarm intelligence: a novel technology for cooperative analysis of big data. ScienceDaily. www.sciencedaily.com/releases/2021/05/210526132126.htm (2021). Accessed 8 Jan. 2022.
2. Agrawal, J., Shikha A.: Acceleration based particle swarm optimization for graph coloring problem. Procedia Comput. Sci. **60**, 714–721 (2015). https://doi.org/10.1016/j.procs.2015.08.223.
3. Tani, L.: Comparison of Bayesian and particle swarm algorithms for... arXiv.Org (2022). arxiv.org/abs/2201.06809.
4. Li, B., et al. Recursive particle swarm optimization applications in radial basis function networks modeling system. In: 2011 4th International Conference on Biomedical Engineering and Informatics (BMEI) (2011). https://doi.org/10.1109/bmei.2011.6098689.
5. Noufaily, A., et al.: An improved algorithm for outbreak detection in multiple surveillance systems. Statistics in Medicine **32**(7), 1206–1222 (2012). https://doi.org/10.1002/sim.5595.
6. Gertler, M., et al.: Outbreak of Cryptosporidium Hominis following river flooding in the City of Halle (Saale), Germany, August 2013. BMC Infect. Dis. **15**(1) (2015). https://doi.org/10.1186/s12879-015-0807-1.
7. Salmon M., Schumacher D., Burmann H., Frank C., Claus H., et al.: A system for automated outbreak detection of communicable diseases in Germany. *Eurosurveillance*, 31 Mar. 2016. Eur. Commun. Dis. Bull. **21**(13) (2016). www.eurosurveillance.org/content/https://doi.org/10.2807/1560-7917.ES.2016.21.13.30180.
8. Stojanović, O., et al.: A Bayesian Monte Carlo approach for predicting the spread of infectious diseases. In: Cathy W.S.C. (ed.) PLOS ONE **14**(12), e0225838 (2019). https://doi.org/10.1371/journal.pone.0225838.
9. Xia, Y., et al. Measles metapopulation dynamics: a gravity model for epidemiological coupling and dynamics. Am. Nat. **164**(2), 267–281 (2004). https://doi.org/10.1086/422341.

10. Anand, S., et al. Prevalence of SARS-CoV-2 antibodies in a large nationwide sample of patients on dialysis in the USA: a cross-sectional study. Lancet **396**(10259), 1335–1344 (2020). https://doi.org/10.1016/s0140-6736(20)32009-2.
11. Haouari, M., Mariem M.: A particle swarm optimization approach for predicting the number of COVID-19 deaths. Sci. Rep. **11**(1) (2021). https://doi.org/10.1038/s41598-021-96057-5.
12. Liu, Y., et al.: Uncovering transmission patterns of COVID-19 outbreaks: a region-wide comprehensive retrospective study in Hong Kong. EClinicalMedicine **36**, 100929 (2021). https://doi.org/10.1016/j.eclinm.2021.100929.
13. Chen, C.W.S., et al.: Markov switching integer-valued generalized auto-regressive conditional heteroscedastic models for dengue counts. J. R. Stat. Soc.: Ser. C (Appl. Stat.) **68**(4), 963–983 (2019). https://doi.org/10.1111/rssc.12344.
14. Callaway, E.: Omicron likely to weaken COVID vaccine protection. Nature **600**(7889), 367–368 (2021). https://doi.org/10.1038/d41586-021-03672-3. Accessed 14 Dec. 2021.
15. Euronews. Booster dose raises protection against Omicron, UK study shows. Euronews. www.euronews.com/2021/12/10/booster-dose-raises-protection-against-omicron-uk-study-shows (2021). Accessed 8 Jan. 2022.
16. Mathrubhumi.: COVID-19: six times increase in 8 days, Omicron variant predominant strain: Union Govt. English.Mathrubhumi (2022). www.english.mathrubhumi.com/news/india/india-1.6332555. Accessed 8 Jan. 2022.
17. hindustantimes.com.: Can you get infected with Omicron twice? White House medical adviser answers. Hindustan Times. www.hindustantimes.com/world-news/can-you-get-infected-with-omicron-twice-white-house-medical-adviser-answers-101642816717127.html (2022). Accessed on 22 Jan. 2022
18. Verde, L., et al.: Exploring the use of artificial intelligence techniques to detect the presence of coronavirus Covid-19 through speech and voice analysis. IEEE Access **9**, 65750–65757 (2021). https://doi.org/10.1109/access.2021.3075571.
19. Kennedy, J., Eberhart R.: Particle swarm optimization. Proceedings of ICNN'95—International Conference on Neural Networks, pp. 1942–1948 (1995). https://doi.org/10.1109/icnn.1995.488968.
20. Euronews.: Omicron COVID variant appears to spread faster than delta, WHO says. Euronews. www.euronews.com/next/2021/12/12/omicron-covid-variant-appears-to-spread-faster-than-delta-who-says (2021).
21. Varadarajan, P.: Omicron spreads faster than delta, data on severity limited: WHO. Businessline. www.thehindubusinessline.com/news/world/omicron-spreads-faster-than-delta-data-on-severity-limited-who/article37944388.ece (2022). Accessed 8 Jan. 2022.
22. Zhan, C. et al.: Optimizing broad learning system hyper-parameters through particle swarm optimization for predicting COVID-19 in 184 Countries. 2020 IEEE International Conference on E-Health Networking, Application & Services (HEALTHCOM) (2021). https://doi.org/10.1109/healthcom49281.2021.9399020.
23. Zreiq, R., et al.: Generalized Richards model for predicting COVID-19 dynamics in Saudi Arabia based on particle swarm optimization algorithm. AIMS Public Health **7**(4), 828–843 (2020). https://doi.org/10.3934/publichealth.2020064.
24. Nagaiah, K., Srimannarayana, G., Phaniraj, G.: Why India should not reopen schools and colleges during COVID-19 pandemic. Downtoearth, downtoearth. www.downtoearth.org.in/blog/governance/why-india-should-not-reopen-schools-and-colleges-during-covid-19-pandemic-74493 (2020). Accessed 26 Dec. 2020.
25. Nagarajan, K., et al.: Social network analysis methods for exploring SARS-CoV-2 contact tracing data. BMC Med. Res. Methodol. **20**(1) (2020). https://doi.org/10.1186/s12874-020-01119-3.
26. Paggi, M.: Simulation of Covid-19 epidemic evolution: are compartmental… *arXiv.Org*, arxiv.org/abs/2004.08207v1 (2020).
27. "COVID-19 tracker for India IN. Google Docs. www.docs.google.com/spreadsheets/d/1swdjquWqq5tjMm9tpxMa-9C8rjCyWVWHs-ODdAXfWDw/edit#gid=936573058 (2022). Accessed 1 Feb. 2022.

28. "COVID live—coronavirus statistics—Worldometer. Worldometer, www.worldometers.info/coronavirus/#countries (2022). Accessed 13 Feb. 2022.
29. Wang, D., et al.: Particle swarm optimization algorithm: an overview. Soft Computing **22**(2), 387–408 (2017). https://doi.org/10.1007/s00500-016-2474.
30. Nist.Gov. In: NIST/SEMATECH e-handbook of statistical methods. NIST. www.itl.nist.gov/div898/handbook/eda/section3/eda35g.htm (2013). Accessed 13 Feb. 2022.
31. Verity, R., et al.: Estimates of the severity of coronavirus disease 2019: a model-based analysis. Lancet Infect. Dis. **20**(6), 669–677 (2020). https://doi.org/10.1016/s1473-3099(20)30243-7.
32. Express News Service. Lakshadweep reports first coronavirus case. The Indian express. www.indianexpress.com/article/india/lakshadweep-coronavirus-covid-first-case-7152071/lite (2021). Accessed on Jan 13, 2022.
33. Pti. Lakshadweep reports 14 COVID-19 positive cases. The Hindu. www.thehindu.com/news/national/lakshadweep-reports-first-covid-19-positive-case/article33606645.ece/amp (2021). Accessed on Jan 13, 2022.
34. Ghosh, A.: How Lakshadweep has managed to be India's only Territory without Coronavirus. ThePrint. www.theprint.in/health/how-lakshadweep-has-managed-to-be-indias-only-territory-without-coronavirus/461444/?amp (2020). Accessed on Jan 15, 2022.

Chapter 3
Optimized Gradient Boosting Tree-Based Model for Obesity Level Prediction from patient's Physical Condition and Eating Habits

Geetanjali Bhoi, Etuari Oram, Bighnaraj Naik, and Danilo Pelusi

Abstract Growing of IoT in healthcare allows tracking and monitoring patient's health through sensors. It allows data analytics to assess immense quantities of data and mining useful information out of it. Nowadays, Obesity is one of the major health problems in most of the industrialized countries. Key factor of obesity lies in patient's physical condition and eating habits. In this paper, an optimized ensemble learning machine-based model has been proposed for obesity level prediction from physical condition and eating habits. Here, gradient boosting decision tree model has been designed and it's hyperparameters are optimized using Artificial physics optimization. In this study, sixteen various factors associated to obesity are analyzed and it is observed that patient's Gender, Age, Height, Weight, and FHWO (Family history with Overweight) are the most influenced factors. This approach has been compared with other similar approaches and found to be efficient in predicting various obesity level of the patients.

Keywords Healthcare · Obesity analysis · Machine Learning · Ensemble learning · Gradient boosting decision tree · Artificial physics optimization

---

G. Bhoi (✉) · E. Oram · B. Naik
Dept. of Computer Application, Veer Surendra Sai University of Technology, Burla, Sambalpur, Odisha 768018, India
e-mail: gbhoi_phdca@vssut.ac.in

E. Oram
e-mail: eoram_mca@vssut.ac.in

B. Naik
e-mail: bighnaraj_naik@ieee.org

D. Pelusi
Faculty of Communication Sciences, University of Teramo, Agostino Campus, Coste Sant', Teramo, Italy
e-mail: dpelusi@unite.it

© The Author(s), under exclusive license to Springer Nature Switzerland AG 2023
J. Nayak et al. (eds.), *Nature-Inspired Optimization Methodologies in Biomedical and Healthcare*, Intelligent Systems Reference Library 233,
https://doi.org/10.1007/978-3-031-17544-2_3

3.1 Introduction

Form the last few decades, Obesity has emerged as major health problem in most of the industrialized countries due to its pervasiveness, economic impact and informal connection with serious medical illnesses. Obesity is defined as a denouncing and chronic disease due to the abnormal and excessive dissemination of body fats. According to World health Organization (WHO), Obesity is defined as the accumulation of excessive fats in the body which results in increased rate of premature deaths and chronic diseases. As per the statistics of WHO, more than 1.9 billion adults were identified with overweight and 650 million individuals are identified with obesity in 2016 across the world. Moreover, the number of malnutrition cases are also cause for increase in the number of obesity cases in Southeast Asian countries in 2016 [1]. It is also estimated that obesity rate increases by 41% in the year 2030, if the growth rate of obesity continues. Therefore, to control the increase in the number of obesity cases, accurate measurement of excessive fat in the body using sophisticated tools is required. The simple index used for the accurate assessment of excessive fats in the body is "Body Mass Index" (BMI), which is assessed by calculating [(weight in kg) / (height in m^2)]. Generally, a BMI $\geq$ 25 kg/m^2 is considered as overweight, whereas BMI $\geq$ 30 kg/m^2 is considered as obesity. It is widely known that obesity and overweight are the major causes of chronic illnesses and premature deaths among individuals in both developed and developing countries.

High obesity in adults i.e., BMI with greater than or equal to 25 kg/m^2 can cause high incidence of cardiovascular disease which results in increase in the mortality rate [2]. Therefore, it is necessary to determine the factors that causes obesity in order to develop the policies and approaches which can be used to control the obesity in both children and adults. Unhealthy habits like smoking, laziness, overeating, excess drinking, not having proper physical exercises are considered as major reasons for obesity and other serious medical illnesses [3]. However, multiple factors can cause obesity. Several researches have been carried out to determine the factors that causes obesity or overweight in children and adults [4–8]. Ishida et al. [9] investigated factors like education level, taking meals at irregular times, not having proper sleep, less satisfaction with personal life, economic status, lack of physical activity, stress and depression are the causes of obesity. The study of Kadouh and Acosta [10] have shown that multiple factors like biological (genetics, pregnancy, physical disability, menopause, medication etc.), environmental (social status, economic status, food abundance, culture etc.) and behavioral factors (smoking, alcohol consumption, lack of physical activity, irregular food habits, laziness etc.) are the causes of obesity and overweight in individuals. The following Fig. 3.1 shows the factors that cause obesity in individuals.

The consequences of obesity in adults leads to a wide range of complications which include cardiovascular diseases, hypertension, type II diabetes, chronic lung disease, cancers, sleep apnea and osteoarthritis [11]. Particularly, the consequences of diseases caused due to obesity is immensely high in lower income people and lower economic countries. The significant pathophysiological links between obesity

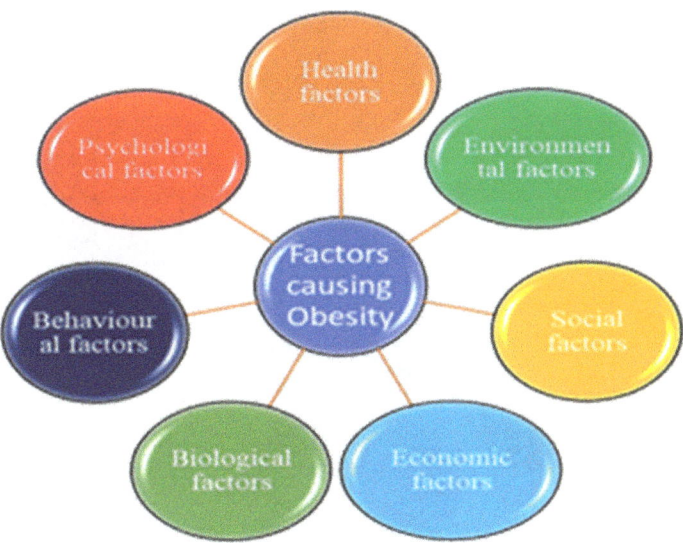

Fig. 3.1 Factors that often cause obesity

and cardiovascular diseases such as coronary heart disease, atrial fibrillation, hypertension and outright heart failure has been provided by Koliaki et al. [12]. Research studies also shows that excessive levels of fats are the major reasons for development of certain types of cancers such as pancreatic, breast, endometrial, colorectal etc. [13, 14]. The following Fig. 3.2 demonstrates the major comorbidities associated with obesity.

In addition to comorbidities, obesity is also responsible for significant increase in the mortality rate particularly with cardiovascular diseases and cancer [11]. According to World Health organization, at least 2.8 million people die each year due to obesity and overweight [15]. Due to increased obesity in individuals, significant increase in the mortality rate of cancer and cardiovascular diseases has been observed particularly in stage 2 or 3 of the EOSS (Edmonton Obesity Staging System) [16]. The following Fig. 3.3 shows the statistics of deaths occurred due to obesity in 2019 [17].

As per the statistics of WHO, it is also estimated that 30% of the deaths in the world will occur due to obesity in 2030. Thus, there is a need to develop suitable approaches and behavioral policies for controlling the risks associated with obesity. Therefore, the development of predictive models to predict one variable from one or more variables plays a vital role in preventing obesity in childhood as well as in adolescents. In addition, predictive models are also used to provide preventive measures for people with high-risk obesity. As predictive models can be used for ranking various risk factors in order of their significance, these models allow design of more cost-effective approaches for weight reduction interferences. Furthermore, these models can also be used to analyze the impact of obesity in specific subpopulation by altering one or

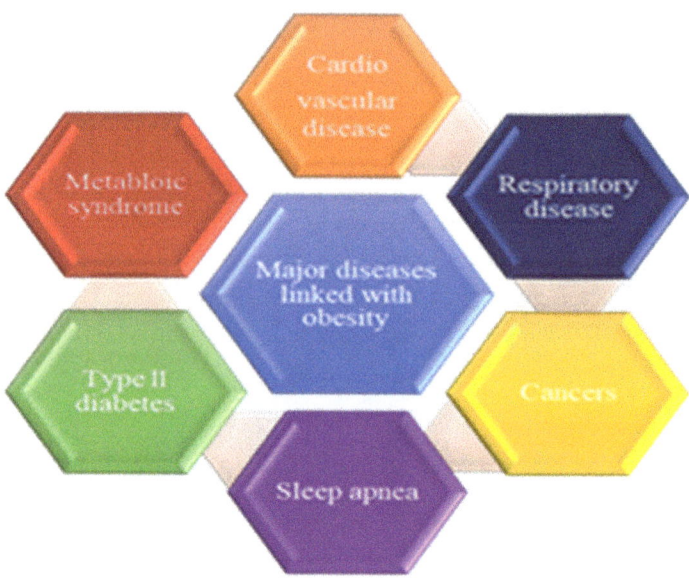

Fig. 3.2 Major diseases associated with Obesity

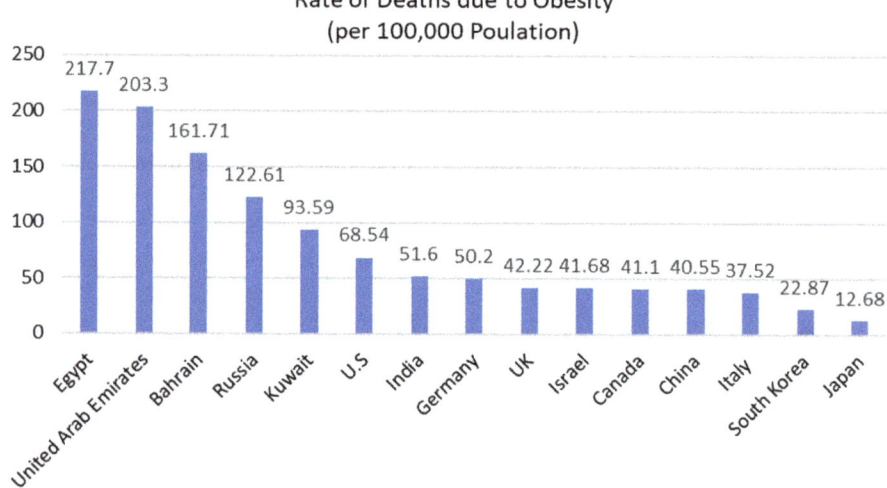

Fig. 3.3 Rate of deaths due to Obesity in 2019 (per 100,000 population)

more predictor variables. In general, conventional statistical approaches like linear models can be used to analyze data having minimum number of predictor variables. As statistical approaches cannot handle high dimensional data, these models cannot provide reliable inferences and thus results in overfitting of the model. Hence, to handle dimensional data having complex relationship between multidomain variable, machine learning (ML) approaches are used. This is basically due to their capability in finding complex and nonlinear relationship between predictor variables in an automated way. Therefore, ML approaches can be easily applied to model datasets having large number of predictor variables when compared to conventional statistical approaches.

Nowadays, ML approaches have been widely used in healthcare sector to predict the existence presence of disease due to their predictive capability, reliability and ease of use. Several research has been carried out in the prediction and diagnosis of disease using ML approaches from the last few decades [18–22]. Shamrat et al. [20] have used different ML approaches such as SVM (Support Vector Machine), NB (Naïve Bayes), KNN (K Nearest Neighbour), RF (Random Forest), DT (Decision Tree) and LR (Logistic Regression) for the early identification of breast cancer. Then the model has been trained on Wisconsin Breast Cancer data and the results indicate that SVM has obtained superior performance of 97.07% classification accuracy in predicting breast cancer as compared to other approaches. For accurate and efficient prediction of heart disease at early stage, various supervised ML approaches has been suggested by Ali et al. [23]. Then the suggested approaches have been trained on heart disease dataset collected from the Kaggle. The empirical results reveal that RF has obtained highest accuracy, sensitivity and specificity of 100% as compared to other approaches. Based on patient's health condition, monitoring the amount of medication required is of utmost important activity in healthcare sector. A combination of distinct ML approaches has been proposed by Khalaf et al. [24] for the accurate prediction of medication dosage needed for inmates suffering with sickle cell disease.

Due to the above advantages, ML approaches have also been used in the early prediction of obesity to curb the risks associated with obesity. Pang et al. [25] have employed several ML approaches for the prediction of childhood obesity in between the age group of 2 to 7 years by considering data from Electronic Healthcare Record (HER) data up to two years age. To efficiently predict the obesity in high school students, enhanced machine learning models known as binary logistic regression, weighted k-nearest neighbor (WKNN), improved decision tree (IDT), and artificial neural network (ANN) has been suggested by Zheng et al. [26]. Moreover, the authors have also discussed about the implications for reducing the obesity in adolescent. To accurately predict the overweight status from a database of 225 overweight and 251 healthy subjects, a novel approach known as extreme learning machine was proposed by Chen et al. [27]. Furthermore, results also reveal that there is a significant difference in the blood indexes of the overweight and healthy individuals. The following are some of the limitations that have been identified in the prediction of obesity using machine learning approaches i) most of the models have been trained by considering data from single healthcare system ii) most of the models have not included environmental and genetic factors in the determination of obesity iii) most of the models have not considered the social and demographic factors that may impact the pervasiveness of obesity.

3.2 Literature Study

In the recent years, Obesity has drawn remarkable significance among the researchers as it is strongly amalgamated with several chronic illnesses which can have negative impact not only on the health of the patients but also on their families. Besides original research carried out using standard scientific approaches, several research works has also been carried out using novel approaches such as machine learning approaches. This section provides a systematic review of the research work carried out in providing quality of life, prevention and treatment to people having obesity using machine learning approaches.

Montañez et al. [28] have proposed machine learning approaches for the prediction of obesity through publicly available genetic profiles and databases that were generated manually. Initially, the determination of genetic variants from the participant profiles has been done by applying data science techniques. These variants are then listed as risk variants in the National Human Genome Research Institute Catalogue are used as input to the ML approaches for the prophecy of obesity. For generating the set of principle variables, dimensionality reduction task has been performed. Further, the performance of the ML approaches such as gradient boosting, generalized linear model, classification and regression trees, k-nearest neighbours, support vector machines, random forest and multilayer perceptron neural network has been evaluated using AUC-ROC (Area Under the Curve- Receiver Operating Characteristics) curve on 6622 variables describing genetic variants. From the experimental outcomes, it was observed that support vector machine obtained better performance of 90.5% AUC value for prediction of obesity when compared with other ML approaches.

For the early prediction of peril of obesity and overweight in young people, a novel approach based on machine learning has been developed by Singh et al. [29]. The suggested model makes use of large amount of data accessible through UK's millennium cohort study. Then the issues related to less prediction accuracy due to imbalance dataset has been addressed through synthetic minority oversampling technique (SMOTE). Furthermore, the suggested ML approaches make use of BMI values of 3, 5, 7 and 11 ages to predict the peril of becoming overweight and obese at the age of 14. From the results, it has been observed that the target class can be predicted with a prediction accuracy of above 90%.

Thamrin et al. [30] have suggested machine learning approaches such as logistic regression, CART (Classification and Regression Trees) and NB (Naïve Bayes) for the detection of obesity in adults in Indonesia using publicly available data namely RISKESDAS survey data. In addition, the authors have applied the synthetic minority oversampling technique to minimize the imbalance in the dataset. Then the model has been evaluated and results indicate logistic regression obtained higher performance in comparison to CART and NB. Moreover, the study also identified set of risk factors such as location, marital status, age groups, education, sweet drinks, fatty/oily foods, grilled foods, preserved foods, seasoning powders, soft/carbonated drinks, alcoholic drinks, mental emotional disorders, diagnosed hypertension, physical activity, smoking, and fruit and vegetables consumptions for identifying the presence of obesity in adults.

Ferdowsy et al. [31] have suggested machine learning approaches for determining the risk and reasons of obesity in adults. For assessing the risk and reasons of obesity, authors have collected more than 1100 data from both the people suffering with obesity and non-obesity as well as people of different ages. Then the performance of the ML approaches such as k-nearest neighbor, naïve Bayes, logistic regression, support vector machine, multilayer perceptron, random forest, adaptive boosting, gradient boosting classifier and decision tree have been evaluated using various performance metrics such as accuracy, sensitivity, specificity, precision and recall. The experimental results shows that logistic regression obtained better performance in terms of 97.09% accuracy as compared to other ML approaches.

A novel clinical decision support system based on machine learning approach has been developed by Dugan et al. [32] for the identification of obesity in children after two years age. For this analysis, authors have collected data from a clinical decision support system known as CHICA for all children having at least one visit prior to the age of 2 and having at least one percentile BMI recorded after the second birthday. Then the ML approaches such as Random Forest, ID3, random tree, Naïve bayes, J48 and Bayes have been trained on CHICA data. The results indicate that ID3 has obtained better performance with an overall accuracy, sensitivity, positive predicted value and negative predicted value of 85%, 89%, 84% and 88% respectively as compared to other ML approaches. The following Table 3.1 represents the other literature works carried on the prediction of obesity using ML approaches.

Major contribution of this chapter is as follows: (i) Obesity prediction model based on Gradient boosting decision tree classifier (GBC) [39] is designed and its hyperparameters are optimized using Artificial physics optimization (APO) [40] and (ii) Various factors associated to obesity are studied and its impact on obesity identification is analyzed. The remaining contents are arranged in to following sections: Sect. 3.3. Understanding Factors associated with Obesity, Sect. 3.4. Proposed Approach, Sect. 3.5. Experimental result and analysis, and Sect. 3.6. Conclusion.

3.3 Understanding Factors Associated with Obesity

Here, the used dataset [41] has been collected from the Science Direct repository. These Datasets are of the residents of Mexico, Peru, and Colombia that contain information about their healthcare and their lifestyle. It consists of seventeen attributes and instances of 2111 patients including 1043 females and 1068 males. All the healthcare and obesity-related information captured are represented by 17 features (Table 3.2). Out of 17 features, 5 features (Gender, Family history with Overweight, SMOKE, FAVC, SCC) is of binary type, 3 features (Height, Weight, CH2O) are of Continuous type, 5 features (Age, FAVC, NCP, FAFA, TUE) are of the discrete type and rest 5

Table 3.1 Other review works performed on the prediction of Obesity using ML approaches

Author and Year	Approach	Dataset	Results	Limitations	Ref.
Ali et al. and 2022	Gradient Boosting	Australia's Pharmaceutical Benefits Scheme (PBS) database	AU-ROC = 0.70 for predicting obesity and 0.71 for predicting smoking	External dataset is not used for validating the model	[33]
Cheng et al. and 2022	LSTM (long short-term memory) model	OPEL database	MAE (mean average error) = 0.98 and R^2 (Pearson's correlation coefficient) = 0.72	Early identification of obesity can be done	[34]
Chatterjee et al. and 2020	SVM, KNN, ANN	CHICA system	Accuracy of ANN = 96.81%., precision of ANN = 96.73%, Recall of ANN = 97.36%, and Specificity of ANN = 92.85%	Considered only 3 to 5 age year group data	[35]
Dunstan et al. and 2020	SVM, random forest and extreme gradient boosting	Euromonitor data set containing food and beverage sales from 79 countries and obesity data estimated by Ng et al. [38]	RMSE of random forest = 0.057	Doesn't considered the role of non-official sales in the predominance of obesity	[36]
Hammond et al. and 2019	Lasso regression and binary classification model	EHR (Electronic Health record) dataset	Predict obesity with AUC-ROC Curve = 81.7% for girls and 76.1% for boys	Noisy and incomplete nature of EHR datasets	[37]

features (CAEC, CALC, MTRANS, NObeyesdad (Type of obesity)) are of categorical type. Here we have computed features importance of all the features out of which Weight is found as an important type and most influencing feature in leading obesity patients. From here we can conclude that overweight people are directly proportional to the more chances of causing obesity. However other important attributes are Height, Age, Gender, FAVC, and SMOKE respectively. During this pre-processing phase, the feature correlation matrix (Fig. 3.4) was also calculated. It represents the correlation coefficient of all features which shows the relationship between the target (Types of obesity) variable and each input variable. In Fig. 3.4 it is observed that the input attributes are less co-related to each other (less than 0.5) except Gender and Height.

The feature importance of all features with respect to Death event has been represented in Fig. 3.5. Further from the Fig. 3.6, in (a) if a patient's weight is high that is here weights 110 to 135 are seems to be more affected by obesity_type_III is followed by obesity type II when the weight is within the range of 112–123 kg and patients are considered as normal weight when the range of weight is within 40–65 kg. Height suppress ones overweight when it is more than normal range and they are more likely to be obese likewise, in the Fig. 3.6, (b) depicts the relation between

Table 3.2 Factors associated with obesity and their details

Factors associated with obesity (essential detail)	Data type
Gender (patient's gender information)	Boolean (0/1)
Age (patient's age)	Discrete variable (range: [14,61], unit: years)
Height (patient's height)	Continuous variable (range: [1.45,1.98], unit: meter)
Weight (patient's weight)	Continuous variable (rRange: [39,173], unit: kilogram)
FHWO (family history with overweight) (patient's family member suffered or suffers from overweight)	Boolean (0/1)
FAVC (frequent consumption of high caloric food)	Boolean (0/1)
FCVC (frequency of consumption of vegetables)	Discrete variable (range: [1, 3])
NCP (number of main meals)	Discrete variable (range: [1, 4])
CAEC (consumption of food between meals)	Categorical variable (no, sometimes, frequently, always)
SMOKE (do patient smoke or not)	Boolean (0/1)
CH2O (consumption of water daily)	Continuous variable (range: [1, 4], unit: liter)
SCC (calories consumption monitoring)	Boolean (0/1)
FAF (physical activity frequency)	Discrete variable (range: [0,3], unit: days)
TUE (time using technology devices)	Discrete variable (range: [0,2], unit: hours)
CALC (consumption of alcohol)	Categorical variable (no, sometimes, frequently, always)
MTRANS (transportation used)	Categorical variable (automobile, motorbike, bike, public transportation, walking)
NObeyesdad(Type of obesity)	Categorical variable (insufficient *weight*, *normal* weight, overweight-level*i*, *overweight-level* ii obesity *type* i, obesity *type* ii, obesity *type* iii)

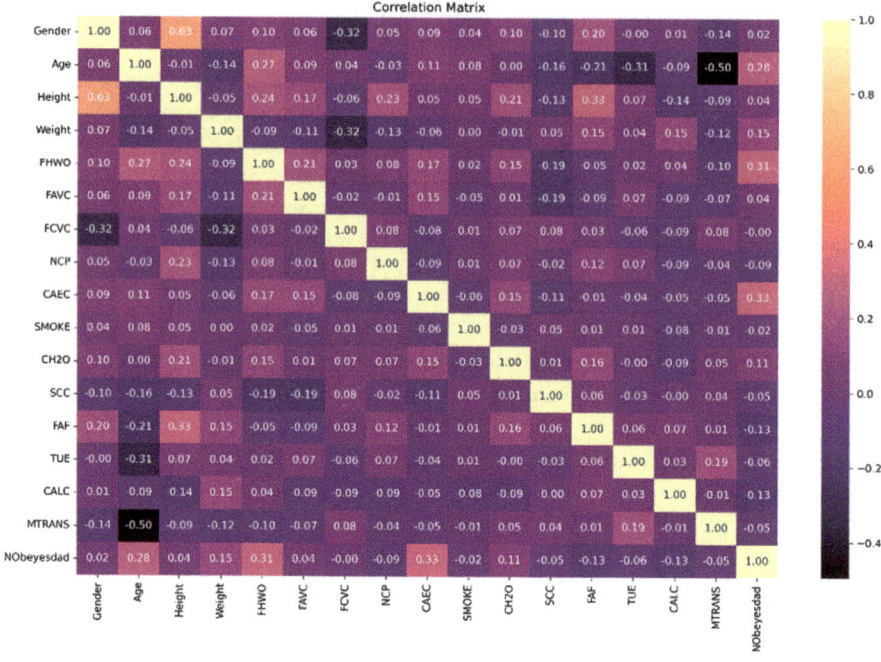

Fig. 3.4 Feature correlation

height and obesity type which shows when a person's height is between 1.3-to-1.9-m then there are chances of obesity type II followed by type I, and when height is 1.64–1.79 there may be a chance of obesity type I. Age is one of the important characteristics of leading obesity as it is shown in Fig. 3.6(c) that when it reaches 30 and above it starts to cause overweight level III, obesity type I, and obesity type II respectively. According to Fig. 3.6(d), male persons are more prone to be overweight level I, obesity type I, and II as compared to females, who may suffer from obesity type I, II, and III respectively. The obesity is related to the feature FAVC (Frequent consumption of high caloric food) that is shown in the Fig. 3.6(e); however, smoke seems less related to obesity types.

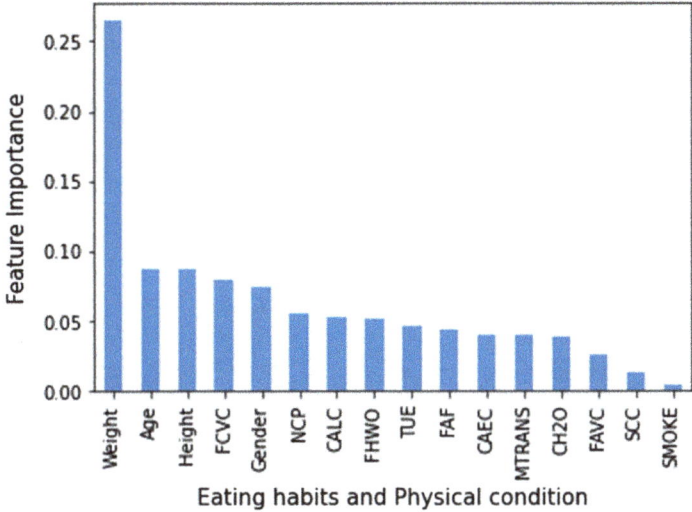

Fig. 3.5 Feature importance of all features w.r.t Death event

3.4 Proposed Approach

The working of the Artificial Physics Optimization and Gradient Boosting approach has been presented in this section.

3.4.1 Artificial Physics Optimization

Artificial physics optimization (APO) [40] is one of the nature-inspired heuristic algorithms analogous to the law of physics. It is motivated by artificial physics and represented based on the physicomimetics framework. The basic terms used in this framework are force, position, velocity, mass, and momentum. Here, the individual solutions are treated as physical particles and possessed these properties. The motion of these particles is controlled by the law of physics and newton's gravitational force. The steps of the APO algorithm are followed by three phases such as initialization, force, and motion calculation. In the initialization phase, particle values are initialized randomly from the n-dimensional search space. For each individual, random velocities are initialized within the particular range. Then, for each particle fitness value is calculated using fitness function in each iteration. The individual with best fitness value is selected each time and stored separately. Prior to the force calculation, the masses of individuals are calculated. The force exerted on each individual is then calculated. Here, the concept is that each individual attracts others with weaker fitness values and repels each other with better fitness values. The best fitness value will not be taking part in the motion means the best individual will neither attracted

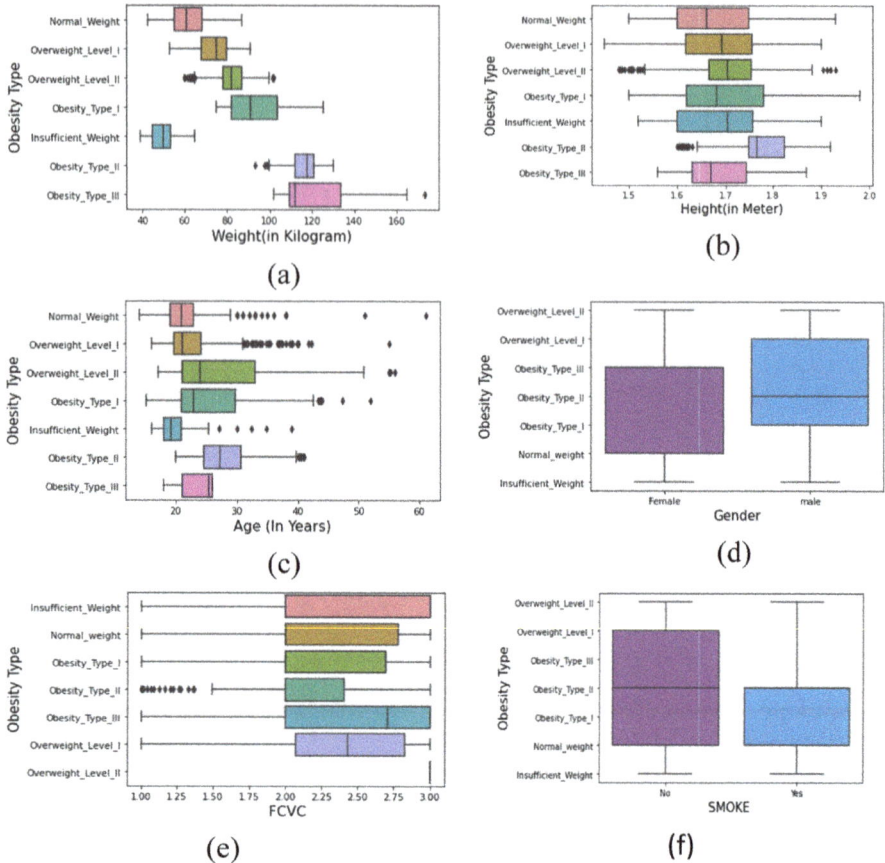

Fig. 3.6 Top influential features and their distribution

nor repelled by other individuals. The total force of each individual is calculated separately and the motion calculation is used to calculate the velocity for each individual. In the next step, the velocity of each individual is updated with the random variable and inertia weight. Finally, the position of each individual is updated. This process of motion and force calculation are repeated until a termination condition is reached.

3.4.2 APO Based GBT for Obesity Prediction

This work proposed a GBC-based model for obesity level prediction from physical condition and eating habits. We have used obesity dataset [41] consisting of patients' physical condition, eating habits with various obesity level. This dataset may be visualized as $D = \{X_i, t_i\}_{i=1}^{n}$, where is X_i is the ith physical condition and eating habit profile and t_i is the 'obesity type' (Normal_Weight, Insufficient_Weight, Overweight_Level_I, Overweight_Level_II, Obesity_Type_I, Obesity_Type_II, Obesity_Type_II). In this work, an optimized GBC [39] has been used to predict obesity type from the patients' physical condition and eating habits. The optimization task in this work has been framed as a search process to get optimal value of various hyperparameters of GBC. The hyperparameters considered for optimization are maximum depth (α), learning rate (β), number of estimators (γ), and subsample size (δ). The hyperparameters' search space is a four-dimensional space in which the range of these hyperparameters are as follows: $\alpha \in (1, 16)$, $\beta \in (0, 1)$, $\gamma \in (1, 100)$, and $\delta \in (0, 1)$. Here, APO [40] has been used for optimizing hyperparameters, which begins with generation of initial population $\psi = \{\psi_1, \psi_2...\psi_n\}$, n is the number of hyperparameter sets. The ith hyperparameter set can be denoted as $\psi_i = \{\alpha_i, \beta_i, \gamma_i, \delta_i\}$. The objective of applying APO is to select the optimal hyperparameter set ψ_i^* that is most suitable for the prediction of obesity level. The complete workflow of the proposed optimization process with integration of GBC can be realized in Fig. 3.7. We have set maximum number of APO iteration to 50.

$$m_i = e^{\frac{f_{\psi_b} - f_{\psi_i}}{fit_{\psi_w} - f_{\psi_b}}} \quad (3.1)$$

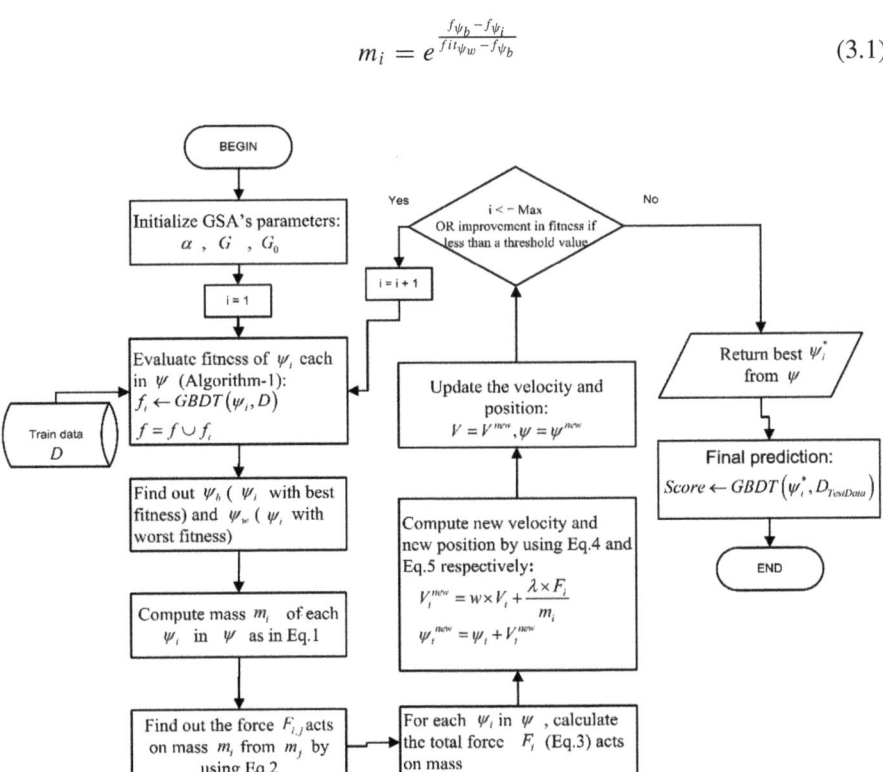

Fig. 3.7 Workflow of the proposed optimization process with integration of GBC

In Eq. 3.1, m_i is the gravitational mass of ψ_i. f_i, f_{ψ_b}, and f_{ψ_w} are fitness of ψ_i, ψ_b (best candidate solution), and ψ_w (worst candidate solution).

$$F_{i,j} = \begin{cases} G \times \frac{m_i \times m_j}{d(\psi_i, \psi_j)^\kappa}(\psi_j - \psi_i) & if\left(f_{\psi_j} < f_{\psi_i}\right) \\ -G \times \frac{m_i \times m_j}{d(\psi_i, \psi_j)^\kappa}(\psi_j - \psi_i) & Otherwise \end{cases} \quad (3.2)$$

In Eq. 3.2, $F_{i,j}$ is force applied on mass of ψ_i by the mass of ψ_j, G is the gravitational constant, $d(\cdot)$ is the Euclidian distance, and κ is a small value constant.

$$F_i = \sum\nolimits_{j=1, j \neq i}^{n} F_{i,j} \forall i \neq best \quad (3.3)$$

In Eq. 3.3, F_i is force applied on mass of ψ_i by the all-other mass of ψ_j.

$$V_i^{new} = w \times V_i + \frac{\lambda \times F_i}{m_i} \quad (3.4)$$

In Eq. 3.4, V_i^{new} is the next velocity of ψ_i, λ is the random variable uniformly distributed in between 0 to 1 and w is the inertia weight in between 0 to 1.

$$\psi_i^{new} = \psi_i + V_i^{new} \quad (3.5)$$

In Eq. 3.5, ψ_i^{new} is the next velocity of ψ_i.

$$F_m(x) \leftarrow F_{m-1}(x) + \beta \times F_m(x) \quad (3.6)$$

In Eq. 3.6, $F_m(x)$ is the mth model and β is the learning rate.

Algorithm-1: *Gradient Boosting Decision Tree*(ψ_i, D)

$\psi_i = \{\alpha_i, \beta_i, \gamma_i, \delta_i\}: i^{t\square}$ hyperparameter set

$D = (X_i, t_i)_{i=1}^N$: Obesity data including physical condition, eating habits, and obesity types. $Y = (y_i)_{i=1}^N$: Predicted obesity types

Step-1: $F_0(X) \leftarrow c_1 = mean(Y)$

Step-2: Create a subsample $S = (X_i, y_i)_{i=0}^{\delta}$ of size δ from D

Step-3: Obtain the additive gradient boosted decision trees

For m in γ

    For each sample X_i in S

        $k_i \leftarrow y_i - F_{m-1}(X_i)$ (computed as in Eq.6)

$$r_i \leftarrow -\left[\frac{\partial L(y, F(X_i))}{\partial F(X_i)}\right]_{F_{m-1}(X)}$$

        Store (X_i, r_i) as instance and create a dataset D'

    $[U, T] \leftarrow DTRegressor(D', \alpha_i)$ (Algorithm-2)

    $TreeSet = TreeSet \cup T$

Step-4: Use $TreeSet$ to make final prediction and calculate prediction score

Step-5: Return Score

Algorithm-2: *DTRegressor*(D', α)

$D' = (X_j, r_j)_{j=1}^{\delta}$: Data includes data samples with their associated gradient

$X_j = (t_i)_{i=1}^{d}$: i^{th} input data sample with d dimension

Cd: Current depth

U_i: Leaf space $U_i = \{U_{i,j}\}_{j=1}^{L}$, where is the number of samples in j^{th} leaf of ith tree

Step-1: $Cd = 1$
Step-2: Find minimum MSE
For each X_j in D'
    For each t_i in X_j
        Find min(MSE)
Step-3: Continue splitting of data samples until the depth α reached
If $Cd < \alpha$
    Split D' in to D_1' and D_2'
    $Cd = Cd + 1$
    $DTRegressor(D_1', \alpha)$
    $DTRegressor(D_2', \alpha)$

Else, Make D' as leaf node
Step-4: Return U and T

3.5 Experimental Result and Analysis

We evaluated the impact of predictors in identifying the obesity type, we have compared the proposed approach with various ML models (DT, LDA, MLP, NB, and LR) and EL models (RF, Bagging, Adaboost, XGBoost, and GBC). Table 3.3 represents the Performance evaluation and comparison of numerous models using several performance metrics such as Recall, Precision, F1 Score, F-beta Score, and Accuracy Score. In Table 3.3, it is observable that the proposed approach GBC + APO has performed better than other models. As an observation on comparison of GBC + APO with GBC + PSO (GBC optimized by PSO [42]) and GBC + GSA (GBC optimized by GSA[43]), it is observed that the proposed approach has remarkable performance over other studied model in the term of Accuracy score. we have attained {0.3088602526333756, 87, 0.6983146840424218, 8}, {0.5451933264379056, 35, 0.9344609911432359, 6} and {0.2495179933715774, 85, 0.7378428825166836, 10}, and as optimal hyperparameters values for the studied hyperparameters $\{lr, ne, sb,$ and $\delta\}$ in GBC + APO, GBC + GSA and GBC + PSO respectively. The performance of various optimization approaches has been depicted in Fig. 3.8. Finally, the overall comparison of models is presented on Fig. 3.9.

Table 3.3 Performance evaluation and comparison

Prediction models	Performance metrics				
	precision	recall	F1 score	Fbeta score	Accuracy score
DT	0.9280072	0.9274447	0.9274782	0.9277383	0.9353312
LDA	0.5944456	0.6009463	0.5925424	0.5924196	0.6009463
MLP	0.9034123	0.9006309	0.9011853	0.9023224	0.9085173
NB	0.6343142	0.6072555	0.5939459	0.6096763	0.6072555
LR	0.5992609	0.6056782	0.5989931	0.5982972	0.6056782
RF	0.9433795	0.9337539	0.9350349	0.9392326	0.9353312
Bagging	0.9396575	0.9384858	0.9386317	0.9391414	0.9400630
Adaboost	0.6383899	0.6246056	0.6215793	0.6288825	0.6246056
XGBoost	0.9549678	0.9542586	0.9542586	0.9545313	0.9542586
GBC	0.9376521	0.9369085	0.9367113	0.9371410	0.9353312
GBC + PSO	0.9523757	0.9511041	0.9512225	0.9517917	0.9621451
GBC + GSA	0.9490857	0.9479495	0.9480539	0.9485602	0.9589905
Proposed model	0.9549673	0.9526813	0.9532966	0.9541798	0.9637223

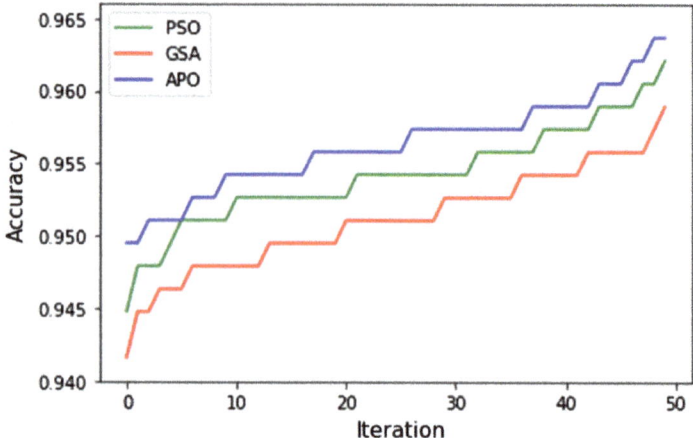

Fig. 3.8 Convergence analysis and comparison

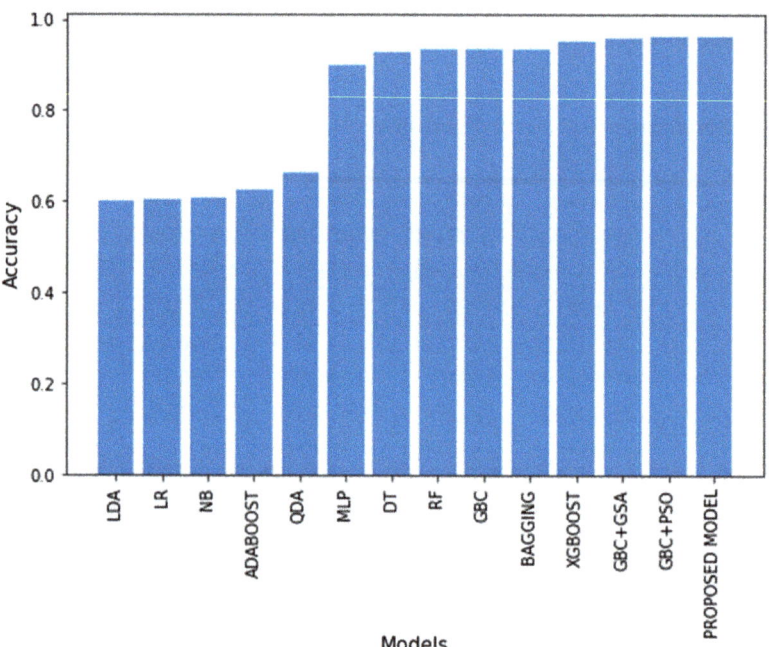

Fig. 3.9 Comparative analysis of accuracy of proposed approach and other similar appraoches

3.6 Conclusion

In this work, optimized GBC-based system obesity detection model has been proposed. This approach is found to be efficient in the considered test problem.

However, there are some potential issues that put a question on acceptability and reliability of these most of the ensemble learning and machine learning based model. Some of the issues are: (i) How much reliable and trustable the model is in terms of prediction of obesity level, (ii) Is the data qualitative and adequate for the target data-driven model, (iii) How the model deals with possible high variance and noise in the data as it is usually collected from diverse and heterogenous sources involve inhomogeneous data collection methods and dissimilar patient groups, and (iv) How the model's prediction results is interpretable by the healthcare practitioners. The first issue could be addressed up to some extent by training and testing the model with real-time data and applications. The collection of data from legitimate source and cross validation from domain experts may overcome the second issue. A proper exploratory data analysis and data integration may be helpful to the address third issue. Further, boosting ensemble learning is known and suitable for handling the data with high variance and noise. In order to address fourth issue, the healthcare practitioners must have adequate basic knowledge on machine learning, ensemble learning, and various exploratory data analysis related to it. Finally, a model or a product is useless if it is not in use. Therefore, it is the healthcare practitioners and AI engineers who can make this possible together. This work is limited to the use of GBC and its hyperparameters optimization for the detection of obesity type.

Acknowledgements This work is supported by Department of Science and Technology (DST), Ministry of Science and Technology, New Delhi, Govt. of India, under Grant no. DST/INSPIREFellowship/2019/IF190611.

References

1. World Health Statistics 2016: Monitoring Health for the SDGs, Sustainable Development Goals. (2016). Available online at: https://www.who.int/about/licensing/copyright_form/en/index.html
2. Chooi, Yu Chung, Cherlyn Ding, and Faidon Magkos. "The epidemiology of obesity." Metabolism 92 (2019): 6–10.
3. Kim, Cheong, et al. "Predicting factors affecting adolescent obesity using general bayesian network and what-if analysis." International journal of environmental research and public health 16.23 (2019): 4684.
4. Singh, Payal, and Sachchida Nand Rai. "Factors affecting obesity and its treatment." Obesity Medicine 16 (2019): 100140.
5. Ross, S.E., Flynn, J.I., Pate, R.R.: What is really causing the obesity epidemic? A review of reviews in children and adults. J. Sports Sci. **34**(12), 1148–1153 (2016)
6. Shukri, Nor Masitah Mohamed, et al. "Awareness in childhood obesity." Research Journal of Pharmacy and Technology 9.10 (2016): 1658.
7. Omer, T.: The causes of obesity: an in-depth review. Adv Obes Weight Manag Control **10**(4), 90–94 (2020)
8. Courtemanche, Charles J., et al. "Can changing economic factors explain the rise in obesity?" Southern Economic Journal 82.4 (2016): 1266–1310.
9. Ishida, Akira, et al. "Factors Affecting Adult Overweight and Obesity in Urban China." Pertanika Journal of Social Sciences & Humanities 28.1 (2020).

10. Kadouh, H.C., Acosta, A.: Current paradigms in the etiology of obesity. Tech. Gastrointest. Endosc. **19**(1), 2–11 (2017)
11. Abdelaal, Mahmoud, Carel W. le Roux, and Neil G. Docherty. "Morbidity and mortality associated with obesity." Annals of translational medicine 5.7 (2017).
12. Koliaki, C., Liatis, S., Kokkinos, A.: Obesity and cardiovascular disease: revisiting an old relationship. Metabolism **92**, 98–107 (2019)
13. Booth, Andrea, et al. "Adipose tissue: an endocrine organ playing a role in metabolic regulation." Hormone molecular biology and clinical investigation 26.1 (2016): 25–42.
14. Steele, C. Brooke, et al. "Vital signs: trends in incidence of cancers associated with overweight and obesity—United States, 2005–2014." MMWR. Morbidity and mortality weekly report 66.39 (2017): 1052.
15. https://www.who.int/news-room/facts-in-pictures/detail/6-facts-on-obesity [accessed on April 9.2022].
16. Kuk, Jennifer L., et al. "Edmonton Obesity Staging System: association with weight history and mortality risk." Applied Physiology, Nutrition, and Metabolism 36.4 (2011): 570–576.
17. https://www.statista.com/statistics/1169479/worldwide-rate-deaths-obesity-related-attributed-country/ [accessed on April 9.2022].
18. Phasinam, Khongdet, et al. "Analyzing the Performance of Machine Learning Techniques in Disease Prediction." Journal of Food Quality 2022 (2022).
19. Ferdousi, Rahatara, M. Anwar Hossain, and Abdulmotaleb El Saddik. "Early-stage risk prediction of non-communicable disease using machine learning in health cps." IEEE Access 9 (2021): 96823–96837.
20. Shamrat, FM Javed Mehedi, et al. "An analysis on breast disease prediction using machine learning approaches." International Journal of Scientific & Technology Research 9.02 (2020): 2450–2455.
21. Mamani, Nibeth Mena. "Machine Learning techniques and Polygenic Risk Score application to prediction genetic diseases." ADCAIJ: Advances in Distributed Computing and Artificial Intelligence Journal 9.1 (2020): 5–14.
22. Bhagwat, Nikhil, et al. "Modeling and prediction of clinical symptom trajectories in Alzheimer's disease using longitudinal data." PLoS computational biology 14.9 (2018): e1006376.
23. Ali, Md Mamun, et al. "Heart disease prediction using supervised machine learning algorithms: performance analysis and comparison." Computers in Biology and Medicine 136 (2021): 104672.
24. Khalaf, Mohammed, et al. "Machine learning approaches to the application of disease modifying therapy for sickle cell using classification models." Neurocomputing 228 (2017): 154–164.
25. Pang, Xueqin, et al. "Prediction of early childhood obesity with machine learning and electronic health record data." International Journal of Medical Informatics 150 (2021): 104454.
26. Zheng, Zeyu, and Karen Ruggiero. "Using machine learning to predict obesity in high school students." 2017 IEEE International Conference on Bioinformatics and Biomedicine (BIBM). IEEE, 2017.
27. Chen, Huiling, et al. "Using blood indexes to predict overweight statuses: An extreme learning machine-based approach." PLoS one 10.11 (2015): e0143003.
28. Montañez, Casimiro Aday Curbelo, et al. "Machine learning approaches for the prediction of obesity using publicly available genetic profiles." 2017 International Joint Conference on Neural Networks (IJCNN). IEEE, 2017.
29. Singh, Balbir, and Hissam Tawfik. "Machine learning approach for the early prediction of the risk of overweight and obesity in young people." International Conference on Computational Science. Springer, Cham, 2020.
30. Thamrin, Sri Astuti, et al. "Predicting Obesity in Adults Using Machine Learning Techniques: An Analysis of Indonesian Basic Health Research 2018." Frontiers in nutrition 8 (2021).
31. Ferdowsy, Faria, et al. "A machine learning approach for obesity risk prediction." Current Research in Behavioral Sciences 2 (2021): 100053.

32. Dugan, Tamara M., et al. "Machine learning techniques for prediction of early childhood obesity." Applied clinical informatics 6.03 (2015): 506–520.
33. Ali, Sitwat, et al. "Predicting obesity and smoking using medication data: A machine-learning approach." Pharmacoepidemiology and Drug Safety 31.1 (2022): 91–99.
34. Cheng, Erika R., Rai Steinhardt, and Zina Ben Miled. "Predicting Childhood Obesity Using Machine Learning: Practical Considerations." BioMedInformatics 2.1 (2022): 184–203.
35. Chatterjee, Kakali, et al. "Early prediction of childhood obesity using machine learning techniques." Advances in Communication and Computational Technology. Springer, Singapore, 2021. 1431–1440.
36. Dunstan, Jocelyn, et al. "Predicting nationwide obesity from food sales using machine learning." Health informatics journal 26.1 (2020): 652–663.
37. Hammond, Robert, et al. "Predicting childhood obesity using electronic health records and publicly available data." PLoS One 14.4 (2019): e0215571.
38. Ng, Marie, et al. "Global, regional, and national prevalence of overweight and obesity in children and adults during 1980–2013: a systematic analysis for the Global Burden of Disease Study 2013." The lancet 384.9945 (2014): 766–781.
39. Friedman, Jerome H. "Greedy function approximation: a gradient boosting machine." Annals of statistics (2001): 1189–1232.
40. Xie, Liping, Ying Tan, and Jianchao Zeng. "Artificial physics optimization algorithm for global optimization." Physicomimetics. Springer, Berlin, Heidelberg, 2011. 565–589.
41. Palechor, Fabio Mendoza, and Alexis de la Hoz Manotas. "Dataset for estimation of obesity levels based on eating habits and physical condition in individuals from Colombia, Peru and Mexico." Data in brief 25 (2019): 104344.
42. Kennedy, James, and Russell Eberhart. "Particle swarm optimization." Proceedings of ICNN'95-international conference on neural networks. Vol. 4. IEEE, 1995.
43. Rashedi, E., Nezamabadi-Pour, H., Saryazdi, S.: GSA: a gravitational search algorithm. Inf. Sci. **179**(13), 2232–2248 (2009)

Chapter 4
Multi-Objective Optimization Algorithms in Medical Image Analysis

Natalia Obukhova, Alexandr Motyko, and Alexandr A. Pozdeev

Abstract Color correction is important part for medical image preprocessing. The proposed method provides color correction with minimum error for the human visual perception. The principal feature of proposed method: the color error is calculated according to perceptual metric CIEDE2000. Using the loss function based on CIEDE2000 metric leads to necessity transfer from least square method using for transformation function parameters identification to multi-objective optimization. Each color of palette is represented as separate target function. As algorithm for palette matching, the 3rd order polynomial with 11 coefficients for each color channel was used. Algorithm of transformation function coefficients estimation based on multi-objective optimization includes three steps: evaluation of starting point by least square method, line search by BFGS (Broyden–Fletcher–Goldfarb–Shanno) algorithm and solution refinement by Nelder—Mead Algorithm. Our experiments show that for all colors from palette error according CIEDE2000 is less than 1. If error of CIEDE2000 for colors after matching is more than 1 the difference between color will be visible for observer.

Keywords Color correction · Pareto front · Palette matching · Color gamut · Perceptual color distance

4.1 Introduction

Color and color contrast play an important role in the analysis of medical images. Specialists are largely guided by color when analyzing an image context. Many signs by which the doctor judges the state of tissues, the development of the disease are expressed in color changes relative to the norm. In the camera-display pipeline of the

---

N. Obukhova (✉) · A. Motyko · A. A. Pozdeev
Saint Petersburg State Electro Technical University «LETI», Professora Popova str. 5, Saint-Petersburg 197022, Russian Federation
e-mail: natalia172419@yandex.ru

A. A. Pozdeev
e-mail: 3puches4@gmail.com

endoscopic system the colors in the resulting image are affected by the applied color correction procedures. Color correction in image processing is understood as a class of methods associated with changing the colors of decomposition elements (pixels) of images. Common to color correction methods is that they do not change the semantics of the image. Color correction is used at various stages of working with video information: it is an obligatory part of the signal processing pipeline when forming an image by a camera, as a rule, it is performed during the processing of graphic information when displayed on a monitor (in this case, correction can be performed in order to match the available graphic information and display capabilities), as a part of processing to enhance the subjective visual quality of the reproduced information, to achieve the desired artistic effect. Color correction procedures are simplistically classified according to their functional purpose:

- Colorimetric;
- Specialized.

Colorimetric procedures ensure color accuracy. They are used to match the spectral characteristics of the camera and the properties of the observer's visual system, white balance, match the color profiles of devices, and so on. Their main function is to ensure colorimetrically correct operation of the camera-display pipeline.

Specialized procedures perform target processing according to the purpose of a particular television system. For example, some algorithm enhances the contrast in the image, resulting in increased subjective visual quality for the operator. Or a certain change in the image palette is carried out, as a result of which the accuracy characteristics of the automatic image analysis procedure by the intelligent system are increased.

The basic use case of a medical video system (in particular endoscopic) is to display a video stream on the monitor that displays what the camera is currently "seeing", without any intelligent specialized processing. Thus, the main color correction here is realized in basic "camera—display" pipeline. The color correction procedures performed within the "camera—display" pipeline, excluding special target processing for the needs of a particular system, are shown in Fig. 4.1.

The most important block in terms of colorimetric color correction is the color space transform block. Here the device depended camera RGB color coordinates are mapped in device independent XYZ (or any other independent coordinates like Pro Photo). To provide this mapping the functions of the Standard Colorimetric Observer is used (Fig. 4.2) and the sensor spectral sensitivities functions (Fig. 4.3).

These Standard Colorimetric Observer functions as shown in Eq. 4.1 define the XYZ coordinates for specific illuminant of the scene reflectances.

$$\begin{aligned} X &= \tfrac{K}{N} \int_\lambda R(\lambda) I(\lambda) \bar{x}(\lambda) d\lambda, \\ Y &= \tfrac{K}{N} \int_\lambda R(\lambda) I(\lambda) \bar{y}(\lambda) d\lambda, \\ Z &= \tfrac{K}{N} \int_\lambda R(\lambda) I(\lambda) \bar{z}(\lambda) d\lambda, \\ N &= \int_\lambda I(\lambda) \bar{y}(\lambda) d\lambda, \end{aligned} \quad (4.1)$$

4 Multi-Objective Optimization Algorithms in Medical Image Analysis

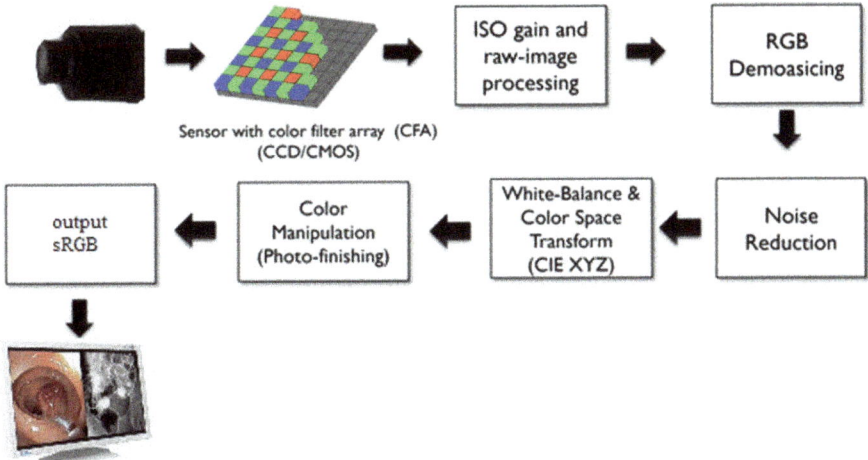

Fig. 4.1 Camera-display pipeline in endoscopic system

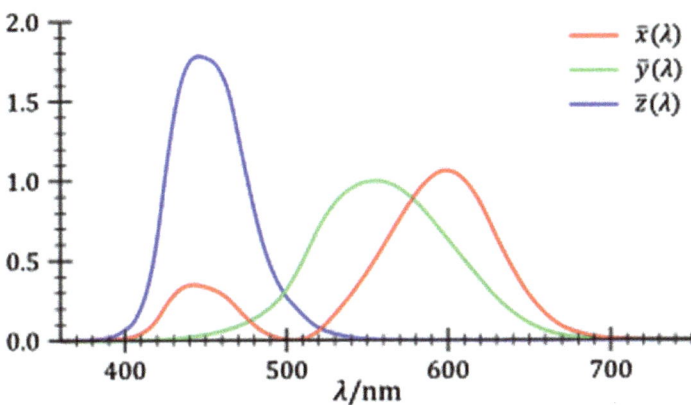

Fig. 4.2 Standard colorimetric observer functions

where $R(\lambda)$—spectral reflection characteristic of the material of the object, $I(\lambda)$—specter of the illuminant, K—scale factor (usually 1, or 100), the integral is usually calculated in range [380, 780] nm.

On the other hand, there are RGB coordinates of the camera. They are depended on sensor spectral sensitivities (example in Fig. 4.3) and the illuminant as shown in Eq. 4.2.

$$\begin{aligned} R &= \int_\lambda R(\lambda)\bar{r}(\lambda)d\lambda, \\ G &= \int_\lambda R(\lambda)\bar{g}(\lambda)d\lambda, \\ B &= \int_\lambda R(\lambda)\bar{b}(\lambda)d\lambda. \end{aligned} \qquad (4.2)$$

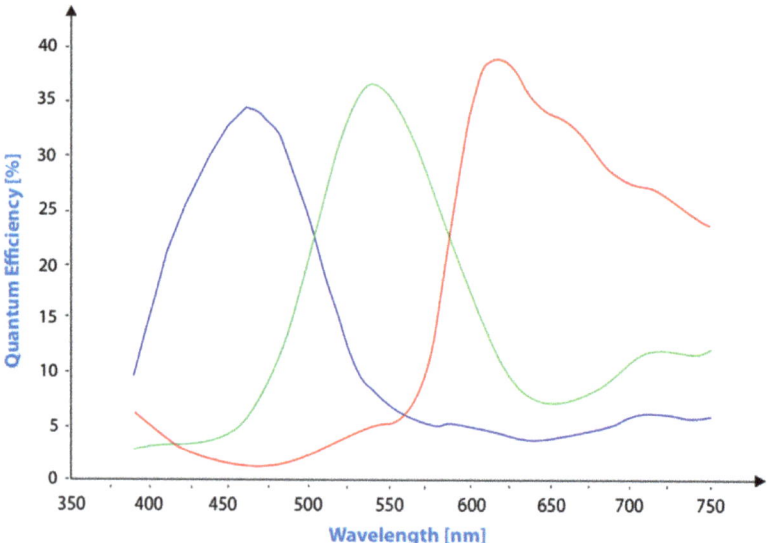

Fig. 4.3 Sensor spectral sensitivities for Micron MT9T031

Obviously, to implement RGB-XYZ mapping, one need to use some test object with known spectral parameters and a specific known illuminant. Which will lead to uniquely defined pairs of RGB and XYZ coordinates of some set of colors and therefore makes it possible to define the parameters of the RGB-XYZ mapping functions. There are many methods for estimating mapping parameters [1]. From the simplest—based on the method of least squares, to complex interpolations using polynomials, splines, etc. But all these methods have a common property. They have a scalar minimization criterion—as a rule the mean error, or squared mean, etc. This leads to the fact that while minimizing the overall error, the error on each specific color can be random and not controlled in any way. However, different colors are important for analysis in different ways.

First, the importance of colors is determined by the specifics of the data. For endoscopic images, it is obvious that shades of red, for example, are more important than shades of blue. Different approaches can be used to determine the most important colors for analysis as based on statistics, as based on priori information. In general, one need to rely on the opinion of doctors and the specifics of the task. Ultimately, it is necessary to ensure the accurate reproduction of the colors of those features that the doctor is guided by when conducting visual analysis.

Second, there is an individual importance of colors. The fact is that the Standard Colorimetric Observer was obtained by averaging data on 21 people [2]. This seemingly rough estimate was quite enough for the monitors with a standard color gamut (sRGB) that existed until recently. Future displays will have ever wider color gamuts (Display-P3, BT.2020) (Fig. 4.4).

Fig. 4.4 Color gamut comparison

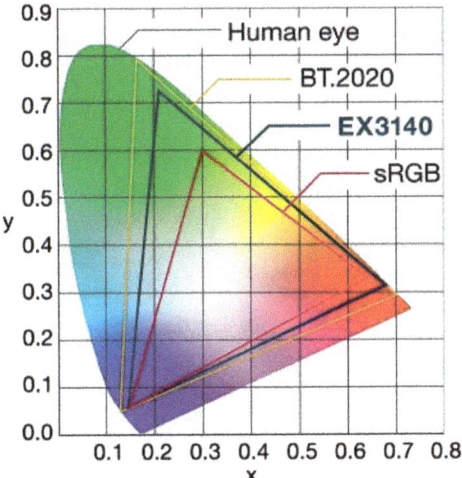

The peculiarity is that the wider the color gamut, the more it will affect the color rendering individually perceived by a person that his own functions differ from the Standard Colorimetric Observer ones. Discrepancies will lead to errors in color perception on certain colors specific to each person. To take into account the individual features of human vision during minimization of color reproduction error, it seems logical to use an individual Color Matching Function (CMF) instead of the Standard Colorimetric Observer. The problem here is that it is impossible to measure an individual CMF without special laboratory equipment. Therefore, there are approaches in which it is proposed to use not an individual CMF, but a categorical one, which approximates the individual more accurately than Standard Colorimetric Observer. Determining the belongings of the users CMF to a certain categorical CMF is much easier. In particular, the works of Sarkar [3] and Asano [4] are devoted to this. In Fig. 4.5 the 8 categorical CMF proposed by Sarkar are presented on a single chart to show their differences.

From this we can draw the following conclusion. Color plays an important role in the analysis of medical images. At the level of constructing the camera-display pipeline, this comes down to the task of color correction. Traditionally, the problem of color correction is solved in a scalar criterion and without taking into account the individual characteristics of human vision and the importance of colors for a particular scene or task. This leads to the fact that the most important colors for color analysis receive, along with the rest, an uncontrolled error. Thus, it is necessary to control the error in the most important colors. One promising approach for this is the transition from a scalar criterion to a multi-objective (vector) one.

In the problem under consideration, it is necessary to estimate the parameters of the transformation function (i.e., color correction function) that transforms the colors of one palette into another. Because of the fact that every color is important for visual perception of an image each color of the palette should be considered as a single objective function in terms of an optimization problem. The multi-objective

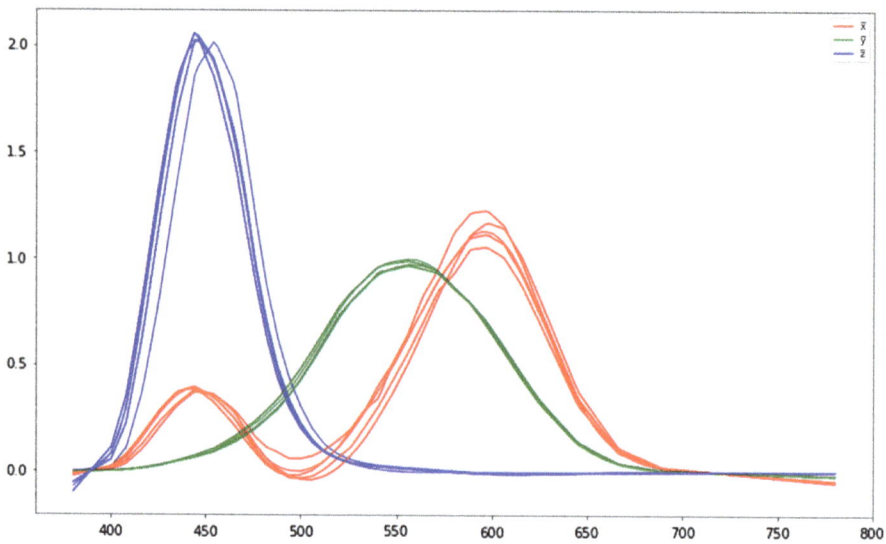

Fig. 4.5 Categorical CMF by Sarkar

optimization task [5] can be formulated as shown in Eq. 4.3:

$$\min(f_1(\boldsymbol{x}), f_2(\boldsymbol{x}), \ldots, f_n(\boldsymbol{x})), \boldsymbol{x} \in X, \quad (4.3)$$

where n—number of objective functions, and the set X is the feasible set of decision vectors.

An element $\mathbf{x} \in X$ is called feasible solution, or feasible decision. In multi-objective optimization, there does not typically exist a feasible solution that minimizes all objective functions simultaneously. Therefore, attention is paid to Pareto optimal solutions; that is, solutions that cannot be improved in any of the objectives without degrading at least one of the other objectives.

The task therefore is to find Pareto optimal solutions [6] (Pareto front, Fig. 4.6) and then choose one of them according to user defined preferences of importance some objectives under others.

In our study we solved the task of multi-objective optimization as main step in color correction procedure based on categorical CMF (8 types, see Fig. 4.5). The main goal was to realized recalculation from RGB space to XYZ space defined by categorical CMF with the high accuracy. The results are presented in this chapter. The chapter is structured as follows. Section 4.2 discusses perceptual method of color correction. Section 4.3 is devoted to experimental investigation of proposed method. In conclusions the main results are summarized and discussed.

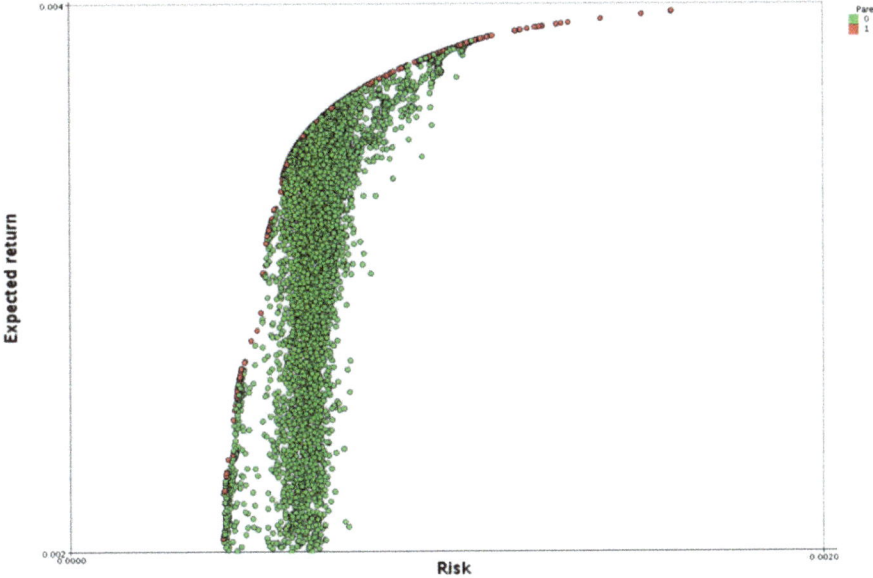

Fig. 4.6 Pareto-front example (red dots)

4.2 Perceptual Method of Color Correction Based on Multi-Objective Optimization

This section describes different perceptual approaches of color correction.

4.2.1 Loss-Function for Perceptual Color Correction

In numerous methods of color correction based on linear or interpolation approach the measure to minimize for identify the parameters of transformation function is sum of errors calculating for all colors of ColorChecker defining spaces XYZ and RGB. All these methods of recalculation suppose that the error between two colors in space RGB and the corresponding color in space XYZ is calculated as Euclidian metric in XYZ or RGB space. In this case the determining of matrix coefficients (linear transformation) or interpolation coefficients can be realized by least square method.

Although the least squares method works well, it suffers from the fact that the quantity being minimized—namely, distance in XYZ—is not the quantity that matters most—namely, distance in a perceptually uniform color space such as CIELAB ΔE or CIEDE2000.

Thus, it is necessary to develop new method of color correction based on minimization of the error between color in reference and recalculated spaces expressed by metric CIEDE2000.

Developing method of space recalculation based on CIEDE2000 and based on multi-objective minimization approach includes next steps:

- To obtain analytic representation of objective function based on CIEDE2000 metric;
- To find the algorithm for multi-objective function minimization, permitting error for each color in CIEDE2000 metric less than 1 (according to literature data if value of CIEDE2000 less than 1, the human vision cannot find error in color mapping).

4.2.2 Multi-Objective Optimization

We realized multi-objective optimization for our task using Nondominated Sorting Genetic Algorithm III (NSGA-III) as a solver [7]. The objective of the NSGA-family algorithms is to improve the adaptive fit of a population of candidate solutions to a Pareto front constrained by a set of objective functions. The algorithm uses an evolutionary process with surrogates for evolutionary operators including selection, genetic crossover, and genetic mutation. The population is sorted into a hierarchy of sub-populations based on the ordering of Pareto dominance. Similarity between members of each sub-group is evaluated on the Pareto front, and the resulting groups and similarity measures are used to promote a diverse front of non-dominated solutions. In our study, we used NSGA-III rather than the no less popular NSGA-II, because the preliminary tests for our specific task already confirmed the prior known conclusions (for example reported in [8] and with some reservations in [9]) that NSGA-III outperforms NSGA-II in case where the number of objectives is quite large.

In our tests we use the achieved precision (sum of CIEDE2000 errors of all colors) of least squares solution as a reference baseline. The example of solution—the pair chart for two objective functions is in Fig. 4.7.

As a result, the solutions belonging to Pareto front, unfortunately, were significantly inferior (almost 10 times) to the estimates obtained by the method of the least squares. We have concluded, that main reasons for this are the following. The large number of target functions, the need to take into account constraints and, most importantly, the complex and nonlinear metrics calculated during optimization lead to a very complex relief of the general objective function containing a lot of local minimums, "plateaus" and "ravines".

The nonlinear character of the CIEDE2000 metrics and the presence of constraints in the problem leads to the occurrence of local minimums (function $y \geq |x|$ with the constraint $y \geq 5 - 4(x-2)^2$ in Fig. 4.8), which also has a negative impact on the finding of the optimum.

4 Multi-Objective Optimization Algorithms in Medical Image Analysis

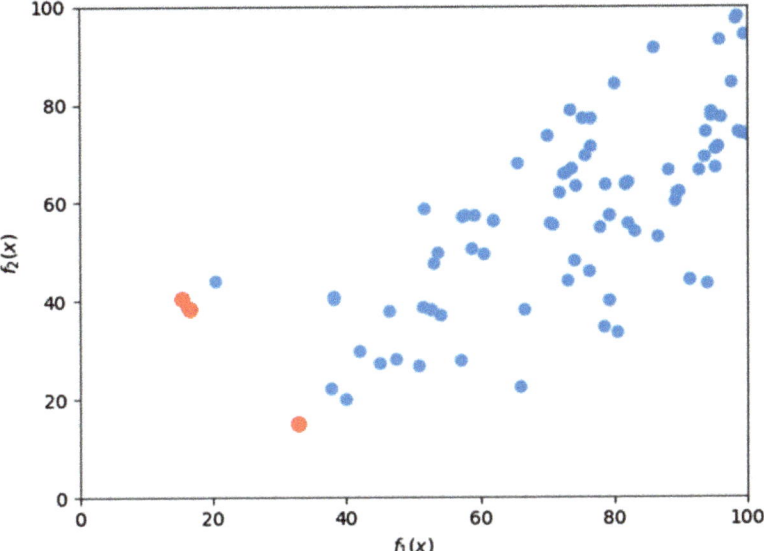

Fig. 4.7 Pareto-front for two (of 24) objective functions

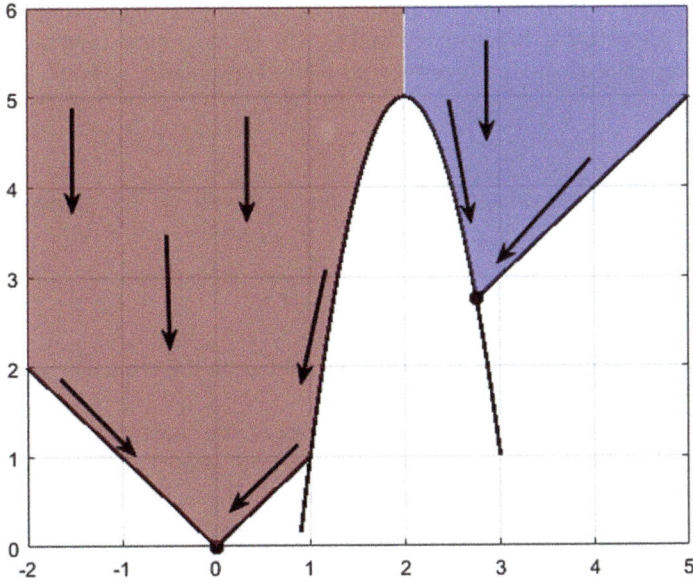

Fig. 4.8 Negative effect of the constraints

The genetics algorithms suitable for multi-objective optimization problems require a huge amount of computational time to produce appropriate solution. Although there are a number of powerful relative fast and precision optimization algorithms designed to solve the scalar optimization problem. Therefore, it is reasonable to scalarize the task. A general formulation for a scalarization of a multi-objective optimization is thus as shown in Eq. 4.4.

$$\min_{x \in X_\theta} g(f_1(x), \ldots, f_k(x), \theta) \qquad (4.4)$$

where θ is a vector parameter, the set $X_\theta \in X$ is a set depending on the parameter θ and g is a function.

The simplest realization is then as shown in Eq. 4.5:

$$\min_{x \in X} \sum_{i=1}^{k} w_i f_i(x) \qquad (4.5)$$

where the weights of the objectives $w_i > 0$ are the parameters of the scalarization.

The more advanced is sequential concessions method that are slightly close to a classical lexicographic method. The lexicographic method assumes that the objectives can be ranked in the order of importance, so that f_1 is the most important and f_k the least important to the decision maker. The lexicographic method consists of solving a sequence of single-objective optimization problems is shown in Eq. 4.6

$$\min f_l(x), \; f_j(x) \leq y_j, \; j = 1, \ldots, l-1, \; x \in X, \qquad (4.6)$$

where y_j is the optimal value of the above problem with $l = j$ as shown in Eq. 4.7. Thus,

$$y_1 := \min_{x \in X} f_1(x) \qquad (4.7)$$

each new problem of the form in the above problem in the sequence adds one new constraint as l goes from 1 to k.

The sequential concessions mean relaxations of the constraints, i.e. each result of previous objective functions optimization can be degraded up to some predefined value to allow next objective function optimization. Thus, for example as shown in Eqs. 4.8 and 4.9 one should solve the following task first:

$$f_1^* = \min_{x \in X} f_1(x), \qquad (4.8)$$

then

$$\begin{cases} f_2^* = \min_{x \in X} f_2(x) \\ f_1(x) \geq f_1^* - \Delta_1 \end{cases}, \qquad (4.9)$$

where Δ_1 and so on for other objectives.

Despite the fact that the method of successive concessions seemed to be the most suitable for the solution of the given task (functions can be ranked according to the importance of colors for the observer, and concessions can be selected accordingly, for example, for Macadam thresholds), the study has shown that adding new constraints to the task significantly complicates the relief of the target function (see Fig. 4.7) and worsens the overall accuracy of the solution. In practice, a satisfactory result was obtained by implementing concessions for no more than two colors.

On the contrary, it was possible to obtain good results and, on the whole, fast and stable convergence of solver algorithms for the scalarized optimization task. Therefore, the final algorithm was built on the base of this approach.

4.2.3 Color Correction Method

The primary task in designing the algorithm was to select the type of transformation for mapping of the palette. Transformations differ in the number of parameters. A large number of parameters provides better accuracy, but makes the optimization process much more complicated. On the basis of the carried-out experiments next transformations were chosen for implementation. The first is a well-known 3 × 4 matrix, that has relatively small number of parameters and has proven itself in color calibration tasks. If $T = [T\_X, T\_Y, T\_Z]$ is the mapped coordinates of some color and $P = [R, G, B]$ are initial coordinates, then O is shown in Eq. 4.10.

$$O = [1 P]A, \qquad (4.10)$$

$$[T\_X, T\_Y, T\_Z] = [R, G, B, 1] \begin{bmatrix} a_{11} & a_{12} & a_{13} \\ a_{21} & a_{22} & a_{23} \\ a_{31} & a_{32} & a_{33} \\ a_{41} & a_{42} & a_{43} \end{bmatrix},$$

where A is described 3 × 4 matrix.

The second is based on the 3rd order polynomial with 11 coefficients for each color channel (i.e. 33 parameters overall). For example, for T_X channel:

$$T\_X = p_1 R + p_2 G + p_3 B + p_4 RG + p_5 RB + p_6 GB$$
$$+ p_7 RR + p_8 GG + p_9 BB + p_{10} RGB + p_{11}$$

It is reported in [1] that this model is a reasonable and achievable compromise between the complexity of the transformation and the stable convergence of the optimization algorithm.

Additionally, we used in investigation polynomial model with 5 coefficients for each color channel.

The result of least squares fitting is used as a baseline for all studies. It is obtained using a trivial approach, the desired vector of coefficients a is shown in Eq. 4.11:

$$\mathbf{a} = \left(\mathbf{P}^T\mathbf{P}\right)^{-1}\mathbf{P}^T\mathbf{b}, \tag{4.11}$$

where P is a factor observation matrix, b—is a vector of responses.

The least square method is used as baseline for parameters estimation, because it gives point of global minimum.

Let the target image T have N color samples, with each color sample being represented using X, Y, and Z coordinates, calculated according to Standard Observer. Organize these target color coordinates into a matrix with N rows $\times 3$ columns as shown in Eq. 4.12.

$$T = \begin{bmatrix} T\_X_1 & T\_Y_1 & T\_Z_1 \\ T\_X_2 & T\_Y_2 & T\_Z_2 \\ \vdots & \vdots & \vdots \\ T\_X_N & T\_Y_N & T\_Z_N \end{bmatrix}, \tag{4.12}$$

Let the transformed image P also have N color samples that correspond to those in the target image as shown in Eq. 4.13.

$$P = \begin{bmatrix} R_1 & G_1 & B_1 \\ R_2 & G_2 & B_2 \\ \vdots & \vdots & \vdots \\ R_N & G_N & B_N \end{bmatrix}, \tag{4.13}$$

What we seek is the optimal linear transformation matrix, for example $\mathbf{A}_{12}$ (4 rows $\times$ 3 columns) that best maps the processed color samples $\mathbf{P}$ into the corresponding original color samples $\mathbf{T}$ as shown in Eq. 4.14.

$$T \approx \hat{T} = [1\ P]A_{12}, \tag{4.14}$$

In the above equation, $\mathbf{1}$ is a column vector of N ones that provides a *DC* offset, or shift, in the brightness level. Thus, each transformed pixel color is a linear combination of a *DC* offset and the processed RGB coordinates. For example, the X color of the first transformed pixel would be equal to Eq. 4.15

$$\widehat{T\_X_1} = A_{11} + A_{21}R_1 + A_{31}G_1 + A_{41}B_1. \tag{4.15}$$

where the two subscripts on the $\mathbf{A}_{12}$ matrix elements denote their row and column positions, respectively. If we have more than twelve independent RGB samples (the number of unknowns in the $\mathbf{A}_{12}$ matrix), then the set of linear equations is overdetermined and the least-squares solution is given by Eq. 4.16

$$\mathbf{A}_{12} = \left([1\,\mathbf{P}]^T[1\,\mathbf{P}]\right)^{-1}[1\,\mathbf{P}]^T\mathbf{T}. \tag{4.16}$$

Last equation is the fundamental equation that we will use to estimate the $\mathbf{A}_{12}$ color correction matrix.

It is important to note that the least squares estimate of matrix $\mathbf{A}_{12}$ is an analytically found global minimum. This position follows from the idea of the least squares method and it is illustrated by the Eq. 4.17, 4.18, 4.19, 4.20, 4.21, 4.22, 4.23, 4.24, 4.25, 4.26, 4.27.

For simple visualization, let us consider in detail obtaining analytical estimation only for one X coordinate (from the RGB triplet). For the Y and Z coordinates, the solution is the same.

As can be seen from the equation, the problem of determining the coefficients vector $\mathbf{a} = (A_1, A_2, A_3, A_4)$ is reduced to minimize the error S.

$$S = \sum_{i=1}^{N} \varepsilon_i^2 = \sum_{i=1}^{N} (T\_X_i - A_1 - A_2 R_i - A_3 G_i - A_4 B_i)^2. \tag{4.17}$$

It is necessary to choose the estimations of A_1, A_2, A_3, A_4 such that their substitution in the equation gives the smallest possible (minimum) value of S. To do this, we differentiate the expressions by A_1, A_2, A_3, A_4

$$\begin{aligned}
\frac{dS}{dA_1} &= -2\sum_{i=1}^{N}(T\_X_i - A_1 - A_2 R_i - A_3 G_i - A_4 B_i) \\
\frac{dS}{dA_1} &= -2\sum_{i=1}^{N} R_i(T\_X_i - A_1 - A_2 R_i - A_3 G_i - A_4 B_i) \\
\frac{dS}{dA_1} &= -2\sum_{i=1}^{N} G_i(T\_X_i - A_1 - A_2 R_i - A_3 G_i - A_4 B_i) \\
\frac{dS}{dA_1} &= -2\sum_{i=1}^{N} B_i(T\_X_i - A_1 - A_2 R_i - A_3 G_i - A_4 B_i)
\end{aligned} \tag{4.18}$$

so, for estimates A_1, A_2, A_3, A_4 we have

$$\sum_{i=1}^{N}(T\_X_i - A_1 - A_2 R_i - A_3 G_i - A_4 B_i) = 0$$

$$\sum_{i=1}^{N} R_i(T\_X_i - A_1 - A_2 R_i - A_3 G_i - A_4 B_i) = 0$$

$$\sum_{i=1}^{N} G_i(T\_X_i - A_1 - A_2 R_i - A_3 G_i - A_4 B_i) = 0 \quad (4.19)$$

$$\sum_{i=1}^{N} B_i(T\_X_i - A_1 - A_2 R_i - A_3 G_i - A_4 B_i) = 0$$

This is a system of so-called normal equations that can be transformed

$$A_1 N + A_2 \sum_{i=1}^{N} R_i + A_3 \sum_{i=1}^{N} G_i + A_4 \sum_{i=1}^{N} B_i = \sum_{i=1}^{N} T\_X_i$$

$$A_1 \sum_{i=1}^{N} R_i + A_2 + A_2 \sum_{i=1}^{N} R_i^2 + A_3 \sum_{i=1}^{N} R_i G_i + A_4 \sum_{i=1}^{N} R_i B_i = \sum_{i=1}^{N} R_i T\_X_i$$

$$A_1 \sum_{i=1}^{N} G_i + A_2 + A_2 \sum_{i=1}^{N} G_i R_i + A_3 \sum_{i=1}^{N} G_i^2 + A_4 \sum_{i=1}^{N} G_i B_i = \sum_{i=1}^{N} G_i T\_X_i$$

$$A_1 \sum_{i=1}^{N} B_i + A_2 + A_2 \sum_{i=1}^{N} B_i R_i + A_3 \sum_{i=1}^{N} B_i G_i + A_4 \sum_{i=1}^{N} B_i^2 = \sum_{i=1}^{N} B_i T\_X_i$$

$$(4.20)$$

We will not obtain specific equations for calculating the coefficients $\mathbf{a} = (A_1, A_2, A_3, A_4)$, but we will find a solution in matrix form. For this, we again write the system of equations in matrix form:

$$\begin{bmatrix} 1 & R_1 & G_1 & B_1 \\ 1 & R_2 & G_2 & B_2 \\ \vdots & \vdots & \vdots & \vdots \\ 1 & R_N & G_N & B_N \end{bmatrix} \begin{bmatrix} A_1 \\ A_2 \\ A_3 \\ A_4 \end{bmatrix} = \begin{bmatrix} T\_X_1 \\ T\_X_2 \\ \vdots \\ T\_X_4 \end{bmatrix}, \quad (4.21)$$

[1 P]a = T_X,

To find a solution, you need to multiply the right and left sides of the equation on the left by the inverse of the $[1\,P]^{-1}$ matrix. However, this matrix is not inverted, since it is not square. Therefore, we will perform the following actions: Let us multiply the matrix $[1\,P]$ by $[1\,P]^T$ on the left:

$$\begin{bmatrix} 1 & 1 & \cdots & 1 \\ R_1 & R_2 & \cdots & R_N \\ G_1 & G_2 & \cdots & G_N \\ B_1 & B_2 & \cdots & B_N \end{bmatrix} \begin{bmatrix} 1 & R_1 & G_1 & B_1 \\ 1 & R_2 & G_2 & B_2 \\ \vdots & \vdots & \vdots & \vdots \\ 1 & R_N & G_N & B_N \end{bmatrix} \qquad (4.22)$$

$$= \begin{bmatrix} N & \sum_{i=1}^{N} R_i & \sum_{i=1}^{N} G_i & \sum_{i=1}^{N} B_i \\ \sum_{i=1}^{N} R_i & \sum_{i=1}^{N} R_i^2 & \sum_{i=1}^{N} R_i G_i & \sum_{i=1}^{N} R_i B_i \\ \sum_{i=1}^{N} G_i & \sum_{i=1}^{N} R_i G_i & \sum_{i=1}^{N} G_i^2 & \sum_{i=1}^{N} G_i B_i \\ \sum_{i=1}^{N} B_i & \sum_{i=1}^{N} R_i B_i & \sum_{i=1}^{N} G_i B_i & \sum_{i=1}^{N} B_i^2 \end{bmatrix}$$

Then multiply the matrix $[1P]^T$ by the vector T_X:

$$\begin{bmatrix} 1 & 1 & \cdots & 1 \\ R_1 & R_2 & \cdots & R_N \\ G_1 & G_2 & \cdots & G_N \\ B_1 & B_2 & \cdots & B_N \end{bmatrix} \begin{bmatrix} T\_X_1 \\ T\_X_2 \\ \vdots \\ T\_X_N \end{bmatrix} = \begin{bmatrix} \sum_{i=1}^{N} T\_X_i \\ \sum_{i=1}^{N} R_i T\_X_i \\ \sum_{i=1}^{N} G_i T\_X_i \\ \sum_{i=1}^{N} B_i T\_X_i \end{bmatrix} \qquad (4.23)$$

Now normal Eq. (4.20) can be written in the following vector–matrix form:

$$[1P]^T [1P]a = [1P]^T T\_X \qquad (4.24)$$

to solve which you need to multiply the right and left sides on the left by the inverse matrix $([1P]^T [1P])^{-1}$, which is square.
Then finally

$$\mathbf{a} = ([1\ \mathbf{P}]^T [1\ \mathbf{P}])^{-1} [1\ \mathbf{P}]^T \mathbf{T\_X}. \qquad (4.25)$$

Generalization of the obtained equation for three coordinates XYZ gives the following expression.

Thus, the recalculation based on the least square method gives point of global minimum, but for Euclidian distance.

Although the least squares method works well, it suffers from the fact that the quantity being minimized—namely, distance in XYZ—is not the quantity that matters most—namely, distance in a perceptually uniform color space such as CIELAB ΔE or CIEDE2000.

Thus, it is necessary to develop new method of space recalculation based on minimization the error between color in reference and recalculated spaces expressed by metric CIEDE2000.

Table 4.1 Ciede2000 errors after least squares fitting

Model	Cat1	Cat2	Cat3	Cat4	Cat5	Cat6	Cat7	Cat8
3 × 4	14.54	11.14	10.90	12.61	11.41	9.34	12.59	10.32
Polynomial	11.32	9.12	8.98	10.80	10.08	8.30	10.98	9.53

The matching error is estimated were as the sum of CIEDE2000 values for all colors from matched (obtained from initial by estimated transform) and target palettes:

$$err = \sum_{i=1}^{n} CIEDE2000(\boldsymbol{T}_i, \boldsymbol{P}_i) \tag{4.26}$$

where $\boldsymbol{T}_i$—is a matched color (input color after transformation).

The described models give the following matching errors after least squares fitting for each categorical observer (Table 4.1).

The optimization of scalarized objective function allows setting different weights $w_i > 0$ for colors.

$$\sum_{i=1}^{k} w_i f_i(\boldsymbol{x}) \rightarrow min. \tag{4.27}$$

Weights can reflect the desired degree of accuracy for specific colors. For example, additional weight may be given to a group of "important" colors for a particular observer. It should be noted that setting unequal weights for different objective functions increases the overall matching error. Selection of the optimal ratio of weights is a rather semi-manual, empirical and poorly automated task (taking into account execution time constraints of the optimization algorithms). Besides, as a result of optimization, "important" weights can have a satisfactory matching error even with equal weights. Therefore, it makes sense to use the weight setting for some "important" color in the manual mode in case of a large error in the course of solving the optimization task.

On the other hand, adding regularization term to the optimized function looks like the reasonable measure for palette matching. The idea of regularization in this task is to provide as uniform distribution of the error as possible across all colors. In addition, solutions where the CIEDE2000 distance exceeds one on some colors should be penalized more, as in this case the difference between the target color and the recalculated color begins to be strongly noticeable.

We studied that most suitable for our task is the use of 2nd–4th order regularization term (Fig. 4.9).

The advantage of this form of regularization is that fact that it significantly penalize the errors greater than 1, has little effect on errors with values close to 1 and non-linearly encourages minor errors with values of 0–0.8.

4 Multi-Objective Optimization Algorithms in Medical Image Analysis

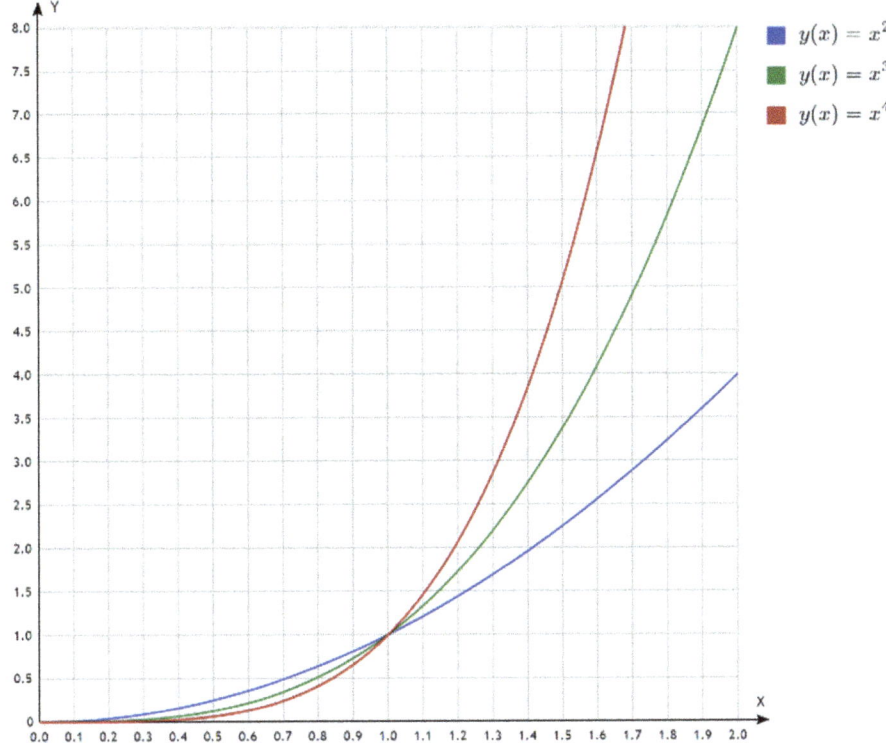

Fig. 4.9 Charts of different regularization terms

In our investigation, we tested different optimization strategies and algorithms. The initial strategy was to use global optimization algorithm and then local optimization with the obtained starting point. Examples of global optimization algorithms, which we have tested, are:

- Dividing rectangles algorithm [10].
- Controlled Random search [11].
- Multi-level single linkage [12].
- Improved Stochastic Ranking Evolution Strategy [13].
- A set of different evolutionary algorithms [14].
    For local optimization we studied:
- Levenberg–Marquardt algorithm [15].
- Constrained optimization by linear approximation [16].
- BFGS and low-storage BFGS [17].
- Nelder-Mead algorithm [18].
- Subplex algorithm [19].

The important point of our investigation is the estimation of initial point. For its estimation we used least square method. Applying of Least square method for estimation of initial point gives us possibility to suppose that we will obtain result of optimization task which is very close to global minimum. Our considerations are next. The least square method gives global minimum, but for Euclidian distance. It was shown above. We are trying to get global minimum, but in CIEDE 2000 metric. This metrics takes in account the features of human vision, so it refining step, but it means that both minimum (according to Euclidian distance and CIEDE 2000 metrics) are rather close each other.

This position is illustrated in Fig. 4.10. On the left chromaticity diagram there are white, green and yellow circles. White circles correspond XYZ coordinate of target colors. Yellow circles correspond XYZ coordinates of colors transformed by LMS. On both figures you can see only 10 colors. These colors have the maximum error after recalculation on the first step. You can see that white and green circles are very close each another. On the right chromaticity diagram there are additional red circles. They correspond XYZ coordinates for the case of matrix A as shown in Eq. 4.28:

$$A = \begin{bmatrix} 1 & 0 & 0 & 0 \\ 0 & 1 & 0 & 0 \\ 0 & 0 & 1 & 0 \\ 0 & 0 & 0 & 1 \end{bmatrix}. \tag{4.28}$$

It is variant without any suggestion about initial value of matrix **A**. You can see that red circles are very far from target circles, sometimes outside of chromaticity diagram. So as initial point we must take the result of recalculation RGB in XYZ by LMS—matrix A_{LS}.

So our task to refine the position of minimum according to properties of human vision. Our investigation of small area around the global minimum according to

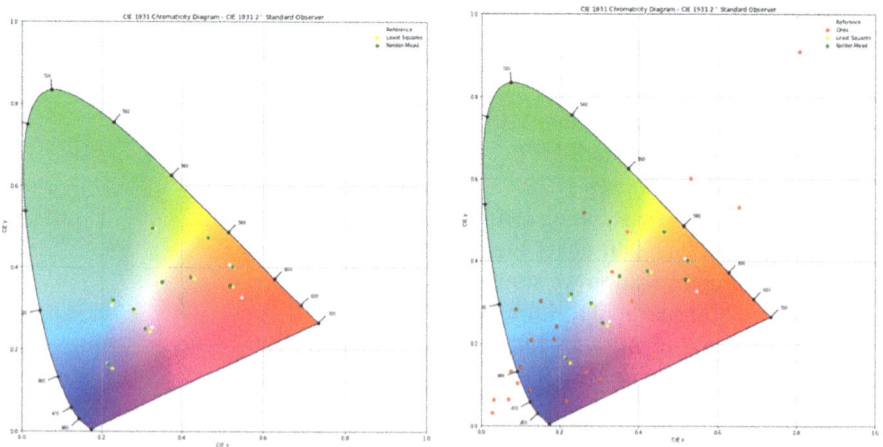

Fig. 4.10 Chromaticity diagrams with target and recalculated colors

Euclidian distance shows that the character of loss function in this small area is unimodal.

That leads to an idea to use the result of least squares fitting as a starting point to optimization routine. The global optimization step is therefore omitted and for the local optimizer the best performance (in terms of speed of finding a satisfactory solution), precision and convergence stability shows the BFGS method, which proved to be one of the most popular line-search methods nowadays.

The general idea of BFGS is the approximation of Hessian (which is necessary for second order optimization methods) by using some information from previously calculated data. The algorithm minimizes the $f(x)$ by the following steps.

1. Initialize the starting point x_0 and set the search accuracy $e > 0$. Determine the initial approximation H_0 which can be identity matrix;
2. Find the point in the direction of which the search will be performed as given in Eq. 4.29:

$$p_k = -H_k \nabla f_k \quad (4.29)$$

3. Calculate through a recurrence ratio as in Eq. 4.30:

$$x_{k+1} = x_k + a_k p_k \quad (4.30)$$

The coefficient a is found using line search, where it meets the Wolfe conditions as given in Eq. 4.31:

$$f(x_k + a_k p_k) \leq c_1 a_k \nabla f_k^T p_k$$
$$\nabla f(x_k + a_k p_k)^T p_k \geq c_2 \nabla f_k^T p_k \quad (4.31)$$

in most implementations $c_1 = 0.0001$ and $c_2 = 0.9$.

4. Evaluate two vectors as given in Eq. 4.32:

$$s_k = x_{k+1} - x_k$$
$$y_k = \nabla f_{k+1} - \nabla f_k \quad (4.32)$$

5. Update the Hessian according to the Eq. 4.33 (here I—identity matrix):

$$H_{k+1} = (I - p_k s_k y_k^T) H_k (I - p_k y_k s_k^T) + p s_k s_k^T$$
$$p_k = \frac{1}{y_k^T s_k} \quad (4.33)$$

6. Check the stopping criteria as given in Eq. 4.34:

$$|\nabla f_k| > e \quad (4.34)$$

Although, despite the fact, that BFGS is reported to achieve high precision, the noise influenced due to numerical calculation of derivatives of CIEDE2000 based

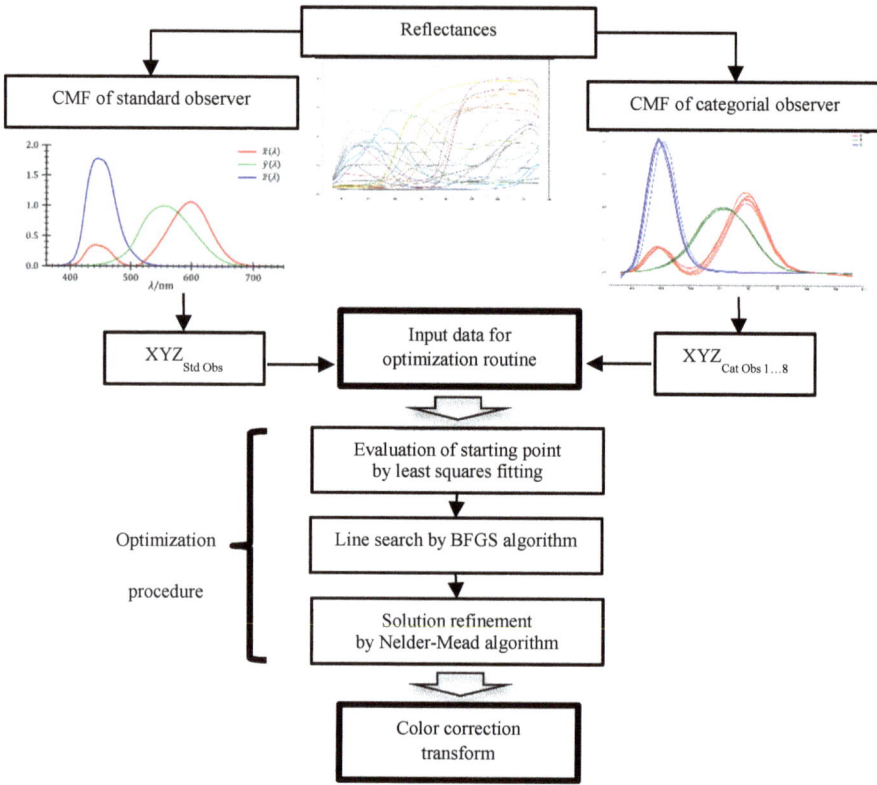

Fig. 4.11 Scheme of optimization procedure

cost function affects the final solution. To overcome this problem, we add a second step of local optimization after BFGS convergence to some solution—a Nelder-Mead algorithm.

Nelder-Mead (also known as Simplex method) is well known derivative-free algorithm and therefore easily applicable to non-smooth or noisy functions. The essence of the method is the sequential movement and deformation of the simplex around the extremum point [12]. In fact, we use this derivative-free algorithm in relatively small surrounding of BFGS solution to "sharp" it.

Therefore, the scheme of developed optimization procedure is presented in Fig. 4.11.

4.3 Experimental Results

The goal of developed method is to process the color mapping that decreases as good as possible visual color difference based on the CIEDE2000 metric.

Table 4.2 Results of least squares fitting and optimization procedure

	Cat1	Cat2	Cat3	Cat4	Cat5	Cat6	Cat7	Cat8
CIEDE2000								
Least squares 3 × 4	14.54	11.14	10.90	12.61	11.41	9.34	12.59	10.32
Least squares polynomial	11.32	9.12	8.98	10.80	10.08	8.30	10.98	9.53
Optimization 3 × 4	10.56	8.24	7.87	8.52	7.94	7.14	10.82	8.63
Optimization polynomial	8.30	6.11	5.60	7.47	7.11	6.12	8.43	6.40
Euclidian								
Least squares 3 × 4	9.24	3.86	3.79	3.14	3.87	3.49	4.43	4.27
Least squares polynomial	6.38	2.77	2.71	2.72	3.14	2.86	3.47	3.33
Optimization 3 × 4	9.15	4.38	4.48	4.53	4.33	4.16	5.11	4.64
Optimization polynomial	6.91	3.06	2.96	3.49	3.46	3.09	3.79	3.49

The least squares fitting procedure is processed in XYZ space using by the fact Euclidian distance between coordinates and then CIEDE2000 color distance is evaluated for each pair of colors from obtained mapped set and given target set. While the optimization routine operates directly with CIEDE2000 metric and does not concern the Euclidian norm discrepancies in the XYZ coordinates.

In Table 4.2 there are resulted Euclidian and CIEDE2000 distances achieved after least squares fitting and optimization procedure by two types of transforms for 8 categorical observers. The given results are obtained without regularization in optimization procedure.

According to the results described in Table 4.2 we can conclude the following.

- The total error in the Euclidian metric according to the optimization results exceeds the error obtained by the least squares method. Nevertheless, the optimization result is better for all observers by the target CIEDE2000 metric.
- A more complex model provides a better match for all categorical observers.

As for increasing the complexity of the model, we tested various options. Of course, in the case of a polynomial model, for example, increasing the number of coefficients and the order of the polynomial increases the mapping accuracy. However, polynomials with an order higher than the third tend to oscillations outside the matching points, besides, the more coefficients, the more difficult it is to achieve the convergence of optimization algorithms, the longer the procedure execution time increases. A detailed overview of the polynomial models for palette mapping is provided in [4]. In Table 4.3 there are optimization results for 5 and 11 coefficients (in each channel) models.

In Table 4.3 we pointed value of color error according in the metric CIEDE 2000. It is the sum which shows us total error obtained for 24 colors of Macbeth Colorchecker. In this case the middle error for per color is in interval from 0.43 to 0.28 for polynomial model with 5 coefficients, and in interval from 0.35 to 23 for polynomial model with 11 coefficients. It means that mean error for both models and

Table 4.3 Optimization results for 5 and 11 coefficients (in each channel) models.

	Cat1	Cat2	Cat3	Cat4	Cat5	Cat6	Cat7	Cat8
Polynomial 5 coeff	10.32	8.07	7.72	8.45	7.84	6.87	10.24	8.17
Polynomial 11 coeff	8.30	6.11	5.60	7.47	7.11	6.12	8.43	6.40

for all types of categorical observers is less than perceptibility threshold. According to state the art investigation in color imaging, if the color error is less than 1 according to CIEDE2000 metric, it cannot be distinguished by human vision. Thus the first conclusion from Table 4.3 means that both model as polynomial model with 5 coefficients, so polynomial model with 11 coefficients gives similar result. But as it mentioned in [4] and proved by our investigation 11-coefficients model is a reasonable trade-off between complexity, stability and provided precision.

However, the low total error for all colors, as a result of optimization, does not guarantee that for each color the error will be less than 1 in CIEDE2000 metrics (perceptibility threshold). Therefore, taking into account the specifics of the CIEDE2000 metric, it is much more important characteristic is the number colors with the error exceeds the perceptibility threshold in comparison with the result obtained for the least squares. The most interesting question from the point of color imaging quality how many colors has error exceeded perceptibility threshold. For this estimation we realized the next variant of investigation. The several color error levels were defined. The fist level is 1 in CIEDE 2000 metrics, the second level is 0.9, the third level is 0.8. The number of colors for each type of categorical observer in which the error exceeds the levels 0.8, 0.9 and 1.0 were calculated. This characteristic is calculated for proposed method based on polynomial model and for least squares method. The proposed method includes the polynomial model with 4th order regularization term was used. These characteristics were obtained for all categorical types. Table 4.4 shows results. First digit is number of colors exceed the level in the case of the least square method applying and the second digit after slash for proposed method based on optimization approach with polynomial model and regularization term.

The results clearly demonstrate that in the case of proposed method for each color in Macbeth ColorChecker the color error in CIEDE metrics is less than perceptibility threshold. The situation is the same for level of threshold 0.9. Only for very high threshold (third row, the threshold level 0.8) for some types of categorical observer there colors with error exceed the level. For the least square method this situation takes place for the first level corresponding perceptibility threshold—1 CIEDE metric, there are colors with high color error for all types of categorical observer. Thus, if

Table 4.4 The number of colors in which the error exceeds the levels

Level	Cat1	Cat2	Cat3	Cat4	Cat5	Cat6	Cat7	Cat8
1.0	3/0	3/0	3/0	2/0	2/0	2/0	3/0	3/0
0.9	4/0	3/0	3/0	2/0	2/0	2/0	3/0	3/0
0.8	5/0	3/2	4/0	3/0	3/0	2/0	3/3	3/3

we apply method of color matching (correction) based on optimization approach with regularization term it gives possibility to get color image with more high color quality than if we use standard methods.

4.4 Conclusion

The principal feature of proposed method: the error between colors from space A and space B is calculated according to metric CIEDE2000. Using the target function based on CIEDE2000 metric leads to necessity transfer from least square method using for transformation function parameters identification to multi objective optimization. Each color of palette is represented as separate target function. The problem of several target functions minimum definition on the set of transformation function parameters must be solved. As algorithm for palette matching, we used the 3rd order polynomial with 11 coefficients for each color channel (i.e., 33 parameters overall), according to our research results it surpasses the accuracy of matching realized by linear transformation with matrix 3×3 and 3×4.

Our investigation was aimed to solve the task of multi objective minimization, where each target function is the distance between colors in space A and space B and set of parameters for fitting—33 coefficients of 3d order polynomial. We have investigated approach based on Pareto front, algorithm of successive concessions and scalarization approach with regularization term. Despite the fact that the method of successive concessions seemed to be the most suitable for the solution of the given task (functions can be ranked according to the importance of colors for the observer, and concessions can be selected accordingly, for example, for Macadam thresholds), the study has shown that adding new constraints to the task significantly complicates the relief of the target function and worsens the overall accuracy of the solution. In practice, a satisfactory result was obtained by implementing concessions for no more than two colors. In our task the genetics algorithms seemed to be the most suitable for multi-objective optimization, but in fact these algorithms require a huge amount of computational time to produce an appropriate solution. For Pareto front defining in our condition the genetics algorithms are the most suitable for multi-objective optimization problems, but these algorithms require a huge amount of computational time to produce appropriate solution. There are a number of powerful relative fast and precision optimization algorithms designed to solve the scalar optimization problem. Therefore, it is reasonable to scalarize the task.

As result we proposed next approach: the task can be solved by scalarization approach for target function creation with consequence adding regularization term in resulting scalar target function. In our work we found that reasonable power of regularization term is 4. We realized research of representative set of minimization algorithms for getting minimum of the target function with regularization term and as result suggest next approach for polynomial transformation function coefficients estimation:

- Evaluation of starting point by least square method.
- Line search by BFGS algorithm.
- Solution refinement by Nelder-Mead Algorithm.

Our experimental research of proposed method includes matching the colors of palette corresponding space A and space B:

- By linear transformation function (matrix 3×4) and 3th order polynomial with coefficients determined by Least Square Method with Euclidian metric in XYZ space;
- By linear transformation function (matrix 3×4) and 3th order polynomial with coefficients determined by our method based on CIEDE2000 metric.

The color space recalculation was realized for all 8 types of categorial observer. We obtained color palettes describing color space of each categorial observer on the base of color matching function and spectral data of Macbeth ColorChecker.

The obtained accuracy of matching palettes of categorical observers with palette, corresponding standard observer, are next. For all 8 types of categorical observers the total error obtained as summarize of error of each color in palette is approximately 30% smaller if we applied our method in comparing with least squares. For example, for categorical observers 7 and 8 with the most remarkable differences between their color space and color space of standard observer the total error in the case of least squares for polynomial function: categorial observer 7—10.98; categorical observer 8—9.53. The total error obtained by optimization (proposed method) for polynomial function: categorical observer 7—8.43; categorical observer 8—6.40. The given results are obtained without regularization in optimization procedure. In the case of categorical observer 1 (the smallest distance between its space and space of standard observer) total error has value 11.32 and 8.3.

Thus, the optimization result is better for all observers by the target CIEDE2000 metric. However, the low total error for all colors, as a result of optimization, does not guarantee that for each color the error will be less than for the least squares. Therefore, taking into account the specifics of the CIEDE2000 metric, it is much more important for how many colors as a result of optimization the error exceeds the visually noticeable threshold in comparison with the result obtained for the least squares. In this case we used optimization with regularization term.

As threshold we used the value 1 for CIEDE2000 metric, if error of CIEDE2000 for colors after matching more than 1 the difference between color will be visible for observer. Our experiments shown that if for color matching method applied estimation of transformation function parameters based on least square, then for each categorical observer the quantity of colors with error hire 1 more is always more than 2, but if we applied our method based on optimization there no any colors pare with error more than 1. The same situation will be saved if the level of threshold will be 0.9. The results clearly demonstrate the advantage of the developed palette matching method based on optimization.

References

1. Guowei, H., Luo, M.R., Rhodes P.A.: A study of digital camera colorimetric characterization based on polynomial modeling. Color research & application: endorsed by Inter-Society Color Council, The Colour Group (Great Britain), Canadian Society for Color, Color Science Association of Japan, Dutch Society for the Study of Color, The Swedish Colour Centre Foundation, Colour Society of Australia, Centre Français de la Couleur **26**(1), 76–84 (2001).
2. Stiles, W.S., Burch, J.M..: NPL colour-matching investigation: final report (1958). Opt. Acta: Int. J. Opt. **6**(1), 1–26 (1959)
3. Sarkar, A., Blondé, L., Morvan, P.: Method for the classification of observers according to their visual characteristics. European Patent Application #10290193.1, filed by Thomson Licensing on April 9, (2010).
4. Asano, Y.: Individual colorimetric observers for personalized color imaging. Rochester Institute of Technology (2015).
5. Miettinen, K.: Nonlinear multiobjective optimization, vol. 12. Springer Science & Business Media, (2012).
6. Fudenberg, D., Tirole J.: Game theory, 1991, vol. 393, 12, pp. 18–23. Cambridge, Massachusetts, 80 (1991)
7. Ciro, G.C., et al.: A NSGA-II and NSGA-III comparison for solving an open shop scheduling problem with resource constraints. IFAC-PapersOnLine **49**(12), 1272–1277 (2016).
8. Ishibuchi, H., et al.: Performance comparison of NSGA-II and NSGA-III on various many-objective test problems. 2016 IEEE Congress on Evolutionary Computation (CEC). IEEE (2016).
9. Campos, G.C., Dugardin, F., Yalaoui, F., Kelly, R.: A NSGA-II and NSGA-III comparison for solving an open shop scheduling problem with resource constraints. 8th IFAC Conference on Manufacturing Modelling, Management and Control MIM 2016, IFAC-PapersOnLine **49**(12), 1272–1277 (2016).
10. Gablonsky, J.M., Kelley, C.T.: A locally-biased form of the DIRECT algorithm. J. Global Optim. **21**(1), 27–37 (2001)
11. Kaelo, P., Ali, M.M.: Some variants of the controlled random search algorithm for global optimization. J. Optim. Theory Appl. **130**(2), 253–264 (2006)
12. Kucherenko, S., Sytsko, Y.: Application of deterministic low-discrepancy sequences in global optimization. Comput. Optim. Appl. **30**(3), 297–318 (2005)
13. Runarsson, T.P., Xin Y.: Search biases in constrained evolutionary optimization. IEEE Trans. Syst., Man, Cybern., Part C (Appl. Rev.) **35**(2), 233–243 (2005).
14. https://platypus.readthedocs.io/en/latest/ (2022). Accessed on March 24, 2022.
15. Kanzow, C., Yamashita, N., Fukushima, M.: Levenberg–Marquardt methods with strong local convergence properties for solving nonlinear equations with convex constraints. J. Comput. Appl. Math. **172**(2), 375–397 (2004)
16. Powell, M.J.D.: Direct search algorithms for optimization calculations. Acta numerica **7**, 287–336 (1998).
17. Nocedal, J.: Updating quasi-Newton matrices with limited storage. Math. Comput. **35**(151), 773–782 (1980)
18. Richardson, J.A., Kuester J.L.: Algorithm 454: the complex method for constrained optimization [E4]. Communications of the ACM **16**(8), 487–489 (1973).
19. Rowan, T.H.: Functional stability analysis of numerical algorithms. The University of Texas at Austin (1990).

Chapter 5
Heart Failure Detection from Clinical and Lifestyle Information using Optimized XGBoost with Gravitational Search Algorithm

Etuari Oram, Bighnaraj Naik, Geetanjali Bhoi, and Danilo Pelusi

Abstract The technological up-gradation in the area of healthcare services is noticeable in the last few decades. This became possible due to the research, development, and application of IoT, which enables sensors, medical devices, and healthcare professionals to connect and provide remote medical services. IoT infrastructure of healthcare components include sensor devices, communication channels, cloud computing, and healthcare suppliers. These advances created scope for data scientists and AI engineers to collect healthcare data and design models for analysis and identification of various diseases. The major contribution of this article is as follows: (i) Understanding the clinical and lifestyle features, and their importance for modeling heart failure detection, (ii) Designing a data-driven heart failure detection model using extreme gradient boosting (XGBoost) ensemble learning technique, and (iii) Optimizing the various hyperparameters of XGBoost such as learning rate, subsample, L2 regularization, L1 regularization, max depth, and max delta step by using Gravitational search algorithm (GSA). The proposed approach has been evaluated by using various performance metrics and compared with other similar approaches.

Keywords Heart failure detection · Extreme gradient boosting machine · Ensemble learning · Gravitational search algorithm

---

E. Oram · B. Naik (✉) · G. Bhoi
Dept. of Computer Application, Veer Surendra Sai University of Technology, Burla, Sambalpur, Odisha PIN: 768018, India
e-mail: bnaik_mca@vssut.ac.in

E. Oram
e-mail: eoram_mca@vssut.ac.in

G. Bhoi
e-mail: pbhoi762@gmail.com

D. Pelusi
Faculty of Communication Sciences, University of Teramo, Coste Sant', Agostino Campus, Teramo, Italy
e-mail: dpelusi@unite.it

© The Author(s), under exclusive license to Springer Nature Switzerland AG 2023
J. Nayak et al. (eds.), *Nature-Inspired Optimization Methodologies in Biomedical and Healthcare*, Intelligent Systems Reference Library 233,
https://doi.org/10.1007/978-3-031-17544-2_5

5.1 Introduction

A good metabolism activity is very essential for the smooth running of the human body. It is processed well when all the organs such as lungs, kidneys, intestine, liver, etc. of a human body function properly. It is the responsibility of the human heart to pump the body parts with nutrient and oxygenated blood properly. Some health issues may be experienced due to improper and insufficient blood supply to body parts. Heart failure is one such type of issue that is mainly associated with the heart. Heart failure is also very often known as cardiovascular or congestive heart failure or myocardial infarction. It is one of the chronic and acute conditions that occurs when blood vessels overload to pump blood to the heart properly and some kind of liquid starts generating in the lungs part for the substitution.

An acute coronary syndrome (ACS) myocardial infarction can be followed by three stages such as ST-segment elevation myocardial infarction (STEMI), Non-ST segment elevation myocardial infarction (NSTEMI), and Coronary spasm/ unstable angina respectively. Heartbeat can be noticeable by the "ST segment", a pattern that developed on the electrocardiogram. STEMI and NSTEMI are the major types of attacks that cause significant loss. When the coronary artery gets blocked entirely and the working muscles around it stop receiving blood supply then STEMI type attack is realized to occur. It arises with the classic type symptoms of chest pain at the center, tightness, or chest discomforts. Other symptoms seem to be shortness of breath, anxiety, dizziness, nausea, breaking out in a cold sweat, pain in both arms, ankle swelling, etc. In contrast to STEMI, NSTEMI occurs when the coronary artery is only partially blocked. On the other hand, coronary artery spasm/coronary spasm is a silent attack that causes one of the heart arteries to tighten and resulting in drastically reduced blood flow. The sign of this heart failure is similar to the STEMI heart attack such as indigestion, muscle pain, jaw pain, and many more. This type of attack doesn't bring any serious loss but it may increase the risk of upcoming heart failure that probably most violent. The main cause of heart failure (HF) is not only the environmental condition but also other challenging factors such as a healthy diet, smoking, physical exercise, blood pressure, cholesterol, glucose control, coronary artery disease, and other malfunctions. A coronary angiography test is conducted to determine the blockage portion of arteries. Similarly, other tests such as clinical examinations, blood sample tests, etc. are also conducted. Based on the test report, immediate medical treatment is provided either in terms of surgery or medication. According to the statistical report of the American Heart Association and the European Society of Cardiology (ESC), nearly about 26 billion people are diagnosed globally in 2021, out of which almost 3.6 billion are diagnosed fresh every year [1]. Approximately 3–5% of hospitalized patients are linked with cardiovascular (2% adults in developed countries and 8% of citizens), out of these, 17–45% died within five years. It had also been observed that after 65 years of age the number of male cases is more than females. In earlier days, medical diagnoses and assessments were conducted manually due to the lack of automation and digitization. Any type of disease could be diagnosed only after rigorous examinations physically and clinically. Various management strategies such as collecting large amounts of healthcare data, monitoring remotely, analyzing the data, assessing severity, and disease early detection are challenging steps in the medical field. The morbidity and mortality rate of HF is high in comparison to other medical issues despite many preventive and therapy measures. Therefore, it needs to be prepared a better action plan for testing, diagnosis, assessment, and prediction process. Healthcare applications, for example, smartwatches, and many more health monitoring devices embedded with body temperature heartbeat, and blood pressure sensors to monitor health issues remotely. XGBoost ensemble learning is one of the most popular ML techniques due to its ability to produce accurate results. It has been witnessed that XGBoost is widely used by industry users, including Alibaba, Google, Tencent, and various start-up companies. Motivated by this fact, in this paper, XGBoost ensemble learning has been used for heart failure prediction and detection where the hyperparameters are optimized using a gravitational search algorithm (GSA).

The major contribution of this article is as follows: (i) Understanding the clinical and lifestyle features, and their importance for modeling heart failure detection, (ii) Designing a data-driven heart failure detection model using extreme gradient boosting (XGBoost) ensemble learning technique, and (iii) Optimizing the various hyperparameters of XGBoost such as learning rate, subsample, lambda, L2 regularization, L1 regularization, max depth, and max delta step by using Gravitational search algorithm (GSA). The proposed approach has been evaluated by using various performance metrics and compared with other similar approaches. The remaining portion of this chapter has been presented by using the following sections: Sect. 5.2 is the literature survey, Sect. 5.3 includes Exploratory data analysis of heart failure data, Sect. 5.4 is representing the Proposed model, followed by Results and analysis, and the Conclusion is Sects. 5.5 and 5.6 respectively.

5.2 Literature Survey

The contribution of IoT and machine learning to the medical domain has a great role. IoT and Machine learning concepts have been amplified widespread on the medical ground as a cloud service, specifically termed the Internet of Medical Things (IoMT). The IoMT is defined as software and hardware smart infrastructure for healthcare applications where medical users are able to control the patients remotely. The main performance of the IoMT is abstracted through the three layers: perception, network, and application layer. The perception layer is responsible for data collection through various devices such as electrocardiogram (ECG) monitoring devices, electromyography (EMG) devices, actuator-based glucometers, and many other sensors. Providing consistent and integrated information through the network is the role of the network layer. Similarly, the application layer represents the interactive interface between the users and IoMT monitoring devices. Also, it deals with the healthcare information repositories to supply customized and personalized healthcare systems. The trend of IoMT design has been increased for decades by machine learning, artificial intelligence, and IoT. The key benefits of IoMT are real-time data processing, optimization, high accuracy in the diagnosis process, high throughput, reduction in hospitalization due to preventive care, etc., and hence cost of the acute diagnosis process is reduced significantly. Now a days, the impact of ML and IoT on medical and heart-related diseases is really more than before. Contributions of Researchers and medical practitioners also have a vital role in it. A ubiquitous IoMT [2, 3] is already being used for processing streaming data in association with machine learning (SVM, DT, RF, etc.) in heart failure diagnosis, determining severity prediction, future adverse conditions, analysis, and assessment. L Ali et al. [4] has developed a support vector machine (SVM) based model, in which a stack of linear and regularised SVM is used to predict heart failure disease in an earlier stage. Further, the model is optimized using a hybrid grid search algorithm. The Cleveland Clinic heart disease dataset has been used for model evaluation, which is collected from the machine learning repository. According to this study, the model gives an accuracy of 92.22%, specificity of 100%, sensitivity of 82.92%, and Mathews correlation coefficients of 0.851. Using the same Cleveland Clinic heart disease dataset, A Javeed et al. [5] have developed a model using Random forests to detect heart disease. In this study, the proposed Random forest-based model is optimized with a Random search algorithm and observed 93.33% accuracy, which is 3.3% more than the conventional Random Forest model. Son et al. [6] have proposed a model based on a Decision tree with a rough set theory to diagnose earlier-stage heart failure. The real dataset has been applied to the model and the output evaluated is in two phases. This approach evaluated and reported an accuracy of 97.5%, a sensitivity of 97.2%, and a specificity of 97.7%. A report by Zerina Masetic et al. [7] includes the implementation of the RF model and other ML models such as C4.5, K-Nearest Neighbour, SVM, etc., for electrocardiography (ECG) signal classification. The authors have used first applied feature extraction on the ECG signal dataset and then used data for model training. In this study, RF has been reported as the best model with an accuracy of 100%. Lal Hussain et al. [8] used heart rate variability (HRV) to predict cardiovascular disease using SVM with the linear kernel and other ensemble learning classifiers. HRV signal is analyzed by extracting multimodal features such as spectral, temporal, complex dynamics, etc. Here, SVM linear kernel providing effective performance than other models.

Ensemble learning models now a days play important role in many research areas and are found efficient. This approach allows the combining of decisions from multiple homogeneous or heterogeneous models. An adaptive boosting ensemble learning is used by Kathleen H. Miao et al. [9] for early diagnosis and prediction of heart disease. This approach is experimented with 4 datasets collected from different sources for coronary heart disease and found better accuracy than previous works. A machine learning-based Logistic Model has been proposed by Dafli K. Plati et al. [10] for chronic disease heart failure. Here, LMT is compared with DT, NB, Logistic regression, Rotation Forest, and KNN. G Lorenzoni et al. [11] has compared the performance of eight ML techniques in the prediction of hospitalization among patients with heart failure, using data from the Gestione Integrata Dello Scompenso Cardiaco (GISC) study. Various models such as logistic regression, random forest, AdaBoost, logit boost, support vector machine, and neural networks are applied to evaluate the feasibility of such techniques in predicting the hospitalization of 380 patients enrolled in the GISC study. As compared to conventional machine learning models, ensemble models are more efficient and robust in the diagnosis and prediction of heart failure diseases. Linyuan Jing et al. [12] have proposed non-linear XGboost and linear logistic regression in the healthcare dataset to predict the mortality rate of patients suffering from chronic heart failure. Various ensemble learning models (Bagging and Boosting) are implemented by Xiao-Yan Gao et al. [13] and compared based on various performance metrics such as precision, recall, f-measure, and Area under the curve (AUC). They claim that bagging classifiers with feature extraction methods (Principal Component Analysis and Linear Discriminant Analysis) out perform machine learning and other ensemble models.

In this paper, XGBoost ensemble learning [14] has been used for heart failure prediction and detection where the hyperparameters are optimized using a gravitational search algorithm (GSA) [15]. The major contribution of this article is as follows: (i) Understanding the clinical and lifestyle features, and their importance for modeling heart failure detection, (ii) Designing a data-driven heart failure detection model using extreme gradient boosting (XGBoost) ensemble learning technique, and (iii) Optimizing the various hyperparameters of XGBoost such as learning rate, subsample, lambda, L2 regularization, L1 regularization, max depth, and max delta step by using Gravitational search algorithm (GSA). The proposed approach has been evaluated by using various performance metrics and compared with other similar approaches.

5.3 Exploratory Data Analysis of Heart Failure Data

In this work, we have used heart failure patients data [16, 17] which includes thirteen clinical and lifestyle information related to heart failure and death events. All these patients had ventricular systolic dysfunction and previous heart failures, and they are put in different class of heart failure [17] based on various stages. This dataset is the collection of clinical and lifestyle information of 299 heart failure patients including

105 women and 194 men. The clinical and lifestyle information of heart failure patients are captured using 13 number of features. Out of 13 features (Table 5.1), six (Anaemia, high blood pressure, diabetes, sex, smoking, and death event (target)) are binary type and other seven (age, creatinine phosphokinase, serum sodium, ejection fraction, serum creatinine, platelets, and time) are of continuous type. We have computed feature importance and it is observed that "time" (Follow-up period) is found to be most dominated and influenced feature as shown in Fig. 5.1. However, other important features are age, creatinine phosphokinase, serum sodium, ejection fraction, serum creatinine, and platelets. It is observed that if patients' follow-up time (Fig. 5.2a) is low (around 30 to 100) then there is a higher chance of heart failure. Similarly, lower values for ejection fraction (Fig. 5.2b) and serum sodium (Fig. 5.2e) may lead to death event due to heart failure. An opposite observation is noticed for the features serum creatinine (Fig. 5.2c), and age (Fig. 5.2d), i.e., death event related to heart failure is high for higher values of serum creatinine and age. However, the platelets (Fig. 5.2f) and creatinine phosphokinase (Fig. 5.2g) has mixed trend towards heart failure.

Table 5.1 Feature name, feature type, and explanation

Feature name with explanation	Feature type
Anaemia (Lack of Haemoglobin or Red blood cells)	Boolean (0/1)
Creatinine phosphokinase (Creatinine phosphokinase enzyme level in blood)	Continuous variable (Range: [23, 7861], Unit: mcg/L)
Sex (Gender information)	Boolean (0/1)
Age (Patient's age)	Discrete variable (Range: [40, 95], Unit: year)
High blood pressure (Patient with/without hypertension)	Boolean (0/1)
Diabetes (Patient with/without diabetes)	Boolean (0/1)
Platelets (Platelets quantity in blood)	Continuous variable (Range: [25.01, 850.00], Unit: kilo platelets/mL)
Ejection fraction (% of blood exit from the heart at each contraction)	Discrete variable (Range: [14, 80], Unit: Percentage)
Smoking (Patient with/without smoking habit)	Boolean (0/1)
Time (Follow-up period)	Discrete variable (Range: [4, 285], Unit: Day)
Serum sodium (Sodium level in blood)	Continuous variable (Range: [114, 148], Unit: mEq/L)
Serum creatinine (Creatinine level in blood)	Continuous variable (Range: [0.50, 9.40], Unit: mg/dL)
Death event (Survival status of the patient during the follow-up period) (Target)	Boolean (0/1)

5 Heart Failure Detection from Clinical and Lifestyle Information … 103

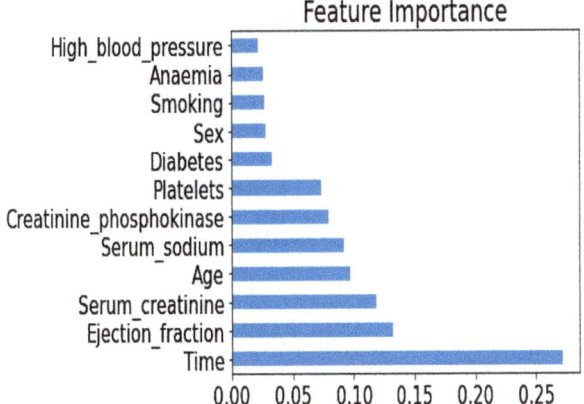

Fig. 5.1 Feature importance of all features w.r.t Death event

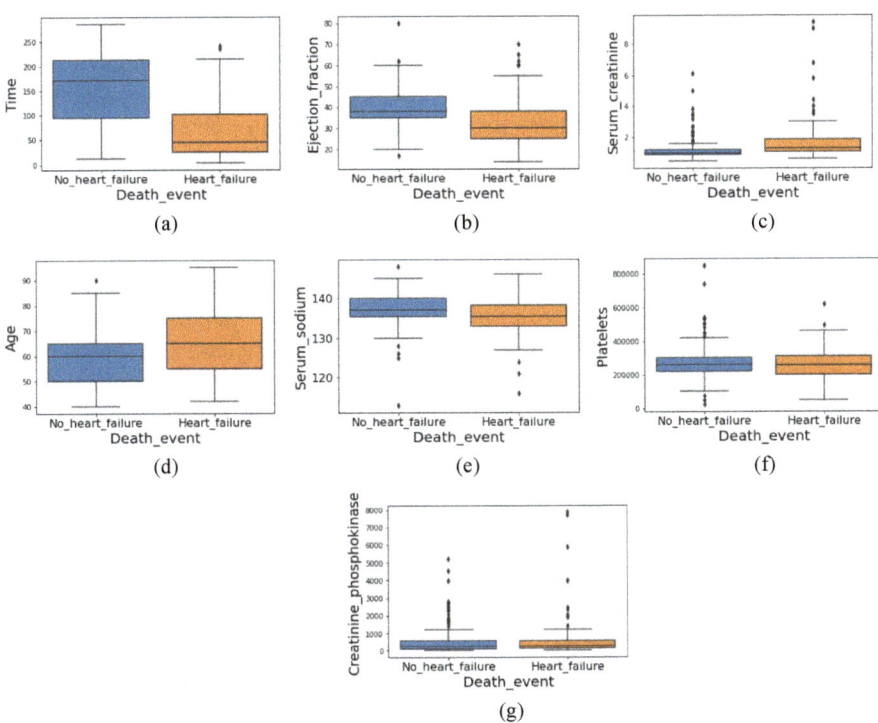

Fig. 5.2 Top influential features and their distribution w.r.t Death event

5.4 Proposed Method

In this section, a detailed description of the proposed GSA and XGBoost has been presented.

5.4.1 Gravitation Search Algorithm

Gravitation Search Algorithm (GSA) [15] is a nature-inspired algorithm that is inspired by Newton's law of gravity and the law of motion. GSA is capable to solve many of the optimization problems more accurately and effectively. Here, candidate solutions (individuals) are treated as objects in the solution space and the performance of each object is determined by its mass. Gravity acts as an attraction between all of these individuals, and this attraction generates an overall movement of all individuals in the direction of the individuals with heavier masses. As a result, gravitational pull serves as a direct channel of communication between masses. The algorithm's exploitation step is ensured by the fact that heavier masses that correspond to good individual solutions move more slowly than lighter ones. Position, inertial mass, active gravitational mass, and passive gravitational mass are the four characteristics that each individual (a feasible solution) has in GSA. The position of the mass is specified by the specific problem, and a fitness function is used to calculate its gravitational and inertial masses. To put it another way, each mass offers a solution, and the algorithm is controlled by correctly adjusting the gravitational and inertia masses. GSA start with random initialization of population containing feasible solutions (individuals), velocities, and GSA's parameters. The fitness function (problem specific) is used to evaluate each individual in the population and the mass of each individual solution is computed based on individual's fitness, best fitness and worst fitness in the population. Then, the force applied on an individual by the other individual is computed. The calculated mass and force are used to compute acceleration of each individual. The next velocity of the object (individual) is determined by the present velocity and acceleration. Finally, the next position of each individual is calculated by using present position and next velocity. These processes are repeated until a termination condition is reached. Finally, the best individual (solution) is return as an output.

5.4.2 GSA-Based XGB for Heart Failure Detection

This work proposed an extreme gradient boosting (XGB) based model for detection of heart failure from clinical and lifestyle information. In this work, the heart failure dataset [17] with 299 instances and 13 features (including target) is used for model construction and testing. Let $H = \{X_i, y_i\}_{i=1}^{n}$ be the heart failure dataset, where X_i is the clinical and lifestyle information of ith patient (with 12 features) (Table 5.1) and y_i is the death event (binary variable representing death/survival of the patient). The proposed work may be summarized into two tasks. First, the XGB has been used to build a prediction model from the clinical and lifestyle information of patients for accurate prediction of heart failure. And, the next task is to obtain optimal values of XGB's hyperparameters. Though XGB is heavy in terms of computation time and space complexity, it is an efficient technique. Therefore, the optimal values of XGB's hyperparameters may solve this issue up to some extent. Here, we have considered the following list of hyperparameters for optimization: learning rate (η)—range (0,1), subsample (s)—range (0.5,1), reg_lambda (λ)—range (0,1), reg_alpha (α)—range (0,1), max_depth (m)—range (1,10), and max_delta_step (δ)—range (1,10). Here, GSA has been used for searching the optimal values of these hyperparameters in the search space. The GSA starts from the initial population (θ), with n number of hyperparameter set $\theta = \{\theta_1, \theta_2...\theta_n\}$. Here, each $\theta_i = \{\eta_i, s_i, \lambda_i, \alpha_i, m_i, \delta_i\}$ represents a randomly generated hyperparameter values set taken from a specific range (0,1), (0.5,1), (0,1), (0,1), (1,10), and (1,10) respectively. The expected final outcome of this search process is to obtain most suitable hyperparameter's values θ_i^* of XGB model for the projected task.

$$m_{\theta_i} = \frac{fit_{\theta_i} - fit_{\theta_{worst}}}{fit_{\theta_{best}} - fit_{\theta_{worst}}} \quad (5.1)$$

In Eq. 5.1, m_{θ_i} is the gravitational mass of θ_i, fit_{θ_i}, $fit_{\theta_{best}}$, and $fit_{\theta_{worst}}$ are fitness of θ_i, θ_{best} (best candidate solution), and θ_{worst} (worst candidate solution).

$$M_{\theta_i} = \frac{m_{\theta_i}}{\sum_{j=1}^{n} m_{\theta_j}} \quad (5.2)$$

In Eq. 5.2, M_{θ_i} is the inertial mass of θ_i.

Algorithm 1: Heart failure detection using optimized XGB based model with Gravitational search algorithm

---

Begin

Set the GSA parameters: α, Gravitational constant G, G_0

iter=1

While (1)

    Calculate fitness of each θ_i in θ:

    For each θ_i in θ

$$fit_{\theta_i} \leftarrow XGB(\theta_i, H)$$
$$fit = fit \cup fit_{\theta_i}$$

    Find out θ_{best} (θ_i with best fitness) and θ_{worst} (θ_i with worst fitness)

    Compute mass M_{θ_i} of each θ_i in θ:

    For each θ_i in θ, Calculate the mass m_{θ_i} as in Eq. 5.1 and M_{θ_i} as in Eq. 5.2.

    Calculate the force F_{θ_i,θ_j} acts on mass M_{θ_i} from M_{θ_j}:

    For $i = 1$ to n

    For $j = 1$ to n

        Calculate the force F_{θ_i,θ_j} using Eq. 5.3.

    For each θ_i in θ, Calculate the total force F_{θ_i} (Eq. 5.4) acts on mass M_{θ_i}

For each in θ_i in θ, Find acceleration a_{θ_i} from mass M_{θ_i} and force F_{θ_i} using Eq. 5.5.

    Find new velocity and new position of each θ_i:

    For $i = 1$ to n

$$V_{\theta_i}{}^{new} = rand(0,1) \times V_{\theta_i} + a_{\theta_i}$$
$$\theta_i{}^{new} = \theta_i + V_{\theta_i}{}^{new}$$

Update: $V = V^{new}, \theta = \theta^{new}$

If (iter==Max OR improvement in fitness if less than a threshold value)

    Exit from While

    Else iter = iter + 1

Return best $\theta_i{}^*$ from θ

$$F_{\theta_i,\theta_j} = \begin{cases} G \times \frac{M_{\theta_i} \times M_{\theta_j}}{d(\theta_i,\theta_j)+\delta}(\theta_j - \theta_i) & i \neq j \\ 0 & i = j \end{cases} \quad (5.3)$$

In Eq. (5.3), F_{θ_i,θ_j} is force applied on mass of θ_i by the mass of θ_j, G is the gravitational constant, $d(\bullet)$ is the Euclidian distance, and δ is a small value constant.

$$F_{\theta_i} = \sum_{j=1, j \neq i}^{n} rand(0,1) \times F_{\theta_i,\theta_j} \quad (5.4)$$

$$a_{\theta_i} = \frac{F_{\theta_i}}{M_{\theta_i}} \quad (5.5)$$

In Eq. (5.4), F_{θ_i} is force applied on mass of θ_i by the all other mass of θ_j. In Eq. (5.5), a_{θ_i} is acceleration of θ_i

---

Algorithm 2: Evaluate the goodness of θ_i in *XGB* using dataset *H*

$$fit_{\theta_i} = XGB(\theta_i, H)$$

Step 1. Create a tree-based ensemble prediction model (Eq. 5.6) with *N* number of functions in additive manner.

$$\hat{y}_i = Pr(X_i) = \sum_{j=1}^{N} f_j(X_i) \quad (5.6)$$

In Eq. 5.6, $\hat{y}_i$ is the predicted output of X_i, $Pr(X_i)$ is the tree-based ensemble model's prediction on X_i, f_j is one of the trees with structure q and weight w from the tree space *F* shown in Fig. 5.3.

Step 2. All the functions f_j, $j = 1$ to N, used in the ensemble model (Eq. 5.1) are learned by minimizing the regularized objective function presented in Eq. 5.7.

$$L(Pr) = \sum_i l(\hat{y}_i, y_i) + \sum_j \Omega(f_j) \quad (5.7)$$

In Eq. 5.7, $l(\cdot)$ is a differentiable loss function and $\Omega(f)$ is the penalty term imposed for model's complexity which can be expressed as $\Omega(f) = \gamma T + \frac{1}{2}\lambda \|w\|^2$. This learning is obtained by adding f_t greedily as depicted in Fig. 5.8 that helps in resulting improved model and this is quickly optimizable function whose second order approximation may be presented as in Eq. 5.9.

$$L^{(t)} = \sum_{i=1}^{n} l(y_i, \hat{y}_i^{(t-1)}) + f_t(X_i) + \Omega(f_t) \quad (5.8)$$

$$L^{(t)} = \sum_{i=1}^{n}[g_i \times f_t(X_i) + 0.5 \times h_i \times f_t^2(X_i)] + \Omega(f_t) \qquad (5.9)$$

In Eq. 5.9, g_i and h_i are first and second gradient expressed as $g_i = \partial_{\hat{y}^{(t-1)}} l(y_i, \hat{y}_i^{(t-1)})$ and $h_i = \partial^2_{\hat{y}^{(t-1)}} l(y_i, \hat{y}_i^{(t-1)})$ respectively.

Letting $I_j = \{i|q(X_i) = j\}$ as the instance set of leaf j, the Eq.9 can be rewritten as Eq. 5.10 by expanding it.

$$L^{(t)} = \sum_{i=1}^{n}[g_i \times f_t(X_i) + 0.5 \times h_i \times f_t^2(X_i)] + \gamma T + 0.5 \times \lambda \sum_{j=1}^{T} w_j^2$$

$$= \sum_{j=1}^{T}[(\sum_{i \in I_j} g_i) \times w_j + 0.5 \times (\sum_{i \in I_j} h_i + \lambda) \times w_j^2] + \gamma T \qquad (5.10)$$

Step 3. The optimal weight w_j of the j leaf for a fixed tree structure is computed as in Eq. 5.11 and the corresponding optimal value has been obtained (Eq. 5.12). The scoring function (impurity score) has been used to evaluate the quality of the structure q.

$$w_j^* = -\frac{\sum_{i \in I_j} g_i}{\sum_{i \in I_j} h_i + \lambda}; \qquad L^t(q) = 0.5 \times$$

$$(5.11)$$

$$\sum_{j=1}^{T} \frac{(\sum_{i \in I_j} g_i^2)}{(\sum_{i \in I_j} h_i + \lambda)} + \gamma T$$

$$(5.12)$$

As it is not possible to evaluate all the possible tress structure q, a greedy procedure is employed to derive optimal tree structure in additive and iterative manner. Assuming $I = IL \cup IR$, where IL and IR are the set of instances of left and right nodes, the reduction of loss after the split is computed as in Eq. 5.13.

$$L_{split} = 0.5 \times \left(\frac{(\sum_{i \in I_L} g_i)^2}{(\sum_{i \in I_L} h_i + \lambda)} + \frac{(\sum_{i \in I_R} g_i)^2}{(\sum_{i \in I_R} h_i + \lambda)} - \frac{(\sum_{i \in I} g_i)^2}{(\sum_{i \in I} h_i + \lambda)}\right) - \gamma$$

$$(5.13)$$

Step 4. The final tree obtained through this iterative and additive procedure is used to distinguish seven different registered varieties of dry beans set of instances.

Return $fit_i = M_K(D)$

5.5 Results and Analysis

In order to evaluate the performance of heart failure identification, we have compared the proposed approach with various ML models (DT, LDA, MLP, NB, SGD, and LR) and EL models (RF, Bagging, Adaboost, GBT, and XGBoost) (Fig. 5.5).

Table 5.2 represents the performance comparison of various studied models by using various performance metrics such as Recall, Precision, F1 Score, and F-beta Score. In Table 5.2, it is noticeable that the proposed approach XGBoost + GSA has better performance and it outperform other models. Under a close observation on comparison of XGBoost + GSA and XGBoost + PSO, it is observed that the both approaches have relatively comparable performance. However, the proposed approach has better convergence rate as compared to XGBoost + PSO (Fig. 5.4).

While tracing the simulation result, we have obtained {0.6486, 0.9874, 0.8370, 0.1932, 8, 3} and {0.4898, 0.9827, 0.1754, 0.2554, 10, 10} as optimal hyperparameters values for the studied hyperparameters $\{\eta, s, \lambda, \alpha, m, \delta\}$

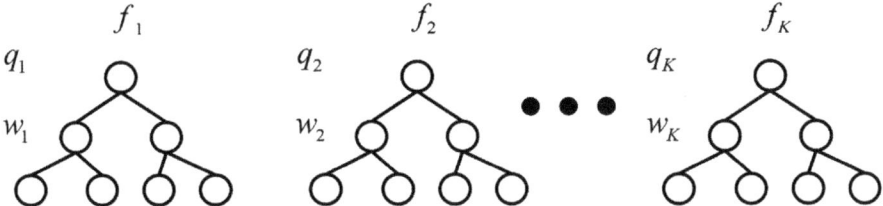

Fig. 5.3 Tree space of K possible tree

Table 5.2 Performance evaluation

Prediction models	Performance metrics			
	Precision	Recall	F1 Score	Fbeta Score
DT	0.7827673	0.788	0.7848436	0.7833480
LDA	0.8059413	0.811	0.8074916	0.8062986
MLP	0.7914285	0.8	0.7914341	0.7902588
NB	0.7689986	0.766	0.7236781	0.7312382
LR	0.8406349	0.844	0.8377821	0.8381843
RF	0.8874034	0.888	0.8859427	0.8862433
Bagging	0.8037888	0.8111	0.8013168	0.8010667
Adaboost	0.8402257	0.844	0.8397382	0.8403198
SGD	0.7364193	0.744	0.7395475	0.7374469
GBT	0.8522199	0.855	0.8505874	0.8506833
XGBoost	0.8754632	0.877	0.8754357	0.8751503
XGBoost + PSO	0.8986372	0.9	0.8980838	0.8981008
Proposed Model	0.9244076	0.922	0.9195470	0.9214497

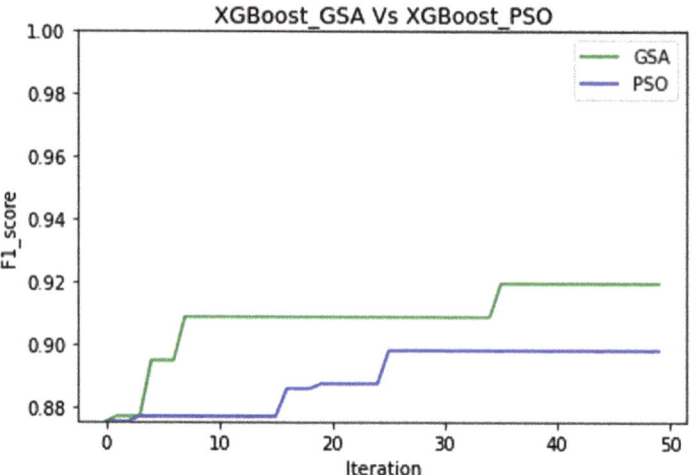

Fig. 5.4 Convergence of studied approaches

in XGBoost + GSA and XGBoost + PSO respectively. Finally, the overall comparison of models is presented on Fig. 5.5.

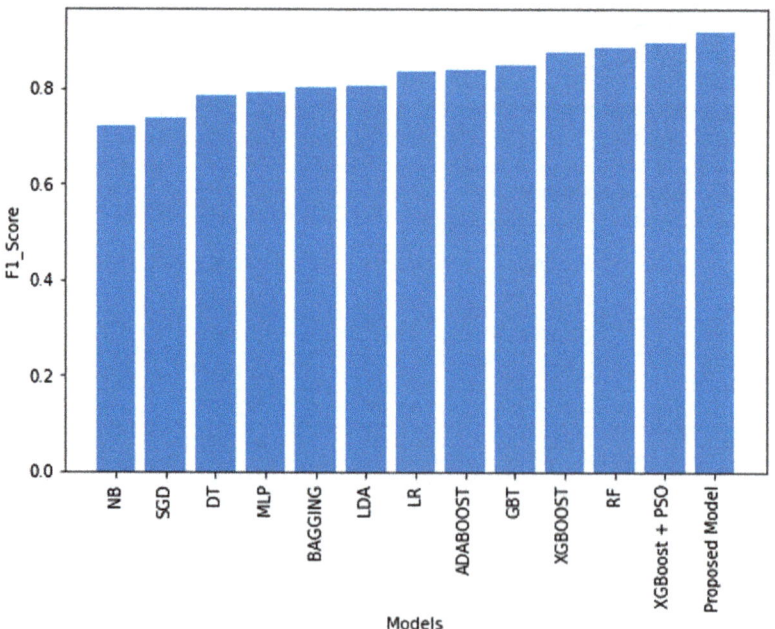

Fig. 5.5 Overall comparison of models' performance

5.6 Conclusion

In this work, EL-based diagnosis system for heart failure management has been reported. This approach is tested and found to be efficient in the considered problem. However, we cannot ignore the issues regarding acceptability and reliability of EL based model in real life application. In this connection, some of the important questions to be answered are: (i) Is the EL-based model reliable and trustable in terms of prediction of heart failure?, (ii) Is the model capable to handle the noise and high variance of the data due to diverse data sources from dissimilar patient groups and heterogenous data collection methods?, (iii) Is the used data adequate, qualitative, and represents all target population?, and (iv) Is the model's output truly interpretable by healthcare professionals?. The rigorous training and testing of the model with realtime data and cross validation may solve the first issue up to some extent. The second issue may be addressed by collecting data from legitimate source with cross checking by domain experts. Use of appropriate data acquisition and sampling (sample selection) method may solve the third issue. Also, proper data integration and exploratory data analysis may offer some solution to this. Making healthcare professional trained with basic knowledge on exploratory data analysis, machine learning and ensemble learning other related concepts. Finally, the product/model is useful if it is in real-life use. So, it is responsibility of the AI expert and healthcare professional to make the model successful in true sense. In this work, an attempt has been made to use an EL-based model for heart failure detection and it is limited to XGBoost with its hyperparameters optimization. In future, this model or modified version may be used and examined on challenging healthcare problem.

Acknowledgements This work is supported by Department of Science and Technology (DST), Ministry of Science and Technology, New Delhi, Govt. of India, under Grant no. DST/INSPIREFellowship/2019/IF190611.

References

1. Tripoliti, E.E., et al.: Heart failure: diagnosis, severity estimation and prediction of adverse events through machine learning techniques. Comput. Struct. Biotechnol. J. **15**, 26–47 (2017).
2. Khan, M.A., Fahad A.: A healthcare monitoring system for the diagnosis of heart disease in the IoMT cloud environment using MSSO-ANFIS. IEEE Access **8**, 122259–122269 (2020).
3. Ahmed, F.: An Internet of Things (IoT) application for predicting the quantity of future heart attack patients. Int. J. Comput. Appl. **164**(6), 36–40 (2017)
4. Ali, L., Niamat, A., Khan, J.A., Golilarz, N.A., Xingzhong, X., Noor, A., Nour, R., Bukhari, S.A.C.: An optimized stacked support vector machines based expert system for the effective prediction of heart failure. IEEE Access **7**, 54007–54014 (2019).
5. Javeed, A., Zhou, S., Yongjian, L., Qasim, I., Noor, A., Nour, R.: An intelligent learning system based on random search algorithm and optimized random forest model for improved heart disease detection. IEEE Access **7**, 180235–180243 (2019).

6. Son, C.S., Kim, Y.N., Kim, H.S., Park, H.S., Kim, M.S.: Decision-making model for early diagnosis of congestive heart failure using rough set and decision tree approaches. J. Biomed. Inform. **45**, 999–1008 (2012).
7. Masetic, Z., Subasi, A.: Congestive heart failure detection using random forest classifier. Comput. Methods Programs Biomed. **130**, 54–64 (2016).
8. Lal, H., Wajid, A., Ishtiaq, K., Monagi, A., Jalal, A.: Detecting congestive heart failure by extracting multimodal features and employing machine learning techniques. BioMed Res. Int. **6**, 1–19 (2020)
9. Miao, K.H., Miao, J.H., Miao, G.J.: Diagnosing coronary heart disease using ensemble machine learning. Int. J. Adv. Comput. Sci. Appl. **7**(10), 1–12 (2016)
10. Plati, D.K., et al.: A machine learning approach for chronic heart failure diagnosis. Diagnostics **11**(10), 1863 (2021).
11. Lorenzoni, G., et al.: Comparison of machine learning techniques for prediction of hospitalization in heart failure patients. J. Clin. Med. **8**(9), 1298 (2019).
12. Jing, L., et al. A machine learning approach to the management of heart failure population. Elseviser (2020).
13. Gao, X.Y., et al.: Improving the accuracy for analyzing heart diseases prediction based on the ensemble method. Complexity **2021** (2021).
14. Chen, T., et al.: Xgboost: extreme gradient boosting. R package version 0.4-2 **1**(4), 1–4 (2015).
15. Rashedi, E., Nezamabadi-Pour, H., Saryazdi, S.: GSA: a gravitational search algorithm. Inf. Sci. **179**(13), 2232–2248 (2009)
16. Ahmad, T., et al.: Survival analysis of heart failure patients: a case study. PloS one **12**(7), e0181001 (2017).
17. Ahmad, T., et al.: Survival analysis of heart failure patients: a case study. Dataset. https://plos.figshare.com/articles/Survival_analysis_of_heart_failure_patients_A_case_study/5227684/1 (2019). Accessed Jan 2022.

Chapter 6
NIANN: Integration of ANN with Nature-Inspired Optimization Algorithms

Soumen Kumar Pati, Ayan Banerjee, Manan Kumar Gupta, and Rinita Shai

Abstract Artificial neural networks (ANNs) are stimulated according to the biological brain's connection of axons and dendrons. These neural networks perform a major part in the advancement of artificial intelligence and learning algorithms. Though initially used for image classification, in modern times applications of ANNs have been useful over numerous fields such as medical data mining, bioinformatics, natural language processing, time series forecasting, and in various optimization problems as well. Nature-inspired algorithms are a set of novel problem-solving approaches that are derived from various incidents occurring in nature around us. Each of the methods such as the BAT, genetic algorithm, or colony optimization methods were created by keeping a specific hard problem in mind. In recent times general purpose use of these nature-inspired algorithms has become widely popular in solving mainly optimization problems derived from the fields of NLP, machine learning, deep learning, classification, and feature selection as well. Nature-inspired algorithms mainly work by mimicking phenomena occurring in nature among various species on a macro scale. A set of nature-inspired algorithms such as the genetic algorithm family mimics the processes that occur in a microorganism such as a cell division, mutation, etc. Since these algorithms are inspired by nature and were developed keeping in mind achieving an optimal solution of a given hard problem, their application in general-purpose problems also yields satisfactory results. If an algorithm fails to achieve a satisfactory solution to a problem, it is easy to modify them

---

S. K. Pati (✉) · M. K. Gupta
Department of Bioinformatics, Maulana Abul Kalam Azad University of Technology, Haringhata, WB 741249, India
e-mail: soumenkrpati@gmail.com

A. Banerjee
Department of Computer Science and Engineering, Jalpaiguri Government Engineering College, Jalpaiguri, WB 735102, India
e-mail: ab2141@cse.jgec.ac.in

R. Shai
Department of Computational and Applied Mathematics, Friedrich-Alexander-Universität, 91054 Erlangen-Nürnberg, Schloßplatz, Germany
e-mail: rinita.shai@fau.de

© The Author(s), under exclusive license to Springer Nature Switzerland AG 2023
J. Nayak et al. (eds.), *Nature-Inspired Optimization Methodologies in Biomedical and Healthcare*, Intelligent Systems Reference Library 233,
https://doi.org/10.1007/978-3-031-17544-2_6

according to the need of the given problem to overcome any obstacle. In this chapter, an approach is introduced that aims to combine the nature-inspired optimization algorithm with the learning model of artificial neural networks to provide a more accurate and streamlined output generation of the neural network. Nature-inspired algorithms can be used as a learning method in the ANN model. In contrast to that, an ANN can also be used as an objective function to a nature-inspired algorithm to improve its capability to generate an optimal solution. This chapter aims to explore both approaches in detail.

Keywords Optimization · ANN · Genetic algorithm · Particle swarm optimization

6.1 Introduction

The gene expression dataset was utilized to observe multiple gene movements for diagnosing and detecting several diseases like cardiovascular diseases, cancer, autism spectrum disorders, tumor, and developmental disorders through gene mutations and structural modifications. To experiment on a wide range of genes microarray analysis has been the most effective way. Microarray analysis is a computational methodology to decipher information obtained by experimenting with a large number of DNAs and RNAs. DNA microarray data analysis [1] shows the efficiency of giving much more accurate results than other methods in disease prediction and cancer classification. In the main medical section microarray analysis plays an important role in extracting medical information. There are a variety of methods for analysing microarray data such as clustering gene expressions, pattern recognition, and so on. Clustering analysis [2] is very commonly used in finding a variety of structural data and deciphering gene expressions. Moreover, it can be classified into several categories like k-means clustering, self-organizing map, and hierarchical clustering. For a very long time Microarray technology plays a vital role even in clinical trials by recognizing the genetic sources and resampling methods.

Artificial Neural Networks (ANNs) [3–5] represent a technology containing a group of connected nodes that perform tasks as a human brain. This has been extensively used to represent various types of data. ANN mainly initiates a bunch of neural networks in multiple domains to solve highly complex real-world problems by developing different models and approaches. It focuses mainly on training, testing of validation sets.

Optimization algorithms [6–8] are well-structured algorithms that are sequentially executed to resolve intricate optimization problems like stochastic optimization, traveling salesmen, discrete optimization, profit maximization, etc. Nature-inspired algorithms are a collective group of analytical approaches and methodologies highly inspired by natural phenomena. There is numerous popular nature-inspired algorithm for optimization like Genetic Algorithm (GA) [9], Differential Evolution (DE) [10], Particle Swarm Optimization (PSO) [11], Ant-Bee Colony Algorithm (ABC) [12], Flower Pollination Algorithm (FPA) [13], Cuckoo Search Algorithm (CS) [14],

Bacterial Foraging Optimization [15], Grey Wolf Optimization [16] and so on. In recent years, several new natural-inspired algorithms were proposed and among them, the t-Social Spider Algorithm [17] is the latest one. These optimizations play a very significant role in solving non-linear complex issues which include fraud detection, image processing, and utilization of improved whale optimization algorithm [6] on Fuzzy clustering algorithm.

6.2 Literature Review

Artificial neural networks [3] use a black-box model and learning algorithms to mimic the behaviour of neurons in a way so that they can learn as they receive input in each layer. In modern times the applications of deep learning using the artificial neural network have improved drastically. They are used in solving problems belonging to almost every scientific and engineering domain.

Luo et al. [18] proposed a method based on ANNs to measure sound insulation performance of the aramid honeycomb sandwich panel. They have used a radial basis function ANN, a backpropagation ANN, and a general region ANN. Their models take as input several parameters (panel thickness, core thickness and density, acoustic frequency, and honeycomb cell diameter). The output of this method is the loss amount of transmission of sound. The experimental outcomes of the general region ANN method give the maximum classification accuracy with the RMS error of 3.45%. The RMS error for the model is 11.48% and prediction quality is poor [18]. Pati and Banerjee [19] proposed an innovative method to identify the possible drugs and target regions based on convolution neural networks and AI to treat the patients of COVID-19. Here, an exhaustive study has been accomplished to obtain the percentage of noncoding, density of gene, and abundances in useful gene classifications utilizing Virus Amplicon Sequencing Assembly Pipeline. Peng et al. [20] proposed a test bench of FPE-LG which is recognized for the ORC scheme with a small scale based on time and displacement strategy. The following properties on FPE-LG are measured- effect of the pressure intake, the motion torque, and outcome efficiency. A prediction method of FPE-LG with an ANN is established based on the evaluation of several learning rates, hidden ANN numbers, and training functions. To optimize the core operating parameters genetic algorithm (GA) has been used here. The experimental dataset is tested by the ANN model based on the mean square error value. By using GA with the ANN structure the extreme power throughput of FPE-LG is optimized [20]. An ANN methodology is offered by Skrypnik et al. [21] to measure the friction factor and the coefficients of heat transmission for the flow turbulent in the tubes. This model was applied on various inner helical tube finning. Saldarriaga et al. [22] used an ANN method to assess the pressure drop in discharged beds of biomass. This ANN model is used to guess the operating and peak pressure drops. A multilayer perceptron model combined with backpropagation was used since the model can simulate non-linear multivariate schemes. The results obtained from the model were significantly superior to the outcomes found in the works. The R square value of 0.92 was obtained for the peak pressure drop situation. Pati et al. [8, 23] proposed chapters which have been given a thorough review on the Analysis of Cancer Disease utilizing Machine Learning methods. This chapter is a survey on different data Analysis procedures with the best outcomes. Hu et al. [24] build a credit risk assessment index method based on the result obtained in the form of previous studies where fourteen financial indicators were selected. Clustering and factor analysis was performed on the sample data to control the definite credit rating. The sample data was used in conjunction with the two most common risk analysis models and three common ANN models to predict the risk assessment [24]. Badura et al. [25] utilized an ANN model to estimate the features of the quaternary ammonium salts alongside Candida albicans. By the serial dilution methodology, the antifungal activity was determined by performing empirical experiments for a sequence of several novel imidazole derivatives. The 3D structures of trial compounds were built where chemical information was transformed to a valuable numeral utilizing computational chemistry. Regression and classification were solved by using ANN. The developed model was categorized by good predictive capability. The classification model yielded the following results: the learning set (91.67%), the testing set (88.57%), and the validation set (95.24%). Gnatowski et al. [26] had shown in their work that the classical mathematical model which numerically simulates the transport phenomenon within a solid oxide fuel cell anode tends to a remarkable inconsistency among computed and projected overpotentials. An ANN is used to change charge transfer coefficients reliant on the active situations and the known data [26]. The gold standard in emergency departments (EDs) to assess mild traumatic brain injury (mTBI) patients is Head computed tomography (CT). Ellethy et al. [27] uses two machine learning methods to find mild Traumatic Brain Injury (mTBI) in a pediatric populace composed as the portion of the pediatric emergency care worked on research network learning. These methods used data from 15,271 patients under 18 years. Firstly, the dimensionality of features was reduced and the highest-ranked features were considered for training an ANN using Random Forests. Secondly, a deep ANN method was used for the classification of the mTBI cases (positive and negative) using the complete set of features. The experimental data were separated in 8:2 format and a five-fold cross-validation method was used for classification [27]. Paul et al. [28] introduces a chaos game representation (CGR) to investigate the pattern of genome sequences. The CGR used a mapping method to portray the DNA sequences that allocate every sequence base into the corresponding location in the 2-D plane. In the study, they had coupled CGR with ANN as a novel method to signify genomes and detect intra-corona virus sequences. Hierarchical clustering was performed to validate the results and the predictions were found to be 90% accurate [28]. Lu et al. [29] analyzed the clinicopathological data of patients from 2010 to 2014 retrospectively. The data of the patients who underwent both surgery and chemotherapy were randomly divided into 70% training and 30% for the validation set. An ANN model was recognized that can forecast the potential advantage of chemotherapy and its correctness was validated using C-index. The potential-CT-benefit-ANN model presented a noble expectation exactness for probable chemotherapy advantage in both training and validation sets.

Squires et al. [30] in their work proposed List Scheduling Wildcard Treatment Genetic Algorithm, which combines heuristic population initialization with an innovative survivor selection policy. The target of the algorithm is to enhance the functioning effectiveness of the medical center through efficient rTMS appointment preparation. Lizhi et al. [31] proposed a multi-objective ant colony optimization method that includes a novel pheromone updating method and 4 novel exploratory evidence. A new method named Enhanced Diversity Particle Swarm Optimization (EDPSO) has been proposed by Fernandes et al. [32], it is a quantum-behaved PSO that accomplishes the route forecasting job of automated mobile robot vehicles in both stationary and dynamic settings. The proposed PSO aims to deliver safe routes, reduce energy surplus, and preserve scheme integrity [32]. Instead of using the general bacterial foraging optimization, Yang et al. [33] proposed a novel discrete foraging algorithm for detecting communities in large networks. They exquisitely embedded the goal of community detection into a redefined distinct framework. Using a topological viewpoint, the evolutionary philosophies of bacterial foraging are established. As novel updating rules, greedy and stochastic approaches are planned to direct the swarm of bacteria to the favored regions [33]. An ensemble method which is a multi-strategy driven shuffled frog leaping method with vertical and horizontal crossover examination is developed by Chen et al. [34] for segmentation of multi-threshold images. Frogs can exchange information by using a horizontal crossover search, thus assuring in persuasive search of every frog. The vertical crossover examination is also instigated to simplify the frogs in stagnation stay in the search actively. The process thus safeguards better equilibrium amid divergence and strengthening [34]. The method proposed by Altabeeb et al. [35] used multiple firefly algorithm populations. The algorithm was hybridized using two variants of local search and a genetic operator. To exchange some solutions, the proposed algorithms, engage in message-passing from time to time. The goal of this hybridization and message passing is to maintain the assortment of the populace to avert down into local optima and to remove the disadvantages of an only swarm. Since classical clustering methodologies like K-means or fuzzy C-means are prone to initial cluster centers and noise, Das et al. [36] proposed an innovative clustering method utilizing Eagle Strategy (two stages) with the help of Stochastic Fractal Search methodology. In the proposed method, morphological reconstruction was applied to the fuzzy clustering algorithm. This sieves the membership matrix to ensure immunity from noise in the data. Furthermore, the Black Hole (BH) optimization is a metaheuristic nature-inspired technique. Deeb et al. [37] modify the classical BH optimization algorithm to introduce a novel approach for generating stars around the black hole that are to be immersed by the black hole. The trajectory of star association has also been modified in their work so that exploration capabilities are increased. The modified algorithm was used to cluster given data without prior knowledge about the nature of the inputs. Standard benchmarks were used to calculate the effectiveness of the proposed method. Moghaddam et al. [1] use a variation of forest optimization algorithm which is multi-objective. The proposed method uses concepts such as grid, archive, and region-based collection. Two versions, one continuous and one binary has been developed to perform wrapper feature selection. The efficiency of the method has been tested using 9 UCI and 2 microarray data. It has been shown that the proposed method was given a similar performance or outperforms the traditional methods in some cases by comparing the results with 7 traditional single techniques and 5 multi-objective techniques. The method proposed by Hao et al. [38] combines chaotic grey wolf optimization and adaptive grey wolf optimization approaches to obtain an algorithm that can estimate solid oxide fuel cell models. Similarly, to achieve higher convergence speed and exploration capability, a recently proposed political optimization (PO) algorithm works well in many cases. However, it has been observed that PO converges prematurely when dealing with some complex problems. Askari et al. [39] proposed some improvements over the existing political optimization algorithm to enhance the exploration ability. Relaxation of the number of equal parties and constituency was performed. Along with that swapping with an arbitrary party member with a random party has been incorporated. Muthusamy et al. [40] proposed an improvement method over the elephant herding optimization (EHO) algorithm utilizing the sine–cosine method. The augmentation is done keeping in mind unremitting function optimization and financial stress forecast problems. The original EHO algorithm has been enhanced by modifying the sine–cosine mechanism and opposition-based knowledge. The sine cosine mechanism has been replaced the separating operator. The modified version was compared with 8 known metaheuristic procedures utilizing 23 standard benchmarks, 10 current CEC2019 benchmarks. Better performance was reported by the methodology compared to the other methods.

ANNs coupled with nature-inspired algorithms play an important role in problem-solving in various domains. Chandar [41] in his work shows ANN coupled with the nature-inspired algorithm for stock market price forecasting. Based on three popular ANNs, a backpropagation ANN combined with a genetic algorithm, radial basis function ANN coupled with PSO, and time delay ANN in conjunction with artificial bee colony method was developed to process stock market data to predict intraday stock prices. For enhancing the parameters of the ANNs, the said nature-inspired algorithms were utilized. Technical key points obtained from the dataset have been taken as input to the proposed hybrid model. Bahiraei et al. [42] used 4 nature-inspired optimization procedures, the system was merged with an MLP network to achieve the best structure designed to predict the total heat transmission coefficient of a ribbed triple-tube heat exchanger. Artificial Bee Colony (ABC), Ant Colony Optimization, Biogeography-Based Optimization, and Ant Lion Optimizer are used in conjunction with the multilayer perceptron model. The input data is provided to the model as a computational solution. The BBO algorithm gives the highest accuracy in predicting the overall heat transfer among other used algorithms. Ghoniem et al. [2] used a genetic artificial bee colony algorithm coupled with an ANN for drug name recognition. In medical information mining, Drug Name Recognition (DNR) is a critical task that involves recognition of a drug name and assigning it a class from the unstructured biomedical data. The structure of the neural network certainly influences the overall process. However neural networks can be disposed to overfitting. This proposed a novel network model which was combined with a hybrid genetic ABC process. This method avoids premature convergence and enables a better exploitation process of ABC, by introducing genetic operators into the artificial bee colony algorithm. The method was compared with other well-known methods and it was shown that it outperforms them in terms of accuracy. Singh et al. [43] proposed a genetic algorithm-based neural network that aims to resolve resource allocation problems in scalable cloud architectures. A neural bio task scheduling approach has been introduced by them. The solution mimics right thinking and making the decision. Effective job scheduling on virtual machines in the cloud environment is a crucial problem. The constructed task scheduler used a genetic approach and an ANN. It performs an optimum arrangement of jobs on the virtual machine. The consistency of the proposed model grows by reducing the number of tasks that failed. Hazas et al. [44] proposed a hypothesis, that some olfactory systems of locusts in Kenyon Cells are more responsive to the stimuli than others. This might indicate that a heterogeneous neural threshold distribution is present in KCs. To study this hypothesis an ANN was constructed that was able to acclimatize with many of the stratagems detected in the locust olfactory systems. A new learning algorithm has also been proposed that can find the best neural verge distribution to solve a classification problem. The proposed method was compared with SVMs and MLP and it outperforms both in the classification segment. Carrillo et al. [45] developed two ANNs, that can estimate the thermal and electrical conductivity. The proposed models have been used as an objective function by MOGA. A good correlation was observed by using the ANN among simulated data and experimental data. Ibrahim [46] proposed a weighted BAT algorithm to train a DNN to classify poisonous plants. The dataset used to train the model contained 3452 samples, each sample having four features, the dataset had two class information. The proposed hybrid bat algorithm-based DNN was used to classify the poisonous plants and the outcomes were compared by the traditional and common classification methods and outperformed most of the traditional methods. A hybrid model based on biased random key GA (BRKGA) was developed by Cicek et al. [47]. The proposed algorithm optimizes an ANN to solve the time series, forecast model. The algorithm was compared against GA-based ANN, backpropagation neural network, support vector, and ARIMA. According to the results, the proposed method can better forecast from time-series data than the other methods. Si et al. [48] uses metaheuristic algorithms to train ANNs to classify fifteen publicly available medical data. A relative experiment is performed using the traditional Levenberg–Marquardt (LM) and other current metaheuristics algorithms. Several assessment standards such as exactness, geometric mean, precision, and sensitivity were measured for performance approximation. The obtained classification accuracies were analyzed using multi-criteria result-based methods and outperformed other methods comprised in the literature.

6.3 Integration of Artificial Neural Network and Optimization Algorithm

This section presents the proposed methodology in detail where the general structure of ANN and different nature-inspired algorithms are combined.

6.3.1 Artificial Neural Network (ANN)

An ANN is a basic model that emulates the working process of a biological nervous system via the means of mathematical modelling. In most general terms a neural network consists of vastly interconnected networks of an enormous number of processing components which are commonly named as nodes in a design motivated by the brain. ANN can become enormously parallel and hence displays the capabilities of distributed parallel processing.

The ANN exhibit features for example mapping, generalization, pattern recognition, fault tolerance, robustness, parallel processing, and high computation speeds. The ANN can also study by example; thus, this model is trained by using various learning algorithms to acquire knowledge. Once trained the model then can be utilized to expect the nature of a given input as per the model has previously learned.

6.3.1.1 A Model of an Artificial Neuron

In its simplest form, an artificial neuron consists of two parts. The first part takes multiple inputs and sends them to a summation unit along with randomly assigned weights to each input. The summation unit sums all the weighted inputs and sends them to the second part which is the thresholding unit. To obtain the outcome, the output of the summation unit is passed through a nonlinear filter named the activation function and it generates the outcome given by the thresholding unit (Fig. 6.1).

An ANN is called a data processing method which is composed of a large number of connected processing components, in a construction that is similar to the arrangement of the cerebral cortex of the human brain. This format can be described as a directed graph.

The simplest neural network is the Single Layer Feedforward Network (Fig. 6.2) formed with two layers, named input layer and output layer. The input and output layer neurons accept the input and output signals respectively. The synaptic links are associated with the weights which are used to link each of the input neurons to the output neuron but not the other way around. Such a network is coined with the term feedforward as it is acyclic. The ANN is also called a single layer as only the neurons of the output layer execute all the necessary computations to generate the results. The input layer merely acts as a transfer module that transfers the input signals to the output layer for the final processing.

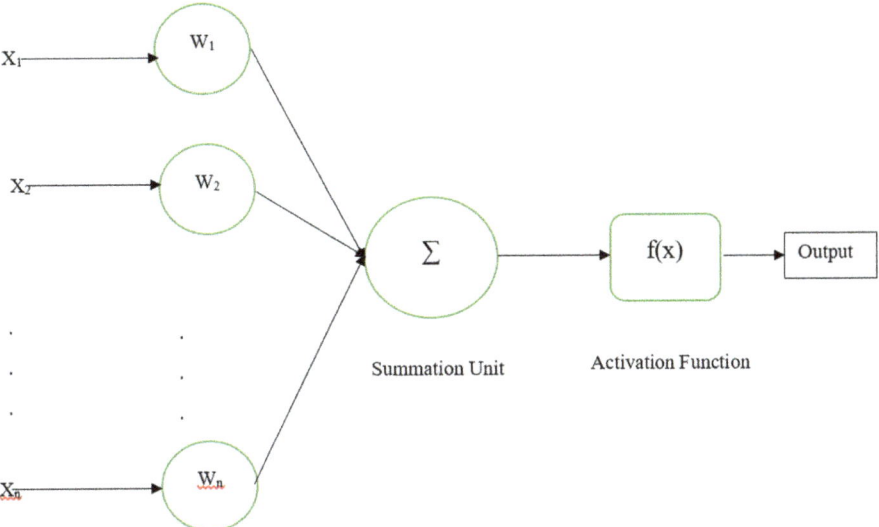

Fig. 6.1 The general structure of an ANN

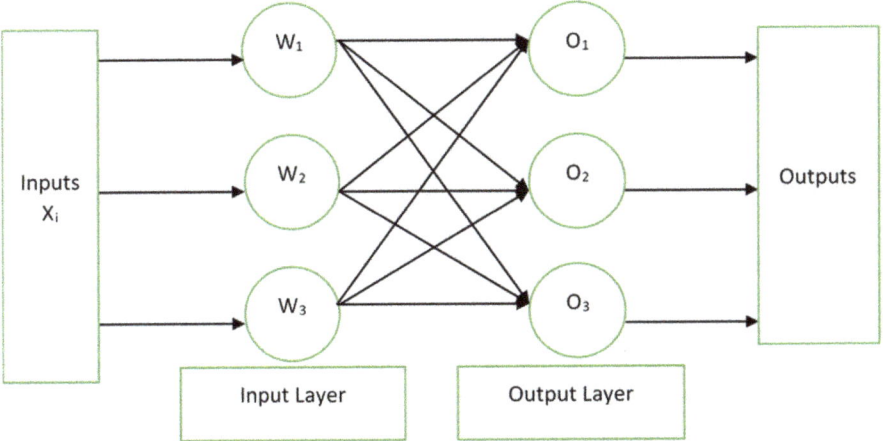

Fig. 6.2 Structure of a simple ANN

Another type of ANN is named the multilayer feedforward network. It is an advanced form of the single-layer network model. In this type of network, one or more than one hidden layer of neurons can be present between the input and output layers. The hidden layers are used for intermediate calculations before sending the input layer to the output layer. The neurons of the input layer are associated with the neurons of the hidden layer. The assigned weights to the input layer are called input-hidden layer weights. Alike, the neurons of the hidden layer are associated with the

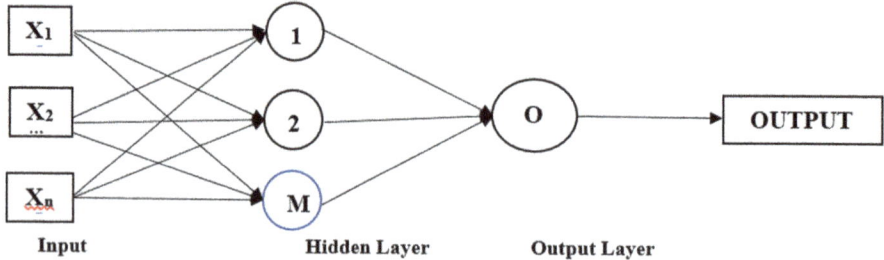

Fig. 6.3 The simple structure of a multilayer ANN

neurons of the output layer, and the weights assigned to the synaptic links are called the hidden-output layer weights. A multilayer feedforward ANN that consists of one-input neurons, m_1 neurons in the 1st hidden layer, m_2 neurons in the 2nd hidden layer, and n is the number of output neurons, described as l-m_1-m_2-n (Fig. 6.3).

6.3.1.2 Learning Methods

A neural network can be put to use with the following learning methods-

- **Supervised Learning**: Every input form has a corresponding output pattern which is the desired output of the given problem in this form of learning. When the network has been trained, the output is matched with the given set of outputs for each pattern to estimate the results of the ANN architecture. The error is calculated by using the actual output and the output produced by the ANN which then can be used to change network parameters for improving the performance of the ANN model.
- **Unsupervised Learning**: Here no target output is present and no observer is required. The ANN simply learns on its own by learning and familiarizing itself with the structural properties of the input forms.
- **Reinforced Learning**: An observer is present only to tell the system whether the output is correct or incorrect in this model. A reward is set for each accurate output and a penalty is given for incorrect ones. Based on rewards and penalties the system gradually learns to predict outputs more efficiently.
- **Hebbian Learning**: This is the oldest form of learning method motivated by biology. Correlative weight adjustment is used on it. The (input, output) pattern pairs (X, Y) are related to the weight matrix W, recognized as the correlation matrix. It is formulated as the Eq. (6.1).

$$W = \sum_{i=1}^{n} X i Y i^t \qquad (6.1)$$

where Yi^t is the transpose of the linked vectors of output.

6.3.2 Optimization Algorithm

This subsection describes the popular well-known nature-inspired algorithms.

6.3.2.1 Genetic Algorithm

Genetic algorithms represent a well-defined tree consisting of a group of computational models evolved by natural processing. The basic model of GA can be introduced both in illustrative as well as pseudo-code form. They are employed by creating a chromosomal strand constituting a parameter of possible solutions. GAs are generally adapted in nature consisting of binary thread-like data structures which are widely utilized to resolve a variety of highly-complex optimization problems. These data structures are chromosomes which are closely bound proteins known as histones forming a DNA structure packed inside the nucleus. Each chromosome comprises a chain of alleles. However, the length of a single chromosome is depended on the quantity of information it's carrying within the phenotype search space. Alleles are genetic variants that depict the speculative artifact expressing the genotype and phenotype chromosomes. In GA Genotypes usually represent a cluster of genes analyzing the genetic framework of a single organism and Phenotypes are perceptible characteristics of an individual such as the color of the iris, height, skin tone, blood group, etc. An organism can easily be identified by only observing hereditary traits, physical development, and appearance.

Genetic algorithms imitate the mechanism of natural selection with changing circumstances of the environment. In the natural selection process, individuals accustom themselves to the environment to survive and reproduce to continue the cycle of generations which is better known as "survival of the fittest". According to the Darwinian Theory of Evolution, there are three significant factors like genetic variation, reproduction, and hereditary transmission which essentially take part a key role in the survival of the offspring. While in natural selection, a progeny inherits the trait from their ancestors and habituate themselves with the environment which improves the prevalence of survival over generations. Genetic algorithms solve highly-complex search problems depending on the biologically influenced operators like Chromosomal Crossover, Mutation, and Gene selection (Fig. 6.4). A genetic algorithm undergoes five stages such as Configuration of Population, Fitness analysis, Chromosomal Crossover, Mutation, Survival Nomination, Population swapping/restoration.

- **Configuration of population**—It is the baby step of the Evolutionary Algorithmic process consisting of a set of chromosomes that works based on the Initialization approaches like randomness and heuristic initialization. This population depends on the area of the population and the length of the chromosome.
- **Fitness analysis**—It measures the fitness ability of a solution to decipher the optimization problems. In fitness analysis, the effectiveness of an individual is chosen for mutation based on their fitness score.

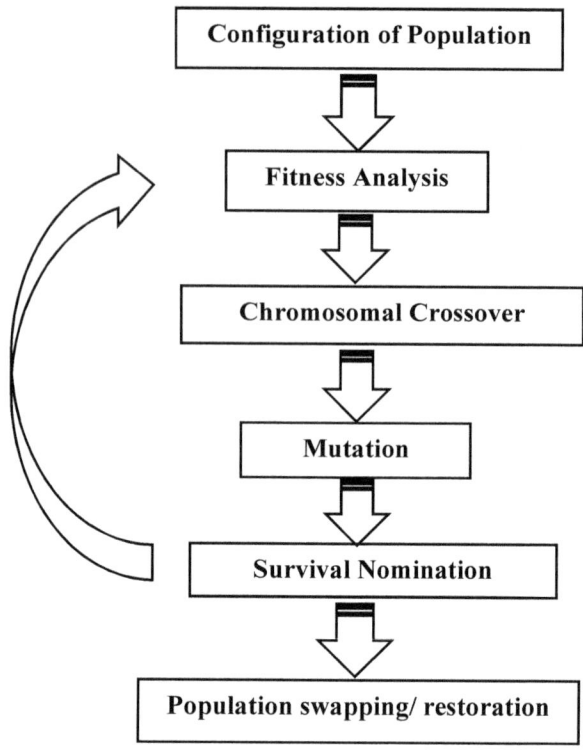

Fig. 6.4 Flow diagram of genetic algorithm

- **Chromosomal crossover**—It happens mostly within two alleles going for a similar genetic code which results in interchanging a part of a chromosome with the other chromosome.
- **Mutation**—Mutation refers to the alteration in a single or multiple DNA nucleotides resulting in genetic variation. When mutation happens genes get replicated. Sometimes genetic mutation undergoes huge changes in DNA sequences leading to genetic disorders.
- **Survival nomination**—In Survival Nomination individuals are chosen from the whole population to transfer to the next generation based on the fitness values.
- **Population swapping**—In the genetic algorithm process population plays a vital role and with the growth in the population increases the chromosome numbers in the optimal solution.
- **Advantages of the genetic algorithm**: It can deliver great answers for different issues including search and improvement. They are quicker and effective when contrasted with the conventional strategies for animal power search. Hereditary Algorithms is demonstrated to have many equal capacities. Upgrades both persistent and discrete capabilities and furthermore multi-objective issues.

- **Disadvantages of genetic algorithm**: GA requires less data about the issue, however planning a goal capability and getting the portrayal and administrators right can be troublesome. GA is computationally costly for example tedious.

6.3.2.2 Particle Swarm Optimization (PSO)

This is a simple bio-inspired optimization algorithm that focuses on searching for the optimal solution from the given space. The only requirement of this algorithm is an objective function that may not be dependent on the gradient or differential form of the actual objective in question. Best in case of finding the maximum and minimum function from a defined multidimensional vector space. Each iteration of PSO improves over a candidate solution found from the given vector space.

The most basic variant of PSO works on a population typically termed as Swarm. The swarm of candidate solutions is termed as particles. The movement of the particles is shown by their best location in the search space, also the total swarm's best location is taken into account for the process. When an improved position is discovered, it is then used to guide the swarm accordingly. Over multiple iterations, this same process is repeated to obtain the best possible candidate result for the problem.

In PSO, the velocity of the particles is regulated by Eq. (6.2). To enable the particles to have a chance at overshooting through the target in the space in half time the random, number generator is multiplied by 2.

$$v \times [i][j] = v \times [i][j] + 2 \times \text{rand}(ij) \times (\text{pBest}[i][j] - \text{presentx}[i][j]) \\ + 2 \times \text{rand}(ij) \times (\text{pBest}[i][\text{gbest}] - \text{presentx}[i][j]) \quad (6.2)$$

A different inertia weight is chosen in each iteration. Equation (6.3) determines the value of the weight. In Eq. (6.3), t is the number of iterations and W is the weight of inertia at the iteration of t.

$$W_t = (W_{max} - W_{min}) \frac{(t_{max} - t)}{t_{max}} + W_{max} \quad (6.3)$$

where the above equation is used for LTV or Linear Time-Varying models, the Eq. (6.4) is a modification over that to facilitate Non-Linear Time-Varying models.

$$W_{t+1} = (W_t - 0.4) \frac{(t_{max} - t)}{t_{max} - 0.4} \quad (6.4)$$

An individual particle converges if the following condition is satisfied. In the condition, Ω is the stochastic factor as in Eq. (6.5).

$$1 > W > \frac{\Omega_1 + \Omega_2}{2} - 1 \geq 0 \quad (6.5)$$

For velocity updating, Eq. (6.6) is used.

$$V_{ij}(t+1) = W \times V_{ij}(t) + r_1(t) \times C_1 \times \left(pbest_{ij}(t) - X_{ij}(t)\right)$$
$$+ r_2(t) \times C_2 \times \left(gbest(t) - X_{ij}(t)\right) \tag{6.6}$$

To update the position of a particle Eq. (6.7) is used.

$$X_{ij}(t+1) = X_{ij}(t) + V_{ij}(t+1) \tag{6.7}$$

- **Advantages of the particle swarm optimization**: The fundamental benefits of the PSO calculation are summed up as: straightforward idea, simple execution, power to control boundaries, and computational effectiveness when contrasted and numerical calculation and other heuristic advancement procedures like most extreme emphasis number, Iter current cycle number.
- **Disadvantages of the particle swarm optimization**: it is difficult to fall into neighbourhood ideal in high-layered space and has a low union rate in the iterative cycle.

6.3.2.3 Differential Evolution (DE)

The DE calculation utilizes the distinction among people to direct the calculation to look in the arrangement space. This fundamentally incorporates populace, transformation activity, hybrid activity, choice activity, etc. The principle thought is to separate and measure between two unique distinct vectors in a similar populace and add another vector in the populace to acquire a change distinct vector, where the parent distinct vector is crossed with a specific likelihood to create an endeavoured distinct vector. At long last, the endeavoured distinct vector and the parent distinct vector are implemented covetous determination, and the improved distinct vector is kept to the future. The essential advancement cycles are portrayed here.

- **Initialization**: The DE calculation utilizes D-layered vectors (M) as the underlying arrangement as defined in Eq. (6.8). Set populace number (N), every individual can be communicated as $g_i(G) = (g_{i1}(G), g_{i2}(G), \ldots, g_{iD}(G))$. The underlying populace is produced in $[G_{min}, G_{max}]$ here, M is the quantity of D-layered vectors, N is the number of populaces, and $g_i(G)$ is the i-th person.

$$g_{iD} = G_{min} + rand(0, 1) \times (G_{max} + G_{min}) \tag{6.8}$$

where G addresses the Gth age, G_{max} dresses the greatest worth of the pursuit space, G_{min} dresses the base worth of the hunt space, rand (0,1) addresses an irregular number that encounters an ordinary dispersion inside (0,1).
- **Mutation operation**: The calculation utilizes the change activity to produce a transformation vector $m_{i,G}$ for every individual $g_{i,G}$ in the present populace (target vector). In every produced target vector, a relating change vector can be created by a specific transformation system. As indicated by the different age techniques

for transformation people, a few different change systems for the DE are shaped. The five most ordinarily utilized change methodologies are portrayed in Eq. (6.9).

$$m_{i,G} = g_i \cdot r_1 - G_{\min} + F \cdot (g_i \cdot r_2 + G_{\max} - g_i \cdot r_3) \quad (6.9)$$

where r_1, r_2, and r_3 are arbitrarily produced selective numbers inside $[1, m]$. The scaling factor F is a positive control boundary to scale distinction vector.

- **Crossover operation**: Every pair of target vector g_i and their relating change vectors $m_{i,G}$ are crossed to create a test vector $U_{i,G} = (u_{1,G}, u_{2,G}, \ldots, u_{i,G})$. In this calculation, a binomial hybrid is characterized as Eq. (6.10).

$$U_{i,G} = g_i \oplus m_{i,G} \quad (6.10)$$

where $\oplus$ implies XOR operation. Now the selection procedure is obtained as follows.

- **Selection**: On the off chance that the upsides of boundaries surpass the relating lower or upper limits, they can be further initialized haphazardly and consistently inside the specified reach. Then, at that point, the goal work upsides of all test vectors are assessed, and the choice activity is completed. The goal work esteem f $(U_{i,G})$ of every test vector is contrasted and the goal works worth of the comparing objective vector in the present populace. Assuming the goal work worth of the test vector is not exactly or equivalent to that of the relating objective vector, then, at that point, the objective vector is swapped by the test vector for the future. In any case, the objective vector has stayed for the future. The determination activity can be communicated as Eq. (6.11).

$$f(U_{i,G}) = U_{i,G}, if U_{i,G} < g_i \text{else} g_i \quad (6.11)$$

However, this selection process is unable to find global optimum works only on local optima which isn't efficient for genetic optimization.

- **Advantages of differential evolution**: It is a populace based metaheuristic search calculation that enhances an issue by iteratively further developing a competitor arrangement in light of a transformative cycle. Such calculations make not many or no suspicions about the basic advancement issue and can rapidly investigate extremely huge plan spaces.
- **Disadvantages of differential evolution**: Combinatorial streamlining issues, for example, a travelling salesperson issue are not by any stretch appropriate for differential development. For this situation you can pick a more qualified hereditary calculation. BTW, Ant settlement enhancement might be a superior counterpart for a mobile sales rep issue as it's more particular for such sort of issues.

6.3.2.4 Colony Optimization Algorithm

Colony Optimization is one of the most standard heuristic algorithms utilized to resolve varied complex optimization problems by detecting the finest optimal paths. It can be categorized into two subdivision algorithms like Ant Colony Optimization (ACO) and Bee Colony Optimization (BCO).

The ACO is a conventional computing methodology (Fig. 6.5). It is widely used for solving intricate optimization problems utilizing a probabilistic mechanism for searching optimal pathways. Ants are the insects who explore the path in search of food after leaving their colonies. Ants can smell the essence of the food and with the increase in the smell of the food, it gets easier for them to locate the food. This is known as the pheromone model. In Ant Colony Optimization a similar thing happens where artificial ants create a communication seeking for the best optimal paths to move on the graphs. In this optimization algorithm, artificial ants try to impersonate the behavioural changes of the real ants.

The obtained ABC calculation begins from an introduced populace and afterward emphasizes the utilized phase, passer-by phase, scout phase, and nearby inquiry phase until an end basis has happened. Mean the populace size of people like P, and the top age of every person as λ. The method of ABC is illustrated below.

It is critical to begin the calculation with a populace described by a significant degree of value and variety. The model is produced three people with the three heuristics separately to guarantee the nature of the populace, and the others are made by the InitializationRAN [49] to ensure the populace with great variety.

It is a not unexpected issue that the arrangement can either be caught in a neighbourhood enhancement or encounter an untimely assembly and even, now and again an underlying arrangement with restricted potential can prompt no enhancement inside various continuous emphases, in all likelihood, a much more regrettable arrangement can be gotten.

- **Advantages of ACO**: They enjoy an upper hand over mimicked tempering and hereditary calculation ways to deal with comparative issues when the chart might

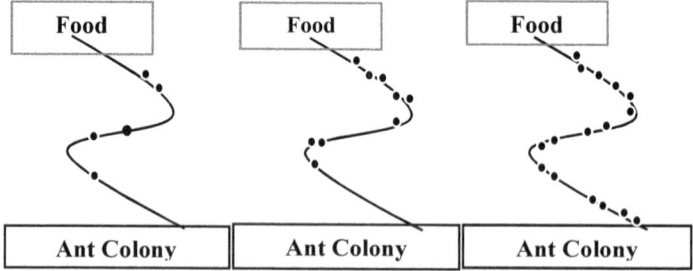

Fig. 6.5 A sample ACO structure

change progressively; the subterranean insect state calculation can be run consistently and adjust to changes continuously. This is of interest in network steering and metropolitan transportation frameworks.
- **Disadvantages of ACO**: Theoretical analysis is difficult; Sequences of random decisions and they are not independent to each other; Probability distribution changes by every iteration i.e. unstable.

6.3.2.5 BAT Algorithm

BAT is a metaheuristic algorithm enthused by the echolocation performance of micro-bats. This algorithm is utilized for global optimization. Echolocation is the property of bats that uses a variation of pulse rates and emissions to convey their locations to other bats within the vicinity.

The algorithm works in the following way. Each virtual bat flies with a random velocity v. Say it has position x. The loudness of emission is denoted by A, the wavelength varies from bat to bat. The goal of the bat is to find prey. When it finds a prey the frequency and loudness of emission changes, it is denoted by r. A locally initialized random walk is used to increase the intensity of the search. This process continues until the best candidate is found by using some predefined stop criteria. A frequency tuning approach is used by this method that controls the dynamic behaviour of the bats. The stability between exploration and exploitation is reached by defining the parameters of the frequency tuning system used by the algorithm (Fig. 6.6).

- **Advantages of BAT algorithm**: Simple, flexible, fast and easy to implement; solve highly non-linear problems efficiently;
- **Disadvantages of BAT algorithm**: quick convergence at early stage, gradually slows down later; no mathematical analysis to link the parameters with convergence rate.

6.3.2.6 Blackhole Algorithm

In this algorithm, an initial set of solutions is generated for an optimization problem. Along with that, an objective function is also defined for the solution. The best candidate is selected in each iteration to become the black hole. The remaining are marked as normal stars orbiting the black hole. Once the initialization process is completed, the black hole as a general phenomenon starts pulling stars near itself to absorb them completely. Once a star gets too close to the black hole it gets absorbed into it. In the place of the stars, a new random candidate is selected which becomes a new star. The new star is placed in the search space and a new search procedure begins its iteration.

- **Advantages of Blackhole algorithm**: simple structure, easy implementation, and freedom from hyper-parameters.

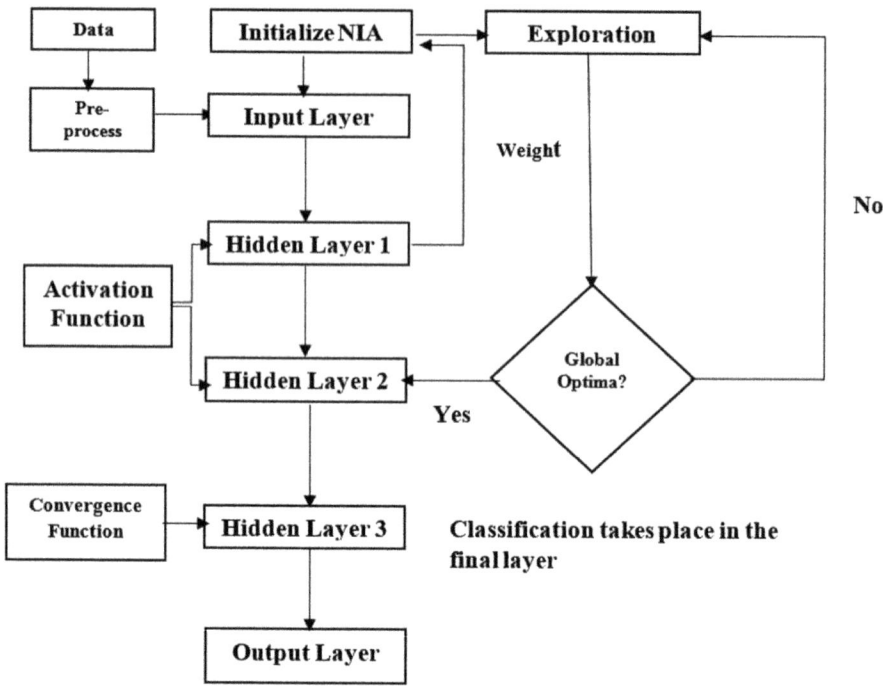

Fig. 6.6 Flow chart of the BAT optimization

- **Disadvantages of Blackhole algorithm**: BH also suffers from many drawbacks that prevent it from solving complex and high-dimensional problems.

6.3.3 Integration of ANN and OA

In this work, a gathering of optimization is applied to take care of this issue. There are no registers in the writing of any endeavour toward utilizing the microarray and the genetic classes (GEO) as an advancement strategy for the best organization engineering issue. Further, we characterize the computational intricacy of a feedforward ANN engineering as an element of the all-out number of loads and predisposition present in its designs and the time expected for organizational learning. We get from this a punishment term that is utilized to assess the goal capacity to keep away from over-complex networks designs. The utilization consolidated of these components is additionally a commitment of this work.

Ideal organization designs can be developed to fit a given job that needs to be done. Both the organization geography portrayal and search administrators utilized in our examinations are the main issues to consider in the development of structures. The most suitable determination of information and secret layer neurons is the advancement issue for this situation. The hereditary calculation is utilized for tracking down the ideal number of neurons in the info and secret layers. The chromosome length is separated into two sets. The first set addresses the number of neurons in the information layer, while the subsequent set addresses the number of neurons in the secret layer.

For demonstrating the non-direct conduct of electrical burden, MLPNN model construction with 8 sources of info and 20 secret neurons is utilized. On account of the brain model, the neuron numbers in the input and secret layer, and their interconnections have been enhanced. The interconnection guide of the organization is coded into the chromosomes of the GA, where every chromosome is made out of 160 qualities and can be addressed as displayed in the following figure. These qualities can be addressed with a worth of either True or False, where True addresses association among neurons and False represents no association.

For tracking down the ideal brain network geography with hereditary control of chromosomes, the mean square mistake (MSE) of the model is utilized as wellness work. The wellness assessment work is characterized in Eq. (6.12).

$$F = \text{MSE} + (1 - \alpha) \times \left(\frac{\omega}{\omega_n}\right) \times 10^{-5} + \alpha \times \left(\frac{n}{n_n}\right) \times 10^{-15} \quad (6.12)$$

where, MSE = mean square error, α = learning rate, ω = no. of weighted interconnections between the input and hidden layer, ω_n = maximum number of all interconnections, n = number of nodes in the ANN activated at each layer and n_n = maximum number of nodes can be activated on the above-mentioned layer.

The mentioned function is treated as a loss function to train the optimized ANN. The following figure depicts how GA optimizes an ANN. The rest of the optimization technique works similarly only the objective function has to be updated.

Below is the generic workflow of integration of NIA with a fully connected multilayer ANN (Fig. 6.7) to resolve the problems of data classification:

The generic workflow of the hybrid model using a combination of NIA and fully connected multilayer ANN (Fig. 6.8) to perform the task of clustering.

6.4 Experimental Results and Discussion

The tests of the obtained combination are done on various benchmark microarray information gathered from the 'Kent Ridge Biomedical Data Set Repository' [50] openly accessible high volume of qualities with unsystematic commotion, and the examples are straight indistinguishable. The test microarray information is recorded with all elements in Table 6.1.

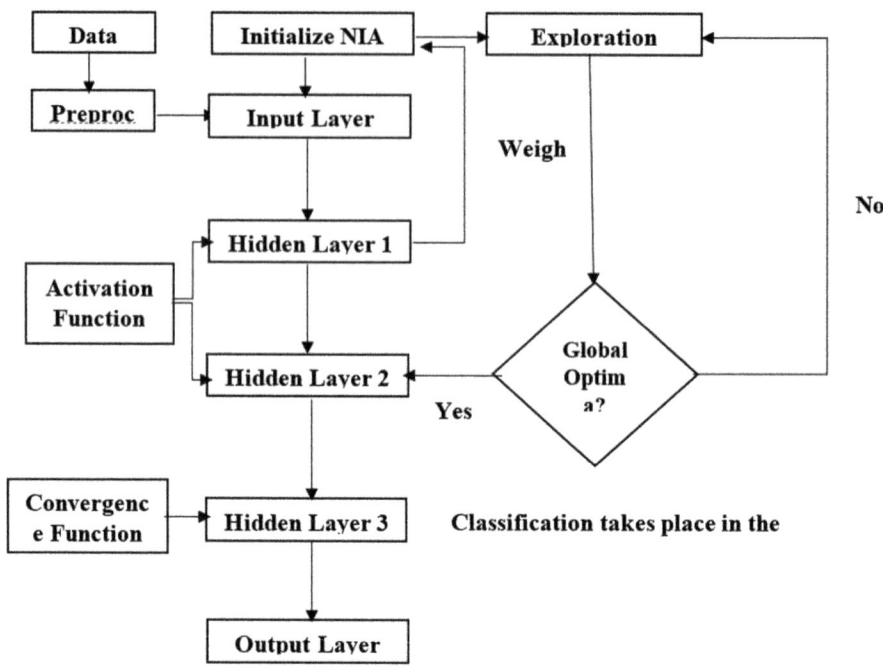

Fig. 6.7 Integration of NIA with a multilayer ANN to resolve data classification

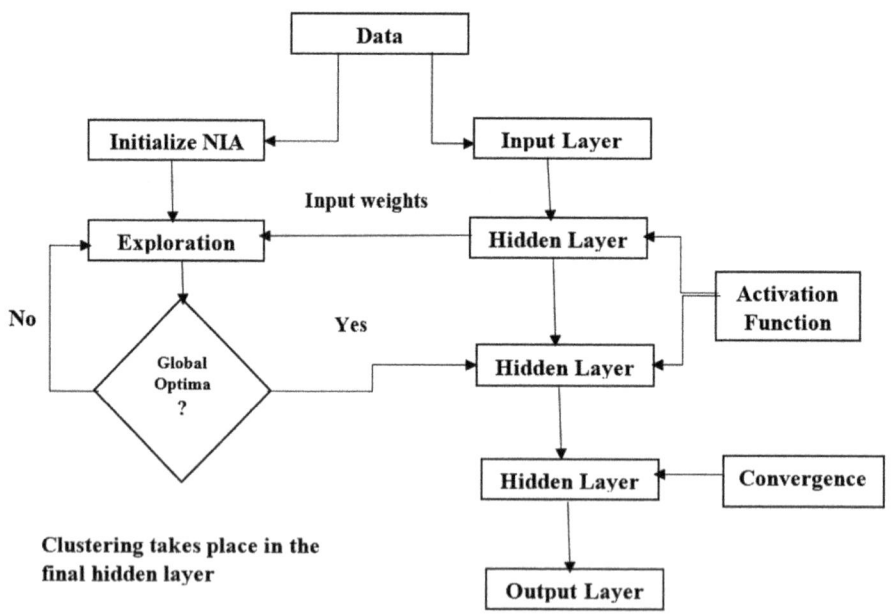

Fig. 6.8 Combination of NIA and multilayer ANN to solve data clustering

Table 6.1 Experimental Dataset Summary

Data	#Genes	Class Name	#Sample (class1/class2)
Prostate	12,600	Normal/Tumor	134 (57/77)
Leukemia	7129	AML/ALL	72 (25/47)
Lung	12,533	Mesothelioma/ADCA	181 (31/150)
Colon	2000	Positive/Negative	62 (22/40)
DLBCL	7129	FL/DLBCL	77 (19/58)

6.4.1 Experimental Setup

The proposed methodology is implemented using the RStudio IDE, Jupyter Notebook, and Spyder (Anaconda-based IDE) dedicated to running the R programming and python programming, respectively. Here, the backbone *Artificial Neural Network* (https://github.com/ayanbabusona/HandsonML/blob/main/bioinformatics/leukemia__Cancer_Classification.ipynb) is implemented by Jupyter Notebook. Similarly, RStudio and Spyder have been used for Nature-inspired optimization applied on pre-trained weights (https://github.com/ayanbabusona/Statistical_Analysis_of_Network_Data/blob/main/Chapter_2:%20Manipulating_Network_data/2.2.3_operations_on_graphs.R). It can run on the desktop (Windows, Linux, and Mac) or in a browser linked to RStudio Server Pro/RStudio Server (Ubuntu, Red Hat, and SUSE Linux). In this paper, the proposed methodology and all the comparative approaches and analysis of the results are performed in Ubuntu-based OS with 4 GB Ram and Intel i3 processor. All the performance analysis is computed on edge with the bio conductor, NumPy, pandas, Keras, and several other python and R packages.

6.4.2 Discussion on ANN

The utilized experimental datasets have a maximum of 12,600 genes (prostate cancer) that's why the proposed ANN has 14 layers ($2^{14} = 16384$) with some zero bias nodes as well as only two nodes in the output layer as it's a binary classification problem. The activation map obtained by ANN is illustrated in Fig. 6.9 in both forward as well as backward propagation for all the experimental datasets.

From Fig. 6.9, it can be concluded that though the ANN can achieve the state of the art accuracy but the parameters are not being converted to any particular points. It indicates that there are no global optima although there are lots of local optimum points. This conclusion depicts the importance of optimization algorithms. But to judge the performance of the ANN quantitative results are equally important. Table 6.2 obtain the statistical analysis of the ANN on the experimental datasets.

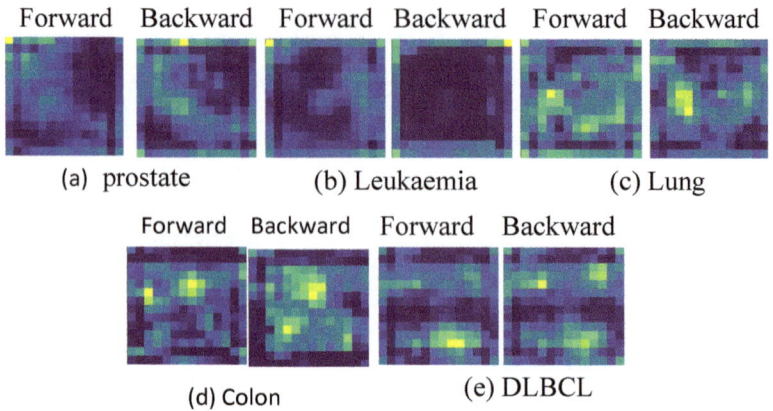

Fig. 6.9 Activation map of the developed ANN

Table 6.2 Performance Evolution of the ANN

Datasets	Precision (%)	Recall (%)	F1-Score (%)	Accuracy (%)
Prostate	80.3	81.8	80.1	83.6
Leukemia	82.7	82.2	82.3	81.4
Lung	77.8	79.4	78.6	82.2
Colon	79.8	81.1	80.7	83.5
DLBCL	82.7	82.2	82.3	84.4

From Table 6.2, it can be concluded that, though the ANN gives state-of-the-art results still its metrics have been fallen for lung cancer. To solve this issue the nature-inspired optimization algorithms have been applied on ANN and their qualitative and quantitative results have been reported in the following subsections.

6.4.2.1 Optimization of ANN with GA

This is the most popular algorithm and best fit with the neural networks as the working principle of the genetic algorithm is similar to ANN. However, it reduces the number of parameters by reducing the number of parameters by surpassing the zero bias node. Figure 6.10 obtained the activation map of this combination to evaluate the strategy.

In comparison, with Fig. 6.9 the yellow spots are more prominent in Fig. 6.10. That indicates the features are more converged to the global optima. The quantitative results are obtained in Table 6.3.

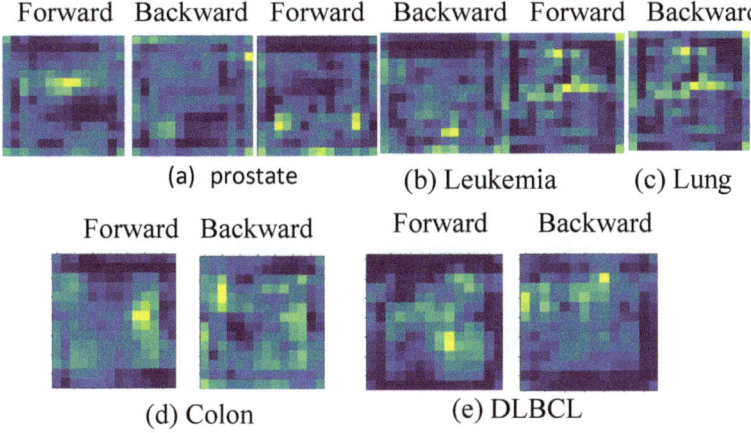

Fig. 6.10 Activation map of the developed ANN with genetic algorithm

Table 6.3 Performance Evolution of the ANN with genetic algorithm

Datasets	Precision (%)	Recall (%)	F1-Score (%)	Accuracy (%)
Prostate	93.0	89.8	91.4	90.6
Leukemia	94.8	89.7	92.2	90.8
Lung	96.0	91.1	93.5	93.6
Colon	95.9	93.0	94.4	95.7
DLBCL	95.8	93.4	94.1	96.6

From Table 6.3, it can be decided that the classification accuracies of this combination are much higher than the ANN due to global convergence. Now to obtain a comparative study, the performance of the other optimization algorithms is obtained as follows.

6.4.2.2 Optimization of ANN with Particle Swarm Optimization

In this combination, ANN has been integrated with PSO. This is a similar type of combination with a genetic algorithm whose activation map is obtained in Fig. 6.11.

In Fig. 6.11 the activation map is exactly similar in forward as well as a backward pass. This indicates the precision the nodes are activated in a similar pattern in both passes. However, it converges to the global optima but local optima's also get the similar priority. The quantitative results are obtained in Table 6.4.

From Table 6.4, it can be stated that the performance of this combination is much higher than the ANN but lower than the GA. Now to obtain a comparative study, the performance of the DE algorithm is obtained as follows.

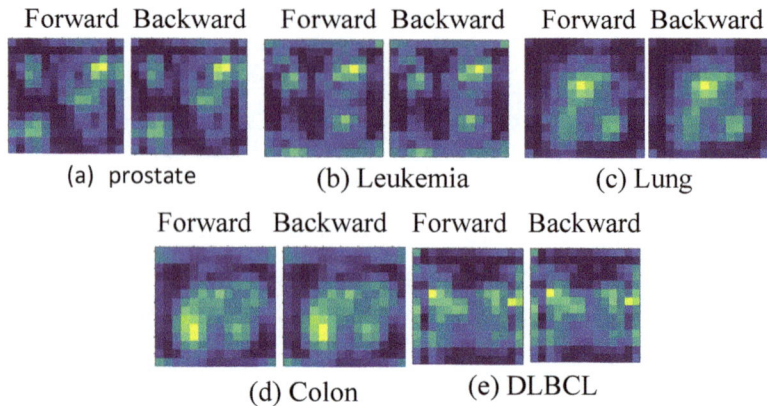

Fig. 6.11 Activation map of the developed ANN with particle swarm optimization

Table 6.4 Performance Evolution of the ANN with PSO

Datasets	Precision (%)	Recall (%)	F1-Score (%)	Accuracy (%)
Prostate	85.6	85.7	85.3	86.6
Leukemia	81.2	89.9	84.6	85.8
Lung	84.0	87.9	85.8	83.6
Colon	87.6	89.9	88.6	84.7
DLBCL	86.5	84.9	85.7	86.6

6.4.2.3 Optimization of ANN with Differential Evolution

Here, it doesn't make not many or no suppositions about the basic streamlining issue and can rapidly investigate exceptionally enormous plan spaces. Figure 6.12 illustrates the activation map of different experimental datasets in forward as well as a backward pass.

From Fig. 6.12, it can be stated that, differential evolution is also unable to converge to a global optimum point as it is iteratively improving the candidate solution space. Table 6.5 depicts the performance evolution of this obtained combination.

From Table 6.5, it is decided that the classification accuracies of this combination are much higher than the ANN but lower than the GA as well as PSO due to the shortcomings of the global optimum. These shortcomings are tried to overcome with the help of colony optimization algorithms.

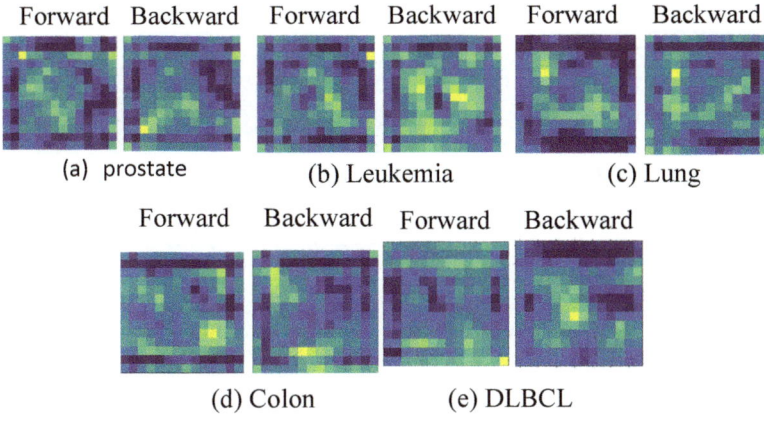

Fig. 6.12 Activation map of the developed ANN with differential evolution

Table 6.5 Performance evolution of the ANN with DE

Datasets	Precision (%)	Recall (%)	F1-score (%)	Accuracy (%)
Prostate	81.4	84.5	83.2	83.4
Leukemia	85.6	86.7	85.9	85.6
Lung	77.8	78.9	78.3	80.9
Colon	80.1	81.2	80.7	87.8
DLBCL	83.2	83.4	83.3	86.2

6.4.2.4 Optimization of ANN with Colony Optimization Algorithm

This province improvement calculation is a probabilistic strategy for tackling computational issues which can be diminished to track down great ways through the graphical pattern of ANN. The activation map of this experiment is shown in Fig. 6.13.

From Fig. 6.13, it is stated that the Colony Optimization technique achieves better than the differential evolution methodology. Not only that, but it is also noticeable that for the Lung cancer dataset there is no significant activation (i.e. zero bias). Here, ANN work as a fully connected network. The quantitative results are obtained in Table 6.6.

From Table 6.6, it can be concluded that the classification performance of this combination is much higher than the ANN and comparable to GA. However, the time complexity of this algorithm has to be considerable.

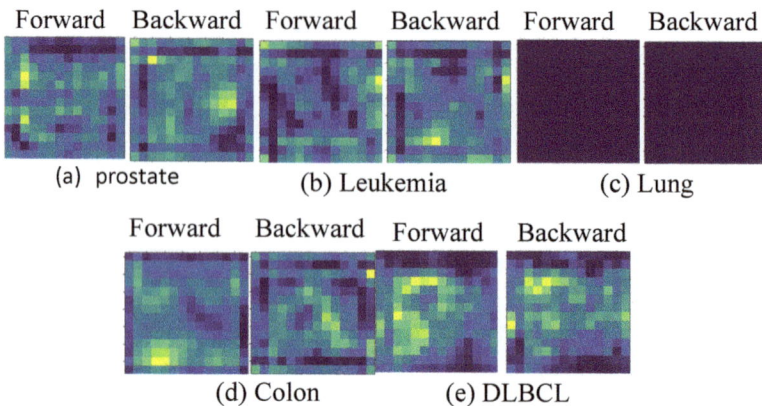

Fig. 6.13 Activation map of the developed ANN with colony optimization

Table 6.6 Performance evolution of the ANN with colony optimization

Datasets	Precision (%)	Recall (%)	F1-Score (%)	Accuracy (%)
Prostate	85.1	91.2	88.2	84.9
Leukemia	87.4	91.8	89.6	86.9
Lung	89.7	91.9	90.5	87.9
Colon	91.2	92.7	91.9	88.9
DLBCL	91.4	92.6	91.4	88.7

6.4.2.5 Optimization of ANN with BAT Algorithm

This combination is a heuristic calculation that works by emulating the echolocation conduct of bats to perform worldwide streamlining. The activation map of this combination is obtained in Fig. 6.14.

The BAT algorithm is a recently developed approach and more powerful than the existing ones as it also tries to find out the global optimum point. The quantitative results of this algorithm are depicted in Table 6.7.

From Table 6.7, it can be concluded that the BAT is the most stabilized optimization algorithm to date. Now to find a comparative study the performance of the other optimization algorithm is obtained as follows.

6.4.2.6 Optimization of ANN with Blackhole Algorithm

Metaheuristics have become well known in tackling enhancement issues. As of late writing has been overwhelmed with part of "novel" streamlining methods. These methods are propelled by different normal peculiarities. One such strategy is the Blackhole Algorithm, which is motivated by the Black Holes. The writer of this

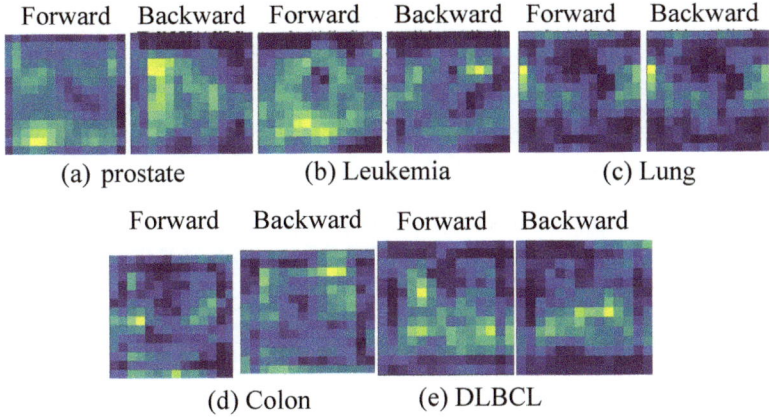

Fig. 6.14 Activation map of the developed ANN with BAT

Table 6.7 Performance evolution of the ANN with BAT algorithm

Datasets	Precision (%)	Recall (%)	F1-Score (%)	Accuracy (%)
Prostate	87.4	91.8	89.6	86.9
Leukemia	89.7	91.9	90.5	87.9
Lung	91.2	92.7	91.9	88.9
Colon	91.4	92.6	91.4	88.7
DLBCL	93.3	93.1	93.1	92.4

method guarantees it to be preferable over other optimization algorithms, yet we have thought that it is the opposite. In this chapter, we analyze the Black Hole Algorithm and another nature-inspired optimization algorithm by assessing them on a standard test suite. The outcomes show that BHA performs inadequately when contrasted with PSO and consequently, distorting the case made by creators of BHA. The activation map of the BHA is obtained in Fig. 6.15 and the quantitative analysis is obtained in Table 6.8.

From Table 6.8 and Fig. 6.14, it is stated that the Blackhole algorithm neither finds the global optimum nor produces good quantitative results compared to the other optimization algorithm. Now the comparative study of all nature-inspired optimization algorithms based on time as well as space complexity is obtained in Fig. 6.15.

From Fig. 6.16 it can be stated that the GA is the best match nature-inspired optimization algorithm while the Blackhole is the worst.

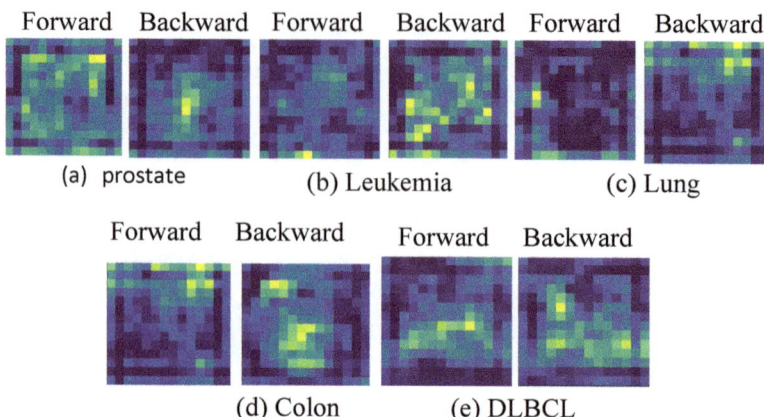

Fig. 6.15 Activation map of the developed ANN with Blackhole optimization

Table 6.8 Performance evolution of the ANN with Blackhole algorithm

Datasets	Precision (%)	Recall (%)	F1-Score (%)	Accuracy (%)
Prostate	82.7	82.2	82.3	82.4
Leukemia	83.6	83.3	83.4	83.3
Lung	83.7	82.2	83.2	85.6
Colon	83.7	82.2	83.2	85.6
DLBCL	87.4	85.2	86.3	84.7

6.5 Conclusion

Nature-inspired optimization has been quite popular in modern days. This chapter represents an extensive analysis of various popular nature-inspired algorithms along with a fully connected ANN showing the convergence hit map of each of the datasets utilizing the algorithms. These hybrid models have been highly utilized to resolve complex optimization problems (here concentrated on the binary classification of the microarray data). It can be concluded that using an optimization algorithm with an ANN produces a better chance of obtaining improved accuracy, precision, and convergence on global optima from the experimental results. In this chapter, the comparison of the different hybrid models will help researchers to select the appropriate model more vividly for their future work. In the case of unsupervised learning methods, such as clustering using such combinations one can improve on the overall learning rate of the given algorithm without adding in much complexity in terms of time. In the future, the proposed work can be extended and tested upon other datasets as well as to solve other supervised or unsupervised learning problems.

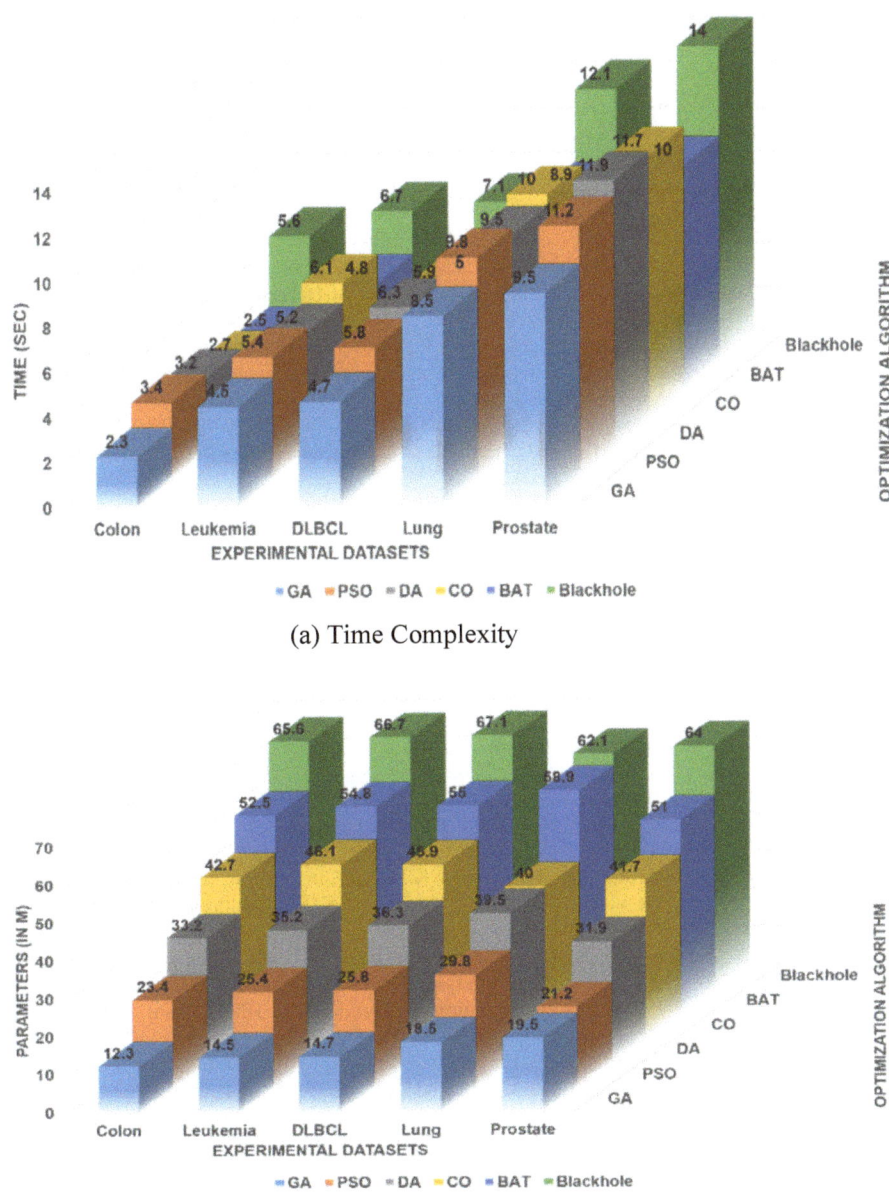

(a) Time Complexity

(b) Space Complexity

Fig. 6.16 Comparative study of the nature-inspired optimization algorithms

References

1. Nouri-Moghaddam, B., Ghazanfari, M., Fathian, M.: A novel multi-objective forest optimization algorithm for wrapper feature selection. Expert Syst. Appl. **175**, 114737 (2021). https://doi.org/10.1016/j.eswa.2021.114737
2. Ghoniem, R.M., Elshewikh, D.L.: A novel genetic artificial bee inspired neural network model for drug name recognition. Procedia Comput. Sci. **189**, 48–60 (2021). https://doi.org/10.1016/j.procs.2021.05.069
3. Abiodun, O.I., Jantan, A., Omolara, A.E., Dada, K.V., Mohamed, N.A., Arshad, H.: State-of-the-art in artificial neural network applications: a survey. Heliyon **4**, e00938 (2018). https://doi.org/10.1016/j.heliyon.2018.e00938
4. Manna, S., Roy, I., Majumder, D., Banerjee, A., Pati, S.K.: Multiple data integration using joint non-negative matrix factorization. In: Computational intelligence in pattern recognition (pp. 667–677). Springer, Singapore (2022)
5. Banerjee, A., Shivakumara, P., Pal, S., Pal, U., Liu, C.L.: DCT-DWT-FFT Based Method for Text Detection in Underwater Images. In: Asian Conference on Pattern Recognition (pp. 218–233). Springer, Cham (2022)
6. Wierzbicki, A.P.: The use of reference objectives in multiobjective optimization - theoretical implications and practical experience [WWW document]. http://pure.iiasa.ac.at/id/eprint/1117/. Accessed 3 July 2022 (1979)
7. Das, A.K., Chakrabarty, S., Pati, S.K., Sahaji, A.H.: Applying restrained genetic algorithm for attribute reduction using attribute dependency and discernibility matrix. In: Venugopal, K.R., Patnaik, L.M. (Eds.) Wireless Networks and Computational Intelligence, Communications in Computer and Information Science, pp. 299–308. Springer Berlin Heidelberg, Berlin, Heidelberg (2012). https://doi.org/10.1007/978-3-642-31686-9_36
8. Mukherjee, R., Pati, S.K., Banerjee, A.: Performance tuning of Android applications using clustering and optimization heuristics. In: Advanced data mining tools and methods for social computing (pp. 27–50). Academic Press (2022)
9. Das, A.K., Pati, S.K., Ghosh, A.: Relevant feature selection and ensemble classifier design using bi-objective genetic algorithm. Knowl. Inf. Syst. **62**, 423–455 (2020). https://doi.org/10.1007/s10115-019-01341-6
10. Ahmad, M.F., Isa, N.A.M., Lim, W.H., Ang, K.M.: Differential evolution: a recent review based on state-of-the-art works. Alex. Eng. J. **61**, 3831–3872 (2022). https://doi.org/10.1016/j.aej.2021.09.013
11. Eberhart, Y.S.: Particle swarm optimization: developments, applications and resources. In: Proceedings of the 2001 Congress on Evolutionary Computation (IEEE Cat. No. 01TH8546). Presented at the 2001 Congress on Evolutionary Computation, IEEE, Seoul, South Korea, pp. 81–86 (2001). https://doi.org/10.1109/CEC.2001.934374
12. Yi, Y., He, R.: A Novel Artificial Bee Colony Algorithm. In: 2014 Sixth International Conference on Intelligent Human-Machine Systems and Cybernetics. Presented at the 2014 6th International Conference on Intelligent Human-Machine Systems and Cybernetics (IHMSC), IEEE, Hangzhou, China, pp. 271–274 (2014). https://doi.org/10.1109/IHMSC.2014.73
13. Khursheed, M.-N., Nadeem, M.F., Khalil, A., Sajjad, I.A., Raza, A., Iqbal, M.Q., Bo, R., Rehman, W. ur: Review of Flower Pollination Algorithm: Applications and Variants. In: 2020 International Conference on Engineering and Emerging Technologies (ICEET). Presented at the 2020 International Conference on Engineering and Emerging Technologies (ICEET), IEEE, Lahore, Pakistan, pp. 1–6 (2020).https://doi.org/10.1109/ICEET48479.2020.9048215
14. Ghose, R., Das, Tiyasha, Saha, A., Das, Tejes, Chattopadhyay, S.P.: Cuckoo search algorithm for speech recognition. In: 2015 International Conference and Workshop on Computing and Communication (IEMCON). Presented at the 2015 International Conference and Workshop on Computing and Communication (IEMCON), IEEE, Vancouver, BC, Canada, pp. 1–5 (2015). https://doi.org/10.1109/IEMCON.2015.7344522

15. Dubuisson, F., Chandra, A., Rezkallah, M., Ibrahim, H.: A bacterial foraging optimization technique and predictive control approach for power management in a standalone Microgrid. In: 2020 IEEE electric power and energy conference (EPEC). Presented at the 2020 IEEE Electric Power and Energy Conference (EPEC), IEEE, Edmonton, AB, Canada, pp. 1–7 (2020). https://doi.org/10.1109/EPEC48502.2020.9320038
16. Guo, M.W., Wang, J.S., Zhu, L.F., Guo, S.S., Xie, W.: An improved grey wolf optimizer based on tracking and seeking modes to solve function optimization problems. IEEE Access **8**, 69861–69893 (2020). https://doi.org/10.1109/ACCESS.2020.2984321
17. Saranya, S., Amudha, T.: Crop planning optimization with social spider optimization algorithm, in: 2017 International Conference on Intelligent Sustainable Systems (ICISS). Presented at the 2017 International Conference on Intelligent Sustainable Systems (ICISS), pp. 776–781. IEEE, Palladam (2017). https://doi.org/10.1109/ISS1.2017.8389281
18. Luo, Z., Li, T., Yan, Y., Zhou, Z., Zha, G.: Prediction of sound insulation performance of aramid honeycomb sandwich panel based on artificial neural network. Appl. Acoust. **190**, 108656 (2022). https://doi.org/10.1016/j.apacoust.2022.108656
19. Banerjee, A., Pati, S.K.: Predicting Antiviral Drugs for COVID-19 Treatment Using Artificial Intelligence Based Approach. In: Nayak, J., Naik, B., Abraham, A. (eds.) Understanding COVID-19: The Role of Computational Intelligence, Studies in Computational Intelligence, pp. 245–269. Springer International Publishing, Cham (2022). https://doi.org/10.1007/978-3-030-74761-9_11
20. Peng, B., Tong, L., Yan, D., Huo, W.: Experimental research and artificial neural network prediction of free piston expander-linear generator. Energy Rep. **8**, 1966–1978 (2022). https://doi.org/10.1016/j.egyr.2022.01.021
21. Skrypnik, A.N., Shchelchkov, A.V., Gortyshov, Yu.F., Popov, I.A.: Artificial neural networks application on friction factor and heat transfer coefficients prediction in tubes with inner helical-finning. Appl. Therm. Eng. **206**, 118049 (2022). https://doi.org/10.1016/j.applthermaleng.2022.118049
22. Saldarriaga, J.F., Cruz, Y., Estiati, I., Tellabide, M., Olazar, M.: Assessment of pressure drop in conical spouted beds of biomass by artificial neural networks and comparison with empirical correlations. Particuology **70**, 1–9 (2022). https://doi.org/10.1016/j.partic.2021.12.004
23. Pati, S.K., Ghosh, A., Banerjee, A., Roy, I., Ghosh, P., Kakar, C.: Data Analysis on Cancer Disease Using Machine Learning Techniques. In: Nayak, J., Favorskaya, M.N., Jain, S., Naik, B., Mishra, M. (eds.) Advanced Machine Learning Approaches in Cancer Prognosis, Intelligent Systems Reference Library, pp. 13–73. Springer International Publishing, Cham (2021). https://doi.org/10.1007/978-3-030-71975-3_2
24. Hu, Y., Su, J.: Research on credit risk evaluation of commercial banks based on artificial neural network model. Procedia Computer Science **199**, 1168–1176 (2022). https://doi.org/10.1016/j.procs.2022.01.148
25. Badura, A., Krysiński, J., Nowaczyk, A., Buciński, A.: Application of artificial neural networks to the prediction of antifungal activity of imidazole derivatives against Candida albicans. Chemom. Intell. Lab. Syst. **222**, 104501 (2022). https://doi.org/10.1016/j.chemolab.2022.104501
26. Gnatowski, M., Buchaniec, S., Brus, G.: The prediction of the polarization curves of a solid oxide fuel cell anode with an artificial neural network supported numerical simulation. Int. J. Hydrog. Energy:S0360319921036028 (2021). https://doi.org/10.1016/j.ijhydene.2021.09.100
27. Ellethy, H., Chandra, S.S., Nasrallah, F.A.: The detection of mild traumatic brain injury in paediatrics using artificial neural networks. Comput. Biol. Med. **135**, 104614 (2021). https://doi.org/10.1016/j.compbiomed.2021.104614
28. Paul, T., Vainio, S., Roning, J.: Detection of intra-family coronavirus genome sequences through graphical representation and artificial neural network. Expert Syst. Appl. **194**, 116559 (2022). https://doi.org/10.1016/j.eswa.2022.116559
29. Lu, J., Xue, Z., Xu, B.-B., Wu, D., Zheng, H.-L., Xie, J.-W., Wang, J.-B., Lin, J.-X., Chen, Q.-Y., Li, P., Huang, C.-M., Zheng, C.-H.: Application of an artificial neural network for predicting the potential chemotherapy benefit of patients with gastric cancer after radical surgery. Surgery. S0039606021008771 (2021). https://doi.org/10.1016/j.surg.2021.08.055

30. Squires, M., Tao, X., Elangovan, S., Gururajan, R., Zhou, X., Acharya, U.R.: A novel genetic algorithm based system for the scheduling of medical treatments. Expert Syst. Appl. **195**, 116464 (2022). https://doi.org/10.1016/j.eswa.2021.116464
31. Chen, L., Liu, W.-L., Zhong, J.: An efficient multi-objective ant colony optimization for task allocation of heterogeneous unmanned aerial vehicles. Journal of Computational Science **58**, 101545 (2022). https://doi.org/10.1016/j.jocs.2021.101545
32. Fernandes, P.B., Oliveira, R.C.L., Fonseca Neto, J.V.: Trajectory planning of autonomous mobile robots applying a particle swarm optimization algorithm with peaks of diversity. Appl. Soft Comput. **116**, 108108 (2022). https://doi.org/10.1016/j.asoc.2021.108108
33. Yang, B., Huang, X., Cheng, W., Huang, T., Li, X.: Discrete bacterial foraging optimization for community detection in networks. Futur. Gener. Comput. Syst. **128**, 192–204 (2022). https://doi.org/10.1016/j.future.2021.10.015
34. Chen, Y., Wang, M., Heidari, A.A., Shi, B., Hu, Z., Zhang, Q., Chen, H., Mafarja, M., Turabieh, H.: Multi-threshold image segmentation using a multi-strategy shuffled frog leaping algorithm. Expert Syst. Appl. **194**, 116511 (2022). https://doi.org/10.1016/j.eswa.2022.116511
35. Altabeeb, A.M., Mohsen, A.M., Abualigah, L., Ghallab, A.: Solving capacitated vehicle routing problem using cooperative firefly algorithm. Appl. Soft Comput. **108**, 107403 (2021). https://doi.org/10.1016/j.asoc.2021.107403
36. Das, A., Namtirtha, A., Dutta, A.: Fuzzy clustering of Acute Lymphoblastic Leukemia images assisted by Eagle strategy and morphological reconstruction. Knowl.-Based Syst. **239**, 108008 (2022). https://doi.org/10.1016/j.knosys.2021.108008
37. Deeb, H., Sarangi, A., Mishra, D., Sarangi, S.K.: Improved Black Hole optimization algorithm for data clustering. J. King Saud Univ. Comput. Inf. Sci. S1319157820306212 (2020). https://doi.org/10.1016/j.jksuci.2020.12.013
38. Hao, P., Sobhani, B.: Application of the improved chaotic grey wolf optimization algorithm as a novel and efficient method for parameter estimation of solid oxide fuel cells model. Int. J. Hydrogen Energy **46**, 36454–36465 (2021). https://doi.org/10.1016/j.ijhydene.2021.08.174
39. Askari, Q., Younas, I.: Improved political optimizer for complex landscapes and engineering optimization problems. Expert Syst. Appl. **182**, 115178 (2021). https://doi.org/10.1016/j.eswa.2021.115178
40. Muthusamy, H., Ravindran, S., Yaacob, S., Polat, K.: An improved elephant herding optimization using sine–cosine mechanism and opposition based learning for global optimization problems. Expert Syst. Appl. **172**, 114607 (2021). https://doi.org/10.1016/j.eswa.2021.114607
41. Kumar Chandar, S.: Hybrid models for intraday stock price forecasting based on artificial neural networks and metaheuristic algorithms. Pattern Recognit. Lett. 147, 124–133 (2021). https://doi.org/10.1016/j.patrec.2021.03.030
42. Bahiraei, M., Kok Foong, L., Hosseini, S., Mazaheri, N.: Neural network combined with nature-inspired algorithms to estimate overall heat transfer coefficient of a ribbed triple-tube heat exchanger operating with a hybrid nanofluid. Measurement **174**, 108967 (2021). https://doi.org/10.1016/j.measurement.2021.108967
43. Rawat, P.S., Dimri, P., Gupta, P., Saroha, G.P.: Resource provisioning in scalable cloud using bio-inspired artificial neural network model. Appl. Soft Comput. **99**, 106876 (2021). https://doi.org/10.1016/j.asoc.2020.106876
44. Lopez-Hazas, J., Montero, A., Rodriguez, F.B.: Influence of bio-inspired activity regulation through neural thresholds learning in the performance of neural networks. Neurocomputing **462**, 294–308 (2021). https://doi.org/10.1016/j.neucom.2021.08.001
45. García-Carrillo, M., Espinoza-Martínez, A.B., Ramos-de Valle, L.F., Sánchez-Valdés, S.: Simultaneous optimization of thermal and electrical conductivity of high density polyethylene-carbon particle composites by artificial neural networks and multi-objective genetic algorithm. Comput. Mater. Sci. **201**, 110956 (2022). https://doi.org/10.1016/j.commatsci.2021.110956
46. Ibrahim, M.H.: WBA-DNN: A hybrid weight bat algorithm with deep neural network for classification of poisonous and harmful wild plants. Comput. Electron. Agric. **190**, 106478 (2021). https://doi.org/10.1016/j.compag.2021.106478

47. Erzurum Cicek, Z.I., Kamisli Ozturk, Z.: Optimizing the artificial neural network parameters using a biased random key genetic algorithm for time series forecasting. Appl. Soft Comput. **102**, 107091 (2021). https://doi.org/10.1016/j.asoc.2021.107091
48. Si, T., Bagchi, J., Miranda, P.B.C.: Artificial neural network training using metaheuristics for medical data classification: an experimental study. Expert Syst. Appl. **193**, 116423 (2022). https://doi.org/10.1016/j.eswa.2021.116423
49. Huang, J.P., Pan, Q.K., Miao, Z.H., Gao, L.: Effective constructive heuristics and discrete bee colony optimization for distributed flowshop with setup times. Eng. Appl. Artif. Intell. **97**, 104016 (2021)
50. Li, J., Liu, H.: Kent ridge bio-medical data set repository. http://datam.i2r.a-star.edu.sg/datasets/krbd (2002)

# Chapter 7
Hybridization of Fuzzy Theory and Nature-Inspired Optimization for Medical Report Summarization

Chirantana Mallick and Asit Kumar Das

Abstract It is becoming increasingly challenging to construct a smart medical system because of the large amount of accumulating information in the scientific literature of the biomedical sector. The current scenario reflects progress in a variety of less known regions as a means of extraction for the understanding of prevention and treatment for significant medical diseases such as COVID-19. Recently, many good scientific research publications in the biomedical arena was released using the MEDLINE/PubMed dataset. In the fields of biomedical research and healthcare, assessing these enormous data sets and extracting valuable information is a critical but difficult endeavour. Here, we attempt to retrieve relevant data from openly accessible text materials, like medical reports, journals, articles, papers, and some other research works, in the medical area. hese types of text data undergo first preprocessing in this chapter using sentence tokenization, then stopword removal, stemming operations, and ultimately vectorization using the BioBERT model. Consequently, a structured data is generated to process each report in feature extraction process and then clustered the similar sentences by Fuzzy C-means clustering. Then, using multiple similarity clustering measures and a bi-objective strength measure, defuzzify the clusters and construct the base summaries. To construct the report summary, en ensemble summarising approach has been employed by using Pareto evolutionary algorithm. The method contains two optimization methods(or functions): one dependent on the produced summary size, which is constant, and the other dependent on the IG (i.e., information gain) of the considering base summaries, which is variable. When the process of evolution converges, the strongest chromosomal solution of the ultimate population offers a desired summary report. This approach is used to generate an efficient summary from biomedical reports publically available in the MEDLINE/PubMed dataset, and finally, its performance comparing with a few similar cutting-edge techniques.

C. Mallick (✉) · A. K. Das
Department of Computer Science and Technology, Indian Institute of Engineering Science and Technology, Shibpur, Howrah 711103, India
e-mail: chirantana9@gmail.com

A. K. Das
e-mail: akdas@cs.iiests.ac.in

© The Author(s), under exclusive license to Springer Nature Switzerland AG 2023
J. Nayak et al. (eds.), *Nature-Inspired Optimization Methodologies in Biomedical and Healthcare*, Intelligent Systems Reference Library 233,
https://doi.org/10.1007/978-3-031-17544-2_7

Keywords MEDLINEPubMed · Bio-medical · BioBERT · Fuzzy ·
Defuzzification · kNN algorithm · Bi-objective nature inspired optimization · Text summarization · Natural language processing · Health care

7.1 Introduction

The amount of text reports in the biomedical scientific literature rises at a rapid rate every day. Millions of blogs and research papers have been publishing per day on the social media. It is now so challenging to separate valuable knowledge from such a vast quantity of information and scientific reports effectively and efficiently. As a means of extracting the important information from these reports, researchers and seekers of information must often study them. As a result, an automated summarising system (i.e., text summarization system) is required to digitally acquire information in the form of a summary of many different offline and internet outlets. As the COVID-19 pandemic progresses, the novel coronavirus disease has drawn the attention of the global scientific community. Researchers from several professions are pooling their resources to improve the worldwide knowledge base for preventing and responding to the COVID-19 pandemic. Researchers and physicians are having a difficult time providing effective health care due to a lack of precise data. Analyzing and extracting meaningful important information from this quickly rising data is a critical and difficult undertaking. Various summarising strategies have been created to lessen the difficulties of collecting reliable information from the big database.

Text summary can be obtained by extracting essential lines or phrases from the original document(s), while another way is by reconstructing the major concepts of the provided document to convey the overall information. Based on these two ways of obtaining a summary, text summarising methods can be divided into extractive summarization and abstractive summarization. TThe primary goal of extractive summarising is to identify the most important sentences in the reports that are provided and to assemble those phrases into the appropriate summary, while in the abstractive summarization, the main information of the given reports is reconstructed in order to generate much more human-like summary. Automatic summarization [1] also builds various mathematical models to get a gist of a given document. Luhn proposed in his work [2], the frequently used terms in a report are important to convey the gist of the report. Many approaches [3, 4] have been created for expressing the intermediate representation of the document by retrieving appropriate information from the given document. To identify the core concepts inside a text, traditional statistical approaches [5, 6] like as inverse document frequency, word frequency, phrase frequency, and many more were employed in the past. According to the input document size (i.e., source size) criterion, summarization system may be divided into two categories: summarising a single document and summarising many documents. One of the earliest cases to emerge was that of a single document [7, 8]. One input document is processed at a time by single document summarization systems. They still utilise only a single document as input, even if they use additional other document for training. A multi-document system, on the other hand, accepts more than one document on the same topic as input. Summarizing many documents (i.e., multi-document system) is more challenging than summarising a single document since issues with duplicate information coherence may occur in the summary. Readers might want a summary that emphasises specific characteristics instead of the primary concept in given document. The summarising technique can also be classified into query-oriented and generic system summary based on the readers' preference. A summary with all the essential details in a input document is provided by generic summarising technique [9], while query-based summarization [10] extracts the parts of a text depending on the specific information required, such as in a search engine where the answer to a question is provided at a predetermined length. If the readers are more interested in the basic idea of a paper than any specific issue, the generic summary is good. When a reader wants a summary of a document that gives attention to a certain character, it certainly include incidents happening the individual not detracting from the central plot. In that situation, the query-oriented summary will be suitable. An automatic text summary can be created from any general text document as well as any domain specific document, and based on this criterion, generic summarising and domain-specific summarization are the two categories. To find out the cue words from the given input document any domain specific concepts (i.e., for an instance MeSH terms for medical document) can be used for some domain specific summarization (i.e., medical, political reports etc.) and generic approaches (i.e., term frequency, word position etc.) have been used in case of generic text summarization. Although general text summarization can be advantageous as they may be used to any area but they will not perform as well as domain-specific ones. In case of domain specific summarization, the performance of the summarizers automatically improve as there the features selection from the given text has been designed for that domain specifically.

In this chapter, we adopted a domain specific extractive summarization technique for single document. It consists of three distinct and separate tasks: (a) Intermediate representation, (b) Sentence scoring, and (c) Selection technique for the summary.

A. Intermediate Representation

Here, the main goal is to find any concealed data in the target report. The "Topic Representation" technique [11] is another name for it because it is often utilised for locating key phrases relevant to a specific report. "Term Frequency-Inverse Document Frequency" (TF-IDF) approach [12], topic signature or word approach [11], frequency-based approach, and so on are examples of this representation style.

B. Sentence Scoring

Following the intermediate representation, the next step is to give each sentence a score depending on its significance in the target report. Sentences containing significant information should, of course, be provided a greater score value than those without. In the graph-based technique, several statistical metrics such as distinct centrality measures, distance between vertices, and vertex similarity are used to score the sentences. For different intermediate representations, the scoring technique may differ.

C. Summary Selection Strategy

The final and most important stage is to choose the summary phrases that will be used to create an effective summary. The sentences from the report that contain essential information are chosen and reassembled in a succinct style here. It is crucial to understand the genre of the reports before putting the sentences into the summary.

7.2 Literature Survey

The major objective of this chapter seems to be thoroughly review recently published biomedical research reports and develop an effective automated summarising approach for quickly extracting information from a large volume of reports. We employed a widely known clustering algorithm, fuzzy C-Means clustering [13, 14], to separate the closely related sentences in a particular report into multiple clusters in this study. Based on recent research, we may divide summarising techniques into four groups: statistics, machine learning, natural language processing, and hybrid approaches. Based on mathematical calculations that employ word frequency and sentence position in the text, the statistical technique [15, 16] provides a rank and a score to each phrase in the document. This approach has been used to find theme words, cue phrases, keywords from any given document. Various text processing approaches [17, 18] have been introduced in natural language processing techniques. Some of these techniques are well-known text processing techniques, like recognition of structural ambiguity (e.g., POS tagging, word meaning disambiguation) [19], lexical knowledge extraction [12], grammatical inference, and semantic relationship [20]. Such techniques are employed to interpret linguistic information since they are processed verbally and in writing. With the use of numerous natural language processing techniques and statistical measurements, D.R. Amancio et al. [21] introduced the usage of complex networks for creating extractive summarizers. In this study, vulnerability, proximity, and betweenness were found to be ineffective for selecting sentences for summarizers, however diversity measures were found to be effective. In the paper [22], the author Mendoza M suggested a boolean optimization method including numerous statistical characteristics such as location, sentence length, and the title of the text material for generating extractive summary. Genetic operators and local search approaches are used to build the summarizer in this work. Tas, Kiyani et al. [23] provided a comparative study of various text summarising approaches. In this survey paper, various text summarization methods namely, Query oriented and Generic Summarization, Neural Networks Based Text Summarization, Hidden Markov Model, Bayesian Classifier, and Fuzzy Logic Based Text Summarization were examined. S. T. Davis and colleagues [24] introduced a combinatorial optimization covering algorithm based multi-document summarization technique to pick sentences that cover the most weighted terms while minimising redundancy. In the paper [25], a multilingual summarization approach based on GA has been presented to generate extractive summaries using different sentence ranking methods. The research [26] introduced a graph-based summarization strategy based on graphical approach to create extractive summaries, where the modified TextRank similarity for all possible pairs of nodes was used to determine the weighting of the edge connecting them. If the summary contains more than one instance of a similar category of high-scoring content, the method's performance may be affected. Another graph-based summarising approach [27] described in constructs an extractive summary by employing infomap clustering of the whole document's visual analysis to discover and choose the most informative words for inclusion in the summary. The performance of the given text document can be improved by fine-tuning the noun-pronoun resolution. René Witte et al. [28] proposed fuzzy clustering based text summarization technique where fuzzy set theory helped to detect common and distinctive topics within a document set. To increase performance in the biomedical domain, any of these general text summarizers can be changed by considering domain specific notions for summarising. To train the summarizer, a variety of machine learning approaches such as neural networks [29], Bayesian topic models [30], and Markov chains [31] are used to extract key phrase segments based on feature vectors. Hybrid approaches are a combination of two or more of the methods outlined above. All these extractive generated summaries usually hold salient information of target reports and have a good performance with respect to human-written summaries. On the other hand, compared to extractive summarising, abstractive summarization is much more exact and effective in retrieving relevant information from many documents. Indicative [32] and informative [4] text summarising are two types of text summarization. An indicative summary highlights a document's main concept, whereas an informative summary provides enough elaboration of the major issues as well as some advice customised to the readers' requirements. The informative summarization technique was utilised to create a general [3] and query-based [33] summary. Generic summaries may communicate the generic theme of a document by incorporating the most content, whereas query-based summaries can answer a series of questions using a limited number of words from the text.

Just-the-news summaries [34] provide the most up-to-date information based on the readers' preferences. Multi-document summarization [35, 36] provides a summary by integrating sentences from numerous papers, whereas single-document summarization [37] creates a summary by using sentences from only one document. A topic-oriented summary [38] is created using the readers' subject of interest and information gathered from specific subjects. The centrality of the sentences is calculated in centrality-based summarization [39] using the importance of words that is largely depended on that clustered text's centroid. The document's core sentences the ones that are closest to the centroid. In current history, graph-based clustering approaches have been researched for automated text summarization.

In medical domain, content accuracy is very crucial. Previous work in biomedical text summarising has been relied on extractive methods, which frequently employ domain-specific criteria to score sentences in the target document. Plaza et al. [40] developed an extractive summarization system that employed machine learning and natural language processing (NLP) approaches to detect salient sentences in biomedical material. The work in [41] introduced an ensemble summurization approach in bio-medical domain. Here, various widely used clustering algorithms have been explored to generate the base summaries for the generation of desired ensemble extractive summary.

The abstracts of the target report and its referenced papers were used as the basis summaries in another ensemble extractive summarization approach [42] in the biomedical domain, and several multi-objective evolutionary algorithms were utilised in order to produce the desire ensemble summary. Previous work in biomedical text summarization has been focused on extractive approaches using domain-specific features such as Unified Medical Language Systems (UMLS) [43] to discover medical concepts and BioBERT [44] embedding to represent any biomedical report. There has been an increasing interest in text summarising approaches in the field of biomedical informatics. Between 1999 and 2005, Afantenos et al. [45] found eight biomedical text summarising approaches that have been published. Numerous freely accessible information sites and sources, including the UMLS [43], PubMed Central [46], and many more tools for natural language, such as cTAKES [47], MetaMap [48], and SemRep [49], have recently contributed to the bio-medical domain.

Rush et al. [50] and Nallapati et al. [51] proposed summarising approaches using words that are not found in the target report and reconstruct sentences to generate abstractive summary. For scientific document summarization, various features (e.g. citation networks) can be used to improve the performance. For tackling any optimization issue, Evolutionary Algorithms (EAs) with single and multi-objective are commonly utilised. In practise, however, most optimization techniques are inherently multi-objective since they demand a large number of competing objectives. Instead of a single best solution, a set of Pareto optimal options is examined in multi-objective optimization issues. NSGA [52], NSGA-II [53], MOEA/D [54], and other multi-objective evolutionary algorithms (MOEAs) efficiently solve multi-objective optimization problems in high-dimensional space. To extract essential elements from Arabic political papers, the paper [55] presented a hybrid, single-document text summary technique with the help of genetic algorithms (GAs), statistical characteristics, and domain knowledge. D.Y. Sakhare et al. [56] proposed a hybrid technique of text summarization that combines Dependency Grammar and the sentence features. M. S. Patil et al. [57] demonstrated a text summarising approach that increased the quality of the summary by cascading the clustering methodology with SVM.

The remaining work is split into three sections: Sect. 7.3 outlines the suggested technique for the proposed summary, and Sect. 7.4 elaborates on the experimental results and performance evaluation on the publicly available MEDLINE/PubMed dataset. Lastly, Sect. 7.5 brings this project to a close.

7.3 Proposed Methodology

In this chapter, an extractive summarization technique has been proposed using a hybrid method of fuzzy logic and nature inspired optimization algorithm. Here, we have considered MEDLINE/PubMed extracted medical reports as the target reports to be summarized. First the extracted reports have been preprocessed using some

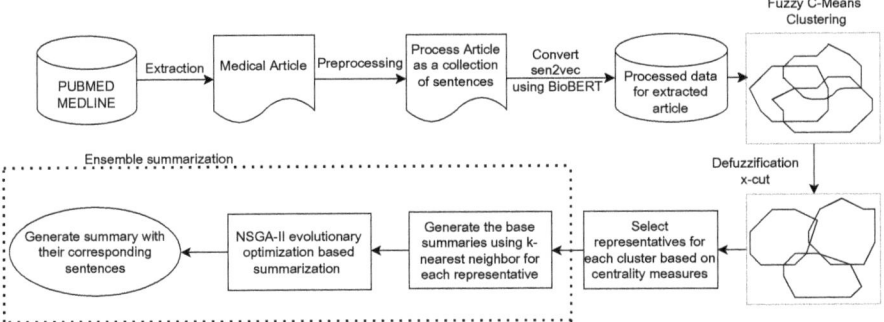

Fig. 7.1 Work flow of the Fuzzy theory based ensemble summarization

domain specific tools to make it easy for analysing the reports. Then, we have used BioBERT model [44] to vectorized the sentences of the processed reports. The entire proposed work has been separated into four different modules: (i) Preprocess the target report and convert each sentence into vector forms (i.e., Sen2Vecs) using BioBERT model [44], (ii) Cluster the sentences (i.e., sentence vectors) of the report into different partitions using Fuzzy C-Means clustering [13, 14], (iii) Apply defuzzification x-cut [58] to reduce the overlapping clustered area(i.e., to help to eliminate the repeated sentences from the summary) (iv) Select the representatives for each cluster using different centrality measures [59] and Generate the base summaries using k-nearest neighbor [60] for each centrality measure, and (vi) Generate ensemble summary sentences using NSGA-II [61] on the base summaries. Figure 7.1 shows the general design of the proposed ensemble summarizer.

7.3.1 Preprocessing

There are several information systems accessible in the biomedical area for data retrieval and reports preparation from the available dataset like MEDLINE/PubMed. To retrieve MEDLINE/PubMed information, this study employs the MEDLINE XML [62] repository and the PubMed Open-Access subset [63]. To begin, this repository has been used to retrieve metadata containing PubMedID. It aids in the extraction of full text of the target report as well as the MeSH [64], keywords for a specific PubMedID. Then, using the Natural Language ToolKit (NLTK) package [65], we lematize the remaining words after removing the stopwords from the collected raw text data. For biomedical reports to properly transmit clinical information, stopword removal and lemmatization are inadequate preparation techniques. It is necessary to examine the concepts for the terminology of medicine and surgery used in the papers. To do so, medical terminology were recognised, and their concepts were extracted using the python UMLS metathesaurus metamap wrapper [66], the 2018AB UMLS [67], and the 2018 version of MetaMap software. Figure 7.2 depicts the extracted

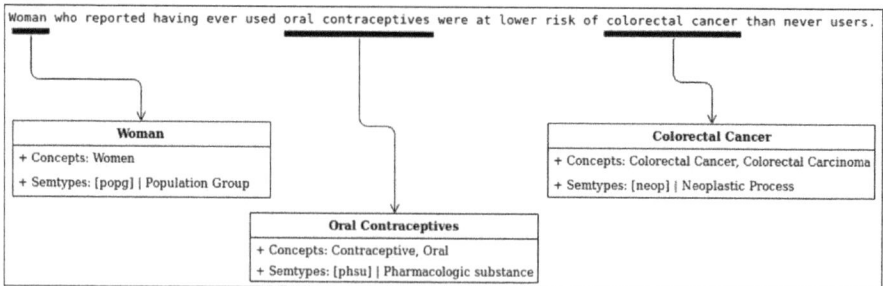

Fig. 7.2 Concepts of MeSH terms present in a report as determined by the UMLS Metathesaurus wrapper

concepts of MeSH words found in a report utilising the UMLS metathesaurus wrapper. Finally, the extracted concepts are substituted for the medical terms, and each phrase of the target report is represented by the set of concepts connected with the medical terms.

Then, the extracted concept vectors of the target report have been embedded using BioBERT representation model based on transfer learning concept. Basically, the BioBERT has been implemented to extract the features from a given report. Using a Bidirectional Encoder Representations from Transformers (BERT) [68] model, the weights of the BioBERT model are pre-trained using English Wikipedia and Books Corpus, as well as biomedical domain corpora such as PMC and MEDLINE/PubMed datasets. It has been used mainly for two different pretraining purposes: One is for Masked language modelling and another is for Next sentence prediction. In this module, we have used this embedding model for mask language modelling (i.e., the model tries to guess the original word contextually by masking a piece of each word). The preprocessed sentences are tokenized before feed into this BioBERT model. Since, the limit of the vocabulary size of BioBERT tokenizer model is 30,000, we have considered WordPiece model that generates a vocabulary with all English characters and the most common words and subwords found in the biomedical domain corpora. After tokenization, some original words have been split into subwords and characters as WordPiece model has been used in the BERT tokenizer. The architecture of the BioBERT has 12 layers with 768 hidden, 16 heads and 340M parameters. To get the embedded vectors for the words as well as for the sentences, we have considered the output of last 2 hidden layers. After embedding, the model generates a fixed size sentence vector for each sentence in the given document. Let, S be the set of the preprocessed sentences of the target report, where each sentence in S is represented by $s_i = (s_{i1}, s_{i2}, s_{i3} \ldots s_{i768})$ $\forall i$ after using BioBERT embedding.

7.3.2 Fuzzy C-Means Clustering

Fuzzy C-Means clustering has been used to discover comparable text vectors and partition the report based on similarity in this suggested work. As there is a possibility to overlap some concepts or medical terms of a sentence to another sentences. The fuzzy C-Means clustering has been taken into account for this work over the hard clustering to consider the overlapping nature of the cluster boundaries. C is the number of classes or clusters in the case of C-Means, and if the considered classes use fuzzy approach, the clustering is termed Fuzzy C-Means clustering. A fuzzy membership value has been assigned as the degree of membership for each class. This approach simplifies the formation of new clusters from the data points(i.e., sentence vectors s_i $\forall i$) that are similar to current classes in terms of membership values using three basic fuzzy operations : the fuzzy membership function, partition matrix and the objective function. Let us assume, S is a set of L number of sentence vectors (i.e., $S = (s_1, s_2, \ldots s_L)$ $2 \leq C \leq L$) for clustering into C classes or clusters. Each vector s_i represented by x real valued measurements (i.e., $s_i \in R^x$) for describing the features of the object s_i. The set of fuzzy partition matrices P_{fm} with dimension (CxL) is defined using Eq. (7.1).

$$P_{fm} = X \in R^{CL} | x_{ij} \in [0, 1] \forall i, j; \quad (7.1)$$

where $\sum_{i=1}^{C} x_{ij} = 1; \forall j$ and $\sum_{j=1}^{L} x_{ij} < L; \forall i$. As a result of this equation, it is evident that a single item may be assigned to several clusters, each with varying membership degrees (i.e., x_{ij}). Now, the objective function for Fuzzy C-Means clustering is defined in Eq. (7.2).

$$O_{fm} = \sum_{j=1; i=1}^{L;C} (x_{ij})^t (d_{ij})^2 \quad (7.2)$$

where $t \in (1, +\infty)$ and $d_{ij} = ||s_j - m_i||$ is the euclidean distance from object s_j to the center of the cluster m_i. So, the minimization of the objective function O_{fm} is performed by an iterative updation of fuzzy cluster centers (m_i) and partition matrix (x_{ij}^k)) defined in Eqs. (7.3) and (7.4).

$$m_i = \frac{\sum_{j=1}^{L} (x_{ij})^t s_j}{\sum_{j=1}^{L} (x_{ij})^t} \quad (7.3)$$

$$x_{ij}^k = \sum_{u=1}^{C} \frac{1}{[\frac{d_{ij}^k}{d_{uj}^k}]^{\frac{2}{t-1}}} \quad (7.4)$$

The step by step process of fuzzy C Means clustering is given by Algorithm (1). Finally, the membership value(μ_{ij}) of jth sample in ith cluster is defined in equation (7.5).

$$\mu_{ij} = [\sum_{k=1}^{C}(\frac{||s_j - m_i||}{||s_j - m_k||})^{\frac{2}{i-1}}]^{-1} \tag{7.5}$$

where C is the number of the cluster, s_j is the jth sample and m_i is the center of ith cluster.

Algorithm 1: Fuzzy C Means clustering

i: Initialize the number of clusters C.
ii: Initialize the set of fuzzy partition matrices P_{fm} with dimension (CxL).
iii: Initialize the cluster prototype Q^0 before the iteration and set iteration counter $count = 0$.
iv: Next calculate the partition matrix x_{ij}^{count} using (7.4).
v: Then calculate the fuzzy cluster centres m_i for $count$ and $count + 1$ using (7.3).
vi: Stop if $||m_i^{count} - m_i^{count+1}|| < \epsilon$ else continue from iii through v.

7.3.3 Defuzzification X-Cut

Defuzzification is the process of converting fuzzy membership to crisp value. In this work defuzzification helps to avoid repeated sentence in the summary by reducing the overlapping area. Here, x-cut method has been considered for defuzzification. In the preceding part, we have got the set of objects with their membership degree for the clusters and x-cut of that set is the subset that consists of the objects that belong to the considering fuzzy set with a membership degree greater or equal than a given value $\in [0, 1]$. Here, experimentally x is set to 0.4. So, the objects with membership degree less than 0.4 for a specific cluster have been removed from that cluster and so on. Gradually, this process reduce the overlapping area among the clusters.

7.3.4 Generate the Base Summaries

After defuzzification, some centrality measurements (graph theory concepts) were explored in order to determine the most influential sentence vector(s) from each cluster as the cluster representative(s). As a result, each cluster provides a set of representative sentence vectors. These representative sentence vectors help to create the base summaries. We employed several centrality measures [41], such as betweenness centrality, proximity centrality, harmonic centrality, node-degree centrality, communicability centrality, and eigenvalue centrality, to choose the representative set of phrase vectors from each cluster. For calculating these centrality measurements all the objects within the cluster have been represented in graph structure.

The betweenness centrality of a node is used to calculate the number of shortest paths in a network that pass through it. The amount of data that is anticipated to transit through the node is represented by this number. Closeness The average of the shortest path lengths from a node to all other nodes in the network is used to determine centrality, which shows how quickly information may pass from one graph node to the next. Closeness centrality is high if a node is close enough to all other nodes in the graph. The centrality of a node in a network is measured by its degree inside the graph. It displays the number of edges (connections) a node has in the graph. The node is more central if the node-degree centrality value is high. It shows which node in the network has the most similarities to other nodes in general. It does not always show which node is in the graph's "middle". Harmonic Centrality is a centrality statistic based on distance. It overcomes the problem of some graph centrality measurements that aren't linked. It gives a centrality metric for disconnected graphs as an alternative to proximity centrality. It also depicts how rapidly information flows from one node to the next in a network. Eigenvalue Centrality is used to determine the structural importance of a node in a network. The structural relevance of a node is connected neighbourhood determines its importance. It is determined by how many other relevant nodes in the graph are connected to that node. Centrality is calculated by counting the number of walks between each pair of nodes in a network. It's a statistic that measures how strongly each node in the network is linked to the others.

After selecting the representative sentence vectors, we apply k-nearest neighbors (i.e., kNN) algorithm [69] within the clusters for each representative using six different centrality measurements. Suppose, R_i is the set of all representatives using ith centrality where i is 1 to 6 for six different centrality measurements. Here, we have considered $k = 7$(experimentally). The target of kNN algorithm is to find the k closest points (min $||s_i - s_j||$) according to some distance metric, like euclidean, manhattan, etc.). Here, euclidean distance has been considered. The objects of the clusters have been sorted in ascending order based on the euclidean distance between the representative and others. Finally seven closest sentence vectors of the representative have been selected from each cluster which altogether form a base summary of the report for each centrality measure. So each centrality measure provides a base summary of the target report.

7.3.5 Nature Inspired Optimization

Selection, Crossover, and Mutation are the three basic genetic operations for most of the Nature Inspired Optimization methods where the solution of the optimisation problem relies on biologically inspired operators. The very first genetic operation is selection, which tries to choose stronger chromosomes from the population to serve as parents for future generations' children. Crossover and mutation operators are frequently employed to drive the population to one of the global optimal solutions by offering exploration and exploitation, respectively. For optimization, we have used the Non-dominated Sorting Genetic Algorithm II (NSGA-II). The goal is to find non-dominated solutions by storing and maintaining previously created non-dominated solutions in a mating pool. First, the original population for NSGA-II was established, as explained in the next subsection. Following population generation, chromosomes were ranked using the Fonseca-Fleming ranking [70] approach based on fitness functions, and non-dominated pareto fronts were formed, with ranked 1 chromosomes in the first front, ranked 2 chromosomes in the second front, and so on. In a Pareto optimization, there is no one objective function that determines the fitness of the several people. As a result, the Fonseca-Fleming ranking technique is adopted to rank the population in Pareto front based on "degree of dominance." These pareto fronts help to create mating pool in every iteration. Let, the first optimal pareto front size (i.e., p) is less than that of mating pool (i.e., m) then the entire front has been put into mating pool and the remaining $(m - p)$ has been filled up by the next pareto front and so on. A truncating procedure [71] has been applied to reduce the number of chromosomes until the front size is equal to the obtainable mating pool space if a front size greater than mating pool size. The next generation population has been created based on the crossover and mutation performed on the mating pool. The entire process has been repeated until it converges. The ultimate optimal solution was found by selecting a solution at random from the first pareto front of the last generation.

7.3.5.1 Creation of Initial Population

Initial population formation is critical in evolutionary algorithms [72]. An initial population of chromosomes is formed by generating a binary string from the base summaries at random. Hence each individual is treated as an individual ensemble summary. The initial population looks like:

$$initial\_population = \begin{bmatrix} & S_1 & S_2 & S_3 & S_4 & \ldots & S_m \\ ch_1 & 0 & 1 & 0 & 1 & \ldots & 0 \\ ch_2 & 1 & 1 & 0 & 0 & \ldots & 0 \\ \vdots & \vdots & & \ddots & & & \\ ch_M & 0 & 1 & 0 & 0 & \ldots & 1 \end{bmatrix}$$

where M is the population size and m is the number of base summaries which have been considered in the initial population creation. Each chromosome reflects the summaries that characterise the ensemble summary, with '0' or '1' in a chromosomal position denoting the lack or existence of the corresponding summary, respectively. These chromosomes were first thought to represent potential solutions for the proposed ensemble summarization technique. For a given iteration, all the '1's in a chromosome reflect summaries that have been taken into account for assessing the chromosomes' strength. After the technique has attained convergence, the best-fit chromosome of the proposed algorithm is the ideal solution. An ensemble summary of the target report is created by combining sentences from those selected summaries that correspond to the best chromosome.

7.3.5.2 Objective Function

This research employs just two objective functions depending on the multi-objective GA to assess the strength of a possible solution. Further down, the goal functions (also known as objective functions) are described.

a. The first objective function (f_{1i}) for i-th chromosomal solution is declared using Eq. (7.6), where L represents the size of summary and ch_i (l_1) indicates the number of '1' in the i-th chromosome (ch_i).

$$f_{1i} = |L - ch_i(l_1)| : ch_i(l_1) \leq L \qquad (7.6)$$

This objective function represents how much the candidate summary size that is close to the model's summary, which is required to be minimum for our proposed desired summarization technique.

b. It is critical to deliver the substance of the intended information without losing the entire context of any summary technique. The first objective function simply cares about the size of generated summary in comparison to the model summary size. As a result, the second objective function is the Information Gain (IG) [73, 74] of base summaries participating in the chromosomal ensemble summary. It indicates how much information about the target item a candidate summary may communicate. The decrease in chromosomal summary entropy relative to the entropy of the target item is used to calculate increasing the Information Gain. The computation of the second fitness function (f_{2i}) for i-th chromosome is defined using using Algorithm 2. The higher the value f_{2i}, the better the chromosome ch (i.e., the corresponding ensemble summary is improved). As a result, our goal is to maximise f_{2i} for more informative ensemble summary corresponding to the i-th chromosomal solution.

7.3.5.3 Pareto Front

The mating pool's chromosomes have been chosen from the non-dominated Pareto optimal front generated through the existing population based on objective functions in each iteration, as illustrated in Fig. 7.3.

In Fig. 7.3, f_1 and f_2 are two objective functions for NSGA-II optimization. This represents the solution space for above mentioned bi-objective optimization problem. In this optimization problem the target is to minimise f_1 and maximize f_2. Considering these two basic criteria, the solutions of B, C, D and E are better with respect to the solution points F and G. These four points (i.e., B, C, D and

Algorithm 2: Information gain of chromosomal ensemble summary

Step 1: Let C is the total number of concepts present in the target report, where d is the distinct unique concepts. Here, only the medical terms and the concepts have been taken into account to provide the medical information regarding the report as we have considered medical reports i.e., domain specific reports.

Step 2: Let, the number of i-th concept in the target report is c_i, for $i = 1, 2, ..., d$. Therefore, $C = \sum_{i=1}^{d} c_i$.

Step 3: The formula of expected information needed to describe the target report based on the extracted concepts is given by eq. (0.7).

$$I(c_1, c_2, \ldots c_d) = -\sum_{j=1}^{d} \frac{c_j}{C} \log_2 \frac{c_j}{C} \qquad (0.7)$$

Step 4: Let i-th chromosome ch_i of the population provides an ensemble of l_1 number of summaries $S_1, S_2, \ldots S_{l_1}$ of the target report.

Step 5: Let, the frequency of concept c_i is t_{ij} in summary S_j, for $j = 1, 2, \ldots l_1$. So, total number of concepts in summary S_j is $C_j = \sum_{i=1}^{d} t_{ij}$. Then the expected information needed to describe the summary S_j based on the available concepts present is given in eq. (0.8).

$$I(t_{1j}, t_{2j}, \ldots t_{dj}) = -\sum_{i=1}^{d} \frac{t_{ij}}{C_j} \log_2 \frac{t_{ij}}{C_j} \qquad (0.8)$$

Step 6: The entropy or expected information needed by the chromosome ch_i to describe the target report considering the summaries $S_1, S_2, \ldots S_{l_1}$ is given by eq. (0.9).

$$E(ch_i) = \sum_{j=1}^{l_1} \frac{\sum_{u=1}^{d} t_{uj}}{C} I(t_{1j}, t_{2j}, \ldots t_{dj}) \qquad (0.9)$$

The term $\frac{\sum_{u=1}^{d} t_{uj}}{C}$ acts as the weight of the summary S_j which is the total number of concepts in S_j divided by the total number of concepts in the target report. The smaller this entropy value, the greater the purity of the chromosome (i.e.; the ensemble summary).

Step 7: The encoding information that would be gained by the chromosome is considered as the second fitness function of the chromosome and is defined by eq. (0.10).

$$f_{2i} = I(t_{1j}, t_{2j}, \ldots t_{dj}) - E(ch_i) \qquad (0.10)$$

Step 8: return(f_{2i})

E) form a Non-dominated set or a Pareto optimal front namely, first Pareto front is shown by a dashed line. However, the solution points F and G are better with respect to the solution point H as the objective function f_1 for the point F much less than that of H similarly, the objective function f_1 for the point G is less than H also the objective function f_2 for the point G is higher than that of H. So, the solution point H is dominated by G and F as well as E, D, C and B. The solution point H represents the worse solution. The points F and G form second Pareto front i.e., a non-dominated Pareto Front with respect to the point H. With respect to two objective functions, solution point A is the strongly dominating solution

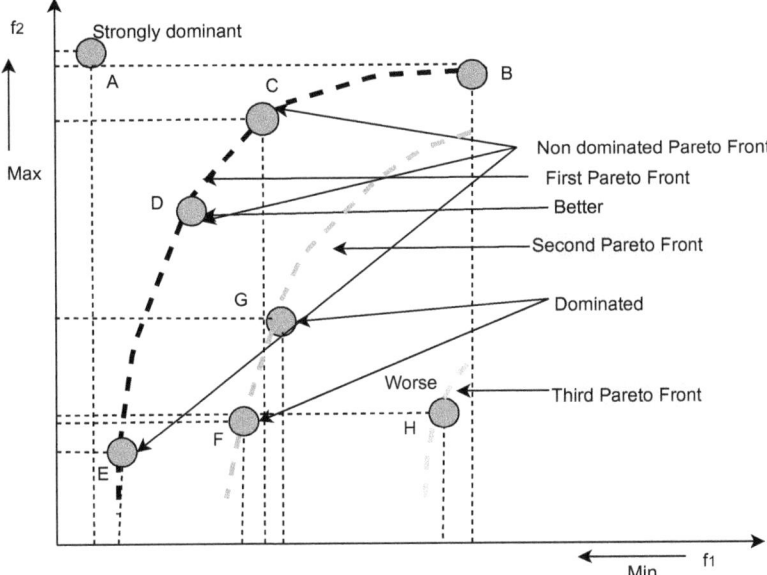

Fig. 7.3 Pareto optimal concept

when compared to all other alternatives. One of the randomly picked chromosomes from the best front of the final population is the ultimate solution. The sentences connected with the final optimal solution chosen and arranged in the target report according to their original arrangement. Finally, a synopsis of the ensemble has been created. Algorithm 3 outlines the proposed NSGA-II Algorithm based ensemble summarization approach.

7.4 Experimental Results

The scientific literature contains a wealth of useful information. Researchers and clinicians can access a number of sources in the biomedical sectors, including Electronic Health Record (EHR) systems, scientific literature databases, web papers, multimedia documents, and e-mailed reports. The proposed strategy has been thoroughly evaluated using citations from biomedical and life sciences journals in the MEDLINE/PubMed database. The US National Library of Medicine, MEDLINE/PubMed database, contains over 25 million references to journal reports in the living sciences, with a focus on biomedicine. For dataset preprocessing, we additionally employed Python 2.7[1] NLTK library [75]. The title, abstract, and metadata for a certain PubMedID can be found in the MEDLINE XML repository. Medical Subject Headings

---

[1] Python 2.7.14 documentation, https://docs.python.org/2/index.html.

Algorithm 3: Ensemble Summarization based on the NSGA-II algorithm

Input: I = the initial population of N binary chromosomes, each of length l; crossover probability Pr_c; mutation probability Pr_m
Output: S_{sum} = Summary of the target report.

1 **begin**
2   **repeat**
3   Rank the chromosomes of I using Fonseca-Fleming method;
4   External population, $E = \emptyset$;
5      $r = 1$;
6   P = Extract all chromosomes of rank R;
7   **repeat**
8   Move all chromosomes from P to E;
9        $r = r + 1$;
10   Extract all chromosomes of rank r to P;
11   **until** *(available space in $E < |P|$)*;
12   **if** *Remaining space in $E > 0$* **then**
13   Truncate P to size L;
14   Move all chromosomes from P to E;
15   **end**
16   I_{new} = Selected 15% chromosomes from E randomly;
17      $E = E - I_{new}$;
18   **repeat**
19   Select two chromosome from E i.e., Selection operation;
20   Generate two offspring chromosomes by performing uniform crossover with Pr_c probability;
21   Choose two best chromosomes among offspring and parent;
22   Put these two newly selected chromosomes into I_{new};
23   **until** I_{new} *contains all N chromosomes*;
24      $I = I_{new}$; /*Replace old population with new one*/
25   **until** *Population is not further modifiable*;
26   Rank the chromosomes of I using Fonseca-Fleming method;
27   ch_{best} = Select chromosome with rank 1 randomly;
28   Select sentences associated with sentence vectors in Ch_{best};
29   Using indices, rearrange sentences in their original order and save them in S_{sum};
30   **return** S_{sum};
31 **end**

(MeSH) terms, PubMedIDs of referenced publications, and other details for the specific report are included in the metadata. We utilised the Python UMLS metathesaurus metamap wrapper to recognise medical words in a report and extract the concepts of those medical terms as well as the MeSH terms. To create a corpus for our research, we used the MEDLINE/PubMed database, PubMed Open-Access subset, and MEDLINE XML repository to randomly choose 1500 biomedical published papers from five distinct classes: oral cancer, genome, heart disease, thalassemia, and brain tumours.

7.4.1 Experimental Setup

For implementing the NSGA-II algorithm with some selected parameters, we have utilised the PyGMO[2] tool. PyGMO was chosen for implementing evolutionary algorithms with lower CPU and memory utilisation during compilation, resulting in improved runtime performance. It also has a better NumPy integration and more widely used Python packages. On top of the Boost Graph Library, PyGMO allows you to construct User-defined topologies. Table lists the parameters of the evolutionary algorithm employed in the proposed approach (FES).

For implementing the NSGA-II algorithm with certain specified parameters, we utilised the PyGMO[3] tool. PyGMO was chosen for implementing evolutionary algorithms with lower CPU and memory utilisation during compilation, resulting in improved runtime performance. It also has a better NumPy integration and more widely used Python packages. On top of the Boost Graph Library, PyGMO allows you to construct User-defined topologies. Table 7.1 lists the parameters of the evolutionary algorithm employed in the proposed technique (FES). After analysing the algorithm on the MEDLINE/PubMed dataset numerous times, the following parameters of our proposed algorithm were chosen. We use the Python programming language to develop the suggested summarization technique, which runs 80 times and 600 generations each time on an HP Pentium core i5 processor PC.

The target size (L_{size}) of the summary is 10%, 15%, 20%, and 25% of the target report size, respectively. A comparative study of several state-of-the-art summarising approaches and the suggested methodology using specific statistical metrics aids the performance evaluation of our proposed method, which is described in the following subsections.

Table 7.1 The parameters of the proposed algorithm that must be satisfied

Parameter	Value
Population size (n)	600
Selection method	Binary tournament
Mutation method	Jumping gene
Crossover probability (Pr_c)	0.75
Mutation probability (Pr_m)	0.02
Maximum Generation	500

---

[2] Pygmo documentation, https://media.readthedocs.org/pdf/pygmo/newdocs/pygmo.pdf.
[3] Pygmo documentation, https://media.readthedocs.org/pdf/pygmo/newdocs/pygmo.pdf.

7.4.2 Performance Evaluation W.r.t ROUGE

(ROUGE) [76] stands for "Recall-Oriented Understudy for Gisting Evaluation" [26] that helps to evaluate the performance of summarising approach. The three ROUGE techniques with the highest usage rates are The ROUGE_N, ROUGE_L, ROUGE_W, and ROUGES_U [26]. In this chapter, we evaluated the effectiveness of the suggested summarising strategy using ROUGE N and ROUGE L.

7.4.2.1 ROUGE_N

ROUGE_N approach is for measuring N-gram ($N \geq 1$) recall between a collection of reference summaries and a system summary is the ROUGE_N approach. It calculates how fluent the summaries are and is defined by an Eq. (7.11).

$$ROUGE\_N = \frac{\Sigma_{serefsum} \Sigma_{gram_N \in S} count_{match}(gram_N)}{\Sigma_{serefsum} \Sigma_{gram_N \in S} count(gram_N)} \quad (7.11)$$

Here, $count(gramN)$ indicates the maximum number of N-grams that can appear simultaneously in a collection of reference summaries and a system summary, and N represents the size of the N-gram.. Because the value of N is regarded as 1 and 2, only ROUGE_1 and ROUGE_2 have been evaluated for assessment. ROUGE_1 and ROUGE_2 stand for the 1-gram and bi-gram overlap between the system and reference summaries.

7.4.2.2 ROUGE_L

The ROUGE_L[77] statistic, which is linked to longest sub sequences, is used to automatically identify the longest co-occurring N-grams. Assume that $G=(g_1, g_2, g_3, \ldots g_T)$ and $R=(r_1, r_2, r_3, \ldots r_S)$ are the system summary and reference summary sentences, respectively. The LCS (Longest Common Sequence) based F-value ($Flcs$) reflects the resemblance between G(of size T) and R(of size S), and according to equations (7.12), (7.13), and (7.14), the sequence of words indicates the resemblance between G(of size T) and R(of size S).

$$R_{lcs} = \frac{LCS(G, R)}{S} \quad (7.12)$$

$$P_{lcs} = \frac{LCS(G, R)}{T} \quad (7.13)$$

$$F_{lcs} = \frac{(1+\beta^2) R_{lcs} P_{lcs}}{(R_{lcs} + \beta^2 P_{lcs})} \quad (7.14)$$

where, LCS(G, R) indicates the size of the LCS of G and R and $\beta = P_{lcs}/R_{lcs}$.

7.4.2.3 Performance Measure

There is no unique corpus for biomedical summarising that we are aware of. The written abstracts provided by the researchers are generally considered as the golden summaries [78] of any scientific study. Therefore, the quality of the suggested technique has been evaluated using the written abstracts of the authors as model reference summaries of the publication. Additionally, we utilised the summary written by the specialist as the benchmark summary of that report to assess our proposed approach. The effectiveness of the summaries is also assessed for each of the 1500 MEDLINE/PubMed biomedical published reports using Eqs. (7.12), (7.13), and (7.14). The average values of performance measurement measures are shown in Tables 7.2 and 7.3, respectively, using an abstract as the model reference summary and a summary created by a specialist as the model reference summary.

For any reasonable summary size, the Rouge scores for Recall and Precision are essentially the same. However, as demonstrated in Tables 7.2 and 7.3, the summary size that includes 20% of the sentences from the reports produces better f-value Rouge scores than other summary sizes. The f-value Rouge score, which is more significant than the individual Recall and Precision Rouge scores, provides the weighted harmonic mean of Recall and Precision. This shows that the recommended FES approach produces a summary with a summary size of 20% that is almost exact to the ground truth summary for the original report.

Table 7.2 Rouge scores derived by the proposed FES approach considering the abstract as reference summary

Size	10%			15%		
ROUGE score	Recall	Precision	f-value	Recall	Precision	f-value
R_1	0.4720	0.4901	0.5180	0.4120	0.5102	0.4490
R_1	0.3580	**0.5121**	0.4303	0.3810	0.4180	0.4020
R_{LCS}	0.3330	0.2009	0.2304	0.3021	0.2300	0.2420
Size	20%			25%		
ROUGE score	Recall	Precision	f-value	Recall	Precision	f-value
R_1	**0.5823**	**0.5894**	**0.5842**	0.5021	0.5199	0.5089
R_2	**0.4113**	**0.4893**	**0.4412**	0.4105	0.4924	0.4312
R_{LCS}	**0.3298**	**0.3114**	**0.3109**	0.3394	0.2393	0.2014

Table 7.3 Rouge scores derived by the proposed FES approach considering specialist written summary as reference summary

Size	10%			15%		
Rouge score	Recall	Precision	f-value	Recall	Precision	f-value
R_1	**0.7801**	0.6521	0.7127	0.6750	**0.7905**	**0.7352**
R_2	0.6730	0.5658	0.6072	0.6596	0.7244	0.6745
R_{LCS}	**0.7556**	0.6334	0.6898	0.5971	0.6887	0.6430
Length	20%			25%		
Rouge score	Recall	Precision	f-value	Recall	Precision	f-value
R_1	0.7319	0.7291	0.7311	0.7056	0.6349	0.6651
R_2	**0.7161**	0.7017	**0.7091**	0.6832	**0.7217**	0.6955
R_{LCS}	0.7234	**0.7483**	**0.7428**	0.6801	0.7109	0.6790

Table 7.4 Comparing FES with different techniques for the reports based on oral cancer while using the abstract as a reference summary

Rouge score		Approaches							
		RS [79]	TTS [80]	CS [81]	WS [82]	FS [83]	CSS [84]	LS [85]	FES
Recall	R_1	0.5610	0.5345	0.3780	0.4610	0.4090	0.4850	0.3830	**0.5791**
	R_2	0.3918	0.3876	0.4320	0.4031	0.4120	**0.4249**	0.3712	0.4024
	R_{LCS}	0.3294	0.3300	0.3120	0.2646	0.2900	0.3004	0.3110	**0.4110**
Precision	R_1	0.5796	0.5893	0.5460	0.5670	0.5630	0.5200	0.5640	**0.6100**
	R_2	**0.4991**	0.4801	0.4570	0.4730	0.4240	0.3670	0.4120	0.4321
	R_{LCS}	0.2983	0.2998	0.2378	0.2787	0.2830	0.2120	0.2039	**0.3230**
f-value	R_1	0.5702	0.5600	0.5288	0.4984	0.5159	0.4976	0.5078	**0.5927**
	R_2	0.4239	0.4237	0.4150	0.4030	0.3890	0.3750	0.4006	**0.4553**
	R_{LCS}	0.3070	0.3010	0.2310	0.2890	0.2270	0.2290	0.2130	**0.3345**

7.4.3 Compare Performance with Different Summarising Approaches W.r.t ROUGE

Some existing state-of-the-art text summarization approaches, such as Lex-Rank summarisation (RS) [79], Textrank summarization (TTS) [80], ClusterRank summarization (CS) [81], Graph-of-words-based summarization (WS) [82], FreqRank summarization (FS) [83], Correlation SumBasic summarization (CSS) [84], and Latent Semantic Analysis for summarization (LS) [85], are considered to assess the efficacy of the proposed FES method. These methods are utilised to generate automatic text summaries for biomedical reports, and Rouge scores are used to compare them to the proposed FES method.

Table 7.4 through Table 7.8 illustrate the Rouge scores of the results obtained by the other approaches, using a summary size of 20% of the size of original report and

Table 7.5 Comparing FES with different techniques for reports based on genome while using the abstract as a reference summary

Rouge score		Approaches							
		RS [79]	TTS [80]	CS [81]	WS [82]	FS [83]	CSS [84]	LS [85]	FES
Recall	R_1	0.5485	0.5600	0.4550	0.3800	0.4210	0.3850	0.4830	**0.5641**
	R_2	0.3896	0.3928	0.4010	0.4020	0.4120	**0.4252**	0.3700	0.4111
	R_{LCS}	0.3294	0.3300	0.3120	0.2646	0.2810	0.3004	0.3110	**0.3450**
Precision	R_1	0.5796	0.5893	0.5460	0.5670	0.5590	0.5200	0.5640	**0.5899**
	R_2	**0.4991**	0.4801	0.4570	0.4730	0.4312	0.3670	0.4120	0.4814
	R_{LCS}	0.2983	0.2998	0.2378	0.2787	0.2960	0.2120	0.2039	**0.3352**
f-value	R_1	0.5702	0.5600	0.5288	0.4984	0.5349	0.4976	0.5078	**0.5937**
	R_2	0.4239	0.4237	0.4150	0.4030	0.3980	0.3750	0.4006	**0.4565**
	R_{LCS}	0.3070	0.3010	0.2310	0.2890	0.2450	0.2290	0.2130	**0.3452**

an abstract as the model summary since it delivers a superior result for the suggested method, as shown in Table 7.2. Tables 7.9, 7.10, 7.11, 7.12 and 7.13 demonstrate the Rouge scores for several summarizers, using a summary size of 20% of the original report and a specialist written summary as the model summary since it delivers a superior result for the proposed technique, as shown in Table 7.3. Tables 7.4, 7.5, 7.6, 7.7, 7.8, 7.9, 7.10, 7.11, 7.12 and 7.13 show the average results of 1500 biomedical published reports on oral cancer, genome, heart disease, thalassemia, and brain tumours, respectively. These tables show that the proposed summarizer (FES) has the highest average Rouge score (marked as bold faced) in the majority of cases, with only a few cases where the Rouge scores for Lex-Rank summarisation (RS) [79] and Latent Semantic Analysis for summarization (LS) [85] are higher than the proposed summarizer, and that all other methods are strictly dominated by the proposed summarizer (FES) based on Rouge scores.

Tables 7.4, 7.5, 7.6, 7.7, 7.8, 7.9, 7.10, 7.11, 7.12 and 7.13 indicate that our proposed FES method outperforms existing summary methods in the majority of summarising approaches, demonstrating the importance of our proposed summarization method. At the time of evaluation, a number of statistical measurement metrics, including recall, precision, and F-value, are examined for accuracy measurement.

7.5 Conclusion and Future Direction

For extractive summarization, the proposed method uses a hybrid way of text summarization technique that combined fuzzy theory followed by a nature-inspired optimization algorithm-based approach. The length of the ensemble summary is one objective function, and the information gain of the candidate chromosome is another objective function in the proposed bi-objective Nondominated Sorting genetic algo-

Table 7.6 Comparing FES with different techniques for reports based on heart disease while using the abstract as a reference summary

Rouge score		Approaches							
		RS [79]	TTS [80]	CS [81]	WS [82]	FS [83]	CSS [84]	LS [85]	FES
Recall	R_1	0.5485	0.5600	0.4550	0.3800	0.4010	0.3850	0.4830	**0.5970**
	R_2	0.3896	0.3928	0.4010	0.4210	0.4020	0.3700	**0.4522**	0.4005
	R_{LCS}	0.3294	0.3300	0.3120	0.2646	0.2870	0.3004	0.3110	**0.3929**
Precision	R_1	0.5796	0.5893	0.5460	0.5670	0.5390	0.5200	0.5640	**0.6010**
	R_2	**0.4991**	0.4801	0.4570	0.4730	0.4430	0.3670	0.4120	0.4931
	R_{LCS}	0.2983	0.2998	0.2378	0.2787	0.2570	0.2120	0.2039	**0.3102**
f-value	R_1	0.5702	0.5600	0.5288	0.4984	0.5439	0.4976	0.5078	**0.5916**
	R_2	0.4239	0.4237	0.4150	0.4030	0.3980	0.3750	0.4006	**0.4430**
	R_{LCS}	0.3070	0.3010	0.2310	0.2890	0.2190	0.2290	0.2130	**0.3091**

Table 7.7 Comparing FES with different techniques for reports based on thalassemia while using the abstract as a reference summary

Rouge score		Approaches							
		RS [79]	TTS [80]	CS [81]	WS [82]	FS [83]	CSS [84]	LS [85]	FES
Recall	R_1	0.5485	0.5600	0.4550	0.3800	0.4010	0.3850	0.4830	**0.5777**
	R_2	0.3896	0.3928	0.4010	0.4120	0.4100	0.3700	**0.4252**	0.4009
	R_{LCS}	0.3294	0.3300	0.3120	0.2646	0.2820	0.3004	0.3110	**0.3340**
Precision	R_1	0.5796	0.5893	0.5460	0.5670	0.5540	0.5200	0.5640	**0.5911**
	R_2	**0.4991**	0.4801	0.4570	0.4730	0.4180	0.3670	0.4120	0.4894
	R_{LCS}	0.2983	0.2998	0.2378	0.2787	0.2710	0.2120	0.2039	**0.3201**
f-value	R_1	0.5702	0.5600	0.5288	0.4984	0.5219	0.4976	0.5078	**0.5840**
	R_2	0.4239	0.4237	0.4150	0.4030	0.3980	0.3750	0.4006	**0.4325**
	R_{LCS}	0.3070	0.3010	0.2310	0.2890	0.2420	0.2290	0.2130	**0.3091**

rithm II. The approach has been tested on MEDLINE/PubMed biomedical reports and has shown to be effective. The suggested technique increases feature extraction in the biomedical field by vectorizing each sentence in the text. In this proposed method, Fuzzy C-Means algorithm helps to consider some common concepts and medical terms while clustering the sentences and it improve the quality of the generated summary. Here, NSGA-II also helps the model in fast and efficient convergence of the considering optimization problem.

Other evolutionary algorithms, such as SPEA2 (i.e., an enhanced SPEA) [71], are capable of combining a compact fitness assignment approach that considers density. In order to summarise biomedical literature, we may additionally include specific lexical links between medical terms, and any graph-based summarising technique may be supplied to boost the accuracy. Healthcare researchers and scientists may find

7 Hybridization of Fuzzy Theory and Nature-Inspired …

Table 7.8 Comparing FES with different techniques for reports based on brain tumors while using the abstract as a reference summary

Rouge score		Approaches							
		RS [79]	TTS [80]	CS [81]	WS [82]	FS [83]	CSS [84]	LS [85]	FES
Recall	R_1	0.5485	0.5600	0.4550	0.3800	0.4010	0.3850	0.4830	**0.5727**
	R_2	0.3896	0.3928	0.4010	0.4120	0.4100	0.3700	**0.4252**	0.4019
	R_{LCS}	0.3294	0.3300	0.3120	0.2646	0.2820	0.3004	0.3110	**0.3341**
Precision	R_1	0.5796	0.5893	0.5460	0.5670	0.5540	0.5200	0.5640	**0.5913**
	R_2	**0.4991**	0.4801	0.4570	0.4730	0.4180	0.3670	0.4120	0.4794
	R_{LCS}	0.2983	0.2998	0.2378	0.2787	0.2710	0.2120	0.2039	**0.3204**
f-value	R_1	0.5702	0.5600	0.5288	0.4984	0.5219	0.4976	0.5078	**0.6011**
	R_2	0.4239	0.4237	0.4150	0.4030	0.3980	0.3750	0.4006	**0.4335**
	R_{LCS}	0.3070	0.3010	0.2310	0.2890	0.2420	0.2290	0.2130	**0.3092**

Table 7.9 Comparing FES with different techniques for reports based on oral cancer while using the specialist written summary as a reference summary

Rouge score		Approaches							
		RS [79]	TTS [80]	CS [81]	WS [82]	FS [83]	CSS [84]	LS [85]	FES
Recall	R_1	0.5485	0.5600	0.4550	0.3800	0.4010	0.3850	0.4830	**0.5777**
	R_2	0.3896	0.3928	0.4010	0.4120	0.4100	0.3700	**0.4252**	0.4009
	R_{LCS}	0.3294	0.3300	0.3120	0.2646	0.2820	0.3004	0.3110	**0.3340**
Precision	R_1	0.5796	0.5893	0.5460	0.5670	0.5540	0.5200	0.5640	**0.5991**
	R_2	**0.4991**	0.4801	0.4570	0.4730	0.4180	0.3670	0.4120	0.4884
	R_{LCS}	0.2983	0.2998	0.2378	0.2787	0.2710	0.2120	0.2039	**0.3301**
f-value	R_1	0.5702	0.5600	0.5288	0.4984	0.5219	0.4976	0.5078	**0.5940**
	R_2	0.4239	0.4237	0.4150	0.4030	0.3980	0.3750	0.4006	**0.4425**
	R_{LCS}	0.3070	0.3010	0.2310	0.2890	0.2420	0.2290	0.2130	**0.3191**

Table 7.10 Comparing FES with different techniques for reports based on genome while using the specialist written summary as a reference summary

Rouge score		Approaches							
		RS [79]	TTS [80]	CS [81]	WS [82]	FS [83]	CSS [84]	LS [85]	FES
Recall	R_1	0.5485	0.5600	0.4550	0.3800	0.4010	0.3850	0.4830	**0.5797**
	R_2	0.3896	0.3928	0.4010	0.4120	0.4100	0.3700	**0.4252**	0.4209
	R_{LCS}	0.3294	0.3300	0.3120	0.2646	0.2820	0.3004	0.3110	**0.4340**
Precision	R_1	0.5796	0.5893	0.5460	0.5670	0.5540	0.5200	0.5640	**0.5961**
	R_2	**0.4991**	0.4801	0.4570	0.4730	0.4180	0.3670	0.4120	0.4394
	R_{LCS}	0.2983	0.2998	0.2378	0.2787	0.2710	0.2120	0.2039	**0.4201**
f-value	R_1	0.5702	0.5600	0.5288	0.4984	0.5219	0.4976	0.5078	**0.5840**
	R_2	0.4239	0.4237	0.4150	0.4030	0.3980	0.3750	0.4006	**0.4525**
	R_{LCS}	0.3070	0.3010	0.2310	0.2890	0.2420	0.2290	0.2130	**0.5091**

Table 7.11 Comparing FES with different techniques for reports based on heart disease while using the specialist written summary as a reference summary

Rouge score		Approaches							
		RS [79]	TTS [80]	CS [81]	WS [82]	FS [83]	CSS [84]	LS [85]	FES
Recall	R_1	0.5485	0.5600	0.4550	0.3800	0.4010	0.3850	0.4830	**0.6777**
	R_2	0.3896	0.3928	0.4010	0.4120	0.4100	0.3700	**0.5252**	0.4009
	R_{LCS}	0.3294	0.3300	0.3120	0.2646	0.2820	0.3004	0.3110	**0.4340**
Precision	R_1	0.5796	0.5893	0.5460	0.5670	0.5540	0.5200	0.5640	**0.6911**
	R_2	**0.4991**	0.4801	0.4570	0.4730	0.4180	0.3670	0.4120	0.4294
	R_{LCS}	0.2983	0.2998	0.2378	0.2787	0.2710	0.2120	0.2039	**0.4201**
f-value	R_1	0.5702	0.5600	0.5288	0.4984	0.5219	0.4976	0.5078	**0.6840**
	R_2	0.4239	0.4237	0.4150	0.4030	0.3980	0.3750	0.4006	**0.5325**
	R_{LCS}	0.3070	0.3010	0.2310	0.2890	0.2420	0.2290	0.2130	**0.4091**

Table 7.12 Comparing FES with different techniques for reports based on thalassemia while using the specialist written summary as a reference summary

Rouge score		Approaches							
		RS [79]	TTS [80]	CS [81]	WS [82]	FS [83]	CSS [84]	LS [85]	FES
Recall	R_1	0.5485	0.5600	0.4550	0.3800	0.4010	0.3850	0.4830	**0.5779**
	R_2	0.3896	0.3928	0.4010	0.4120	0.4100	0.3700	**0.4252**	0.4009
	R_{LCS}	0.3294	0.3300	0.3120	0.2646	0.2820	0.3004	0.3110	**0.3390**
Precision	R_1	0.5796	0.5893	0.5460	0.5670	0.5540	0.5200	0.5640	**0.5991**
	R_2	**0.4991**	0.4801	0.4570	0.4730	0.4180	0.3670	0.4120	0.4899
	R_{LCS}	0.2983	0.2998	0.2378	0.2787	0.2710	0.2120	0.2039	**0.3291**
f-value	R_1	0.5702	0.5600	0.5288	0.4984	0.5219	0.4976	0.5078	**0.5890**
	R_2	0.4239	0.4237	0.4150	0.4030	0.3980	0.3750	0.4006	**0.4395**
	R_{LCS}	0.3070	0.3010	0.2310	0.2890	0.2420	0.2290	0.2130	**0.3099**

Table 7.13 Comparing FES with different techniques for reports based on brain tumors while using the specialist written summary as a reference summary

Rouge score		Approaches							
		RS [79]	TTS [80]	CS [81]	WS [82]	FS [83]	CSS [84]	LS [85]	FES
Recall	R_1	0.5485	0.5600	0.4550	0.3800	0.4010	0.3850	0.4830	**0.5787**
	R_2	0.3896	0.3928	0.4010	0.4120	0.4100	0.3700	**0.4252**	0.4089
	R_{LCS}	0.3294	0.3300	0.3120	0.2646	0.2820	0.3004	0.3110	**0.3380**
Precision	R_1	0.5796	0.5893	0.5460	0.5670	0.5540	0.5200	0.5640	**0.5981**
	R_2	**0.4991**	0.4801	0.4570	0.4730	0.4180	0.3670	0.4120	0.4884
	R_{LCS}	0.2983	0.2998	0.2378	0.2787	0.2710	0.2120	0.2039	**0.3281**
f-value	R_1	0.5702	0.5600	0.5288	0.4984	0.5219	0.4976	0.5078	**0.5880**
	R_2	0.4239	0.4237	0.4150	0.4030	0.3980	0.3750	0.4006	**0.4385**
	R_{LCS}	0.3070	0.3010	0.2310	0.2890	0.2420	0.2290	0.2130	**0.3098**

the suggested automated summarizer valuable in keeping up to speed on new study findings with the least amount of work necessary. Clinical researchers and clinicians may raise the standard of their laboratories and develops intelligent healthcare system as a result of this.

References

1. Mehta, F.: Machine learning techniques for document summarization: A survey (2016)
2. Yadav, C.S., Sharan, A: Hybrid approach for single text document summarization using statistical and sentiment features. Int. J. Inf. Retr. Res. (IJIRR) **5**(4), 46–70 (2015)
3. Gong, Y., Liu, X.: Generic text summarization using relevance measure and latent semantic analysis. In: Proceedings of the 24th Annual International ACM SIGIR Conference on Research and Development in Information Retrieval, pp. 19–25. ACM (2001)
4. Saggion, H., Lapalme, G.: Generating indicative-informative summaries with sumum. Comput. Linguist. **28**(4), 497–526 (2002)
5. Dunning, T.: Accurate methods for the statistics of surprise and coincidence. Comput. Linguist. **19**(1), 61–74 (1993)
6. Eduard, H., Lin, C.Y.: Automated text summarization and the summarist system. In Proceedings of a Workshop on held at Baltimore, Maryland, 13–15 October 1998, pp. 197–214. Association for Computational Linguistics (1998)
7. Christian, H., Agus, M.P., Suhartono, D.: Single document automatic text summarization using term frequency-inverse document frequency (TF-IDF). ComTech: Comput. Math. Eng. Appl. **7**(4), 285–294 (2016)
8. Nagwani, N.K., Verma, S.: A frequent term and semantic similarity based single document text summarization algorithm. Int. J. Comput. Appl. **17**(2), 36–40 (2011)
9. Sarkar, K.: Using domain knowledge for text summarization in medical domain. Int. J. Recent Trends Eng. **1**(1), 200 (2009)
10. Rai, A., Sangwan, S., Goel, T., Verma, I., Dey, L.: Query specific focused summarization of biomedical journal articles. In: 2021 16th Conference on Computer Science and Intelligence Systems (FedCSIS), pp. 91–100. IEEE (2021)
11. Lin, C.Y., Hovy, E.: The automated acquisition of topic signatures for text summarization. In: Proceedings of the 18th Conference on Computational Linguistics, vol. 1, pp. 495–501. Association for Computational Linguistics (2000)
12. Mallick, C., Dutta, M., Das, A.K., Sarkar, A., Das, A.K: Extractive summarization of a document using lexical chains. In: Soft Computing in Data Analytics, pp. 825–836. Springer (2019)
13. Nayak, J., Naik, B., Behera, H.S.: Fuzzy c-means (fcm) clustering algorithm: a decade review from 2000 to 2014. In: Computational Intelligence in Data Mining, vol. 2, pp. 133–149 (2015)
14. Deng, J., Hu, J.L., Chi, H., Wu, J.: An improved fuzzy clustering method for text mining. In: 2010 Second International Conference on Networks Security, Wireless Communications and Trusted Computing, vol. 1, pp. 65–69. IEEE (2010)
15. Knight, K., Marcu, D.: Statistics-based summarization-step one: Sentence compression. AAAI/IAAI **2000**, 703–710 (2000)
16. Jing, H., McKeown, M.: Cut and paste based text summarization. In: *1st Meeting of the North American Chapter of the Association for Computational Linguistics* (2000)
17. Navigli, R., Velardi, P.: Structural semantic interconnections: A knowledge-based approach to word sense disambiguation. IEEE Trans. Pattern Anal. Mach. Intell. **27**(7), 1075–1086 (2005)
18. Pustejovsky, J., Anick, P., Bergler, S.: Lexical semantic techniques for corpus analysis. Comput. Linguist. **19**(2), 331–358 (1993)
19. Wacholder, N., Ravin, Y., Choi, M.: Disambiguation of proper names in text. In: Fifth Conference on Applied Natural Language Processing, pp. 202–208 (1997)

20. Chowdhary, K.R.: Natural language processing. In: Fundamentals of Artificial Intelligence, pp. 603–649. Springer (2020)
21. Amancio, D.R., Nunes, M.G.V., Oliveira Jr., O.N., Costa, L.D.F.: Extractive summarization using complex networks and syntactic dependency. Phys. A Stat. Mech. Appl. **391**(4), 1855–1864 (2012)
22. Mendoza, M., Bonilla, S., Noguera, C., Cobos, C., León, E.: Extractive single-document summarization based on genetic operators and guided local search. Expert Syst. Appl. **41**(9), 4158–4169 (2014)
23. Tas, O., Kiyani, F.: A survey automatic text summarization. PressAcademia Procedia **5**(1), 205–213 (2007)
24. Davis, S.T., Conroy, J.M., Schlesinger, J.D.: Occams–an optimal combinatorial covering algorithm for multi-document summarization. In: 2012 IEEE 12th International Conference on Data Mining Workshops, pp. 454–463. IEEE (2012)
25. Litvak, M., Last, M., Friedman, M.: A new approach to improving multilingual summarization using a genetic algorithm. In: Proceedings of the 48th Annual Meeting of the Association for Computational Linguistics, pp. 927–936. Association for Computational Linguistics (2010)
26. Mallick, C., Das, A.K., Dutta, M., Das, A.K., Sarkar, A.: Graph-based text summarization using modified textrank. In: Soft Computing in Data Analytics, pp. 137–146. Springer (2019)
27. Dutta, M., Das, A.K., Mallick, C., Sarkar, A., Das, A.K.: A graph based approach on extractive summarization. In: Emerging Technologies in Data Mining and Information Security, pp. 179–187. Springer (2019)
28. Witte, R., Bergler, S.: Fuzzy clustering for topic analysis and summarization of document collections. In: Conference of the Canadian Society for Computational Studies of Intelligence, pp. 476–488. Springer (2007)
29. Kaikhah, K.: Automatic text summarization with neural networks. In: Proceedings of the 2004 2nd International IEEE Conference Intelligent Systems, vol. 1, pp. 40–44 (2004)
30. Daumé III, H.: Bayesian query-focused summarization. Preprint at arXiv:0907.1814 (2009)
31. Nenkova, A., Maskey, S., Liu, Y.: Automatic summarization. In Proceedings of the 49th Annual Meeting of the Association for Computational Linguistics: Tutorial Abstracts of ACL 2011, HLT '11, pp. 3:1–3:86, Stroudsburg, PA, USA (2011). Association for Computational Linguistics
32. Kan, M.Y., McKeown, K.R., Klavans, J.L.: Applying natural language generation to indicative summarization. In: Proceedings of the 8th European Workshop on Natural Language Generation, vol. 8, pp. 1–9. Association for Computational Linguistics (2001)
33. Tang, J., Yao, L., Chen, D.: Multi-topic based query-oriented summarization. In: Proceedings of the 2009 SIAM International Conference on Data Mining, pp. 1148–1159. SIAM (2009)
34. Yeh, J.Y., Ke, H.R., Yang, W.P., Meng, I.H.: Text summarization using a trainable summarizer and latent semantic analysis. Inf. Process. Manag. **41**(1), 75–95 (2005)
35. Goldstein, J., Mittal, V., Carbonell, J., Kantrowitz, M.: Multi-document summarization by sentence extraction. In: *Proceedings of the 2000 NAACL-ANLP Workshop on Automatic Summarization*, pp. 40–48. Association for Computational Linguistics (2000)
36. Wan, X., Yang, J., Xiao, J.: Using cross-document random walks for topic-focused multi-document. In: 2006 IEEE/WIC/ACM International Conference on Web Intelligence (WI 2006 Main Conference Proceedings)(WI'06), pp. 1012–1018. IEEE (2006)
37. Litvak, M., Last, M.: Graph-based keyword extraction for single-document summarization. In: Proceedings of the Workshop on Multi-source Multilingual Information Extraction and Summarization, pp. 17–24. Association for Computational Linguistics (2008)
38. Harabagiu, S., Lacatusu, F.: Topic themes for multi-document summarization. In: *Proceedings of the 28th Annual International ACM SIGIR Conference on Research and Development in Information Retrieval*, pp. 202–209. ACM (2005)
39. Nenkova, A., McKeown, K.: A survey of text summarization techniques. In: Mining Text Data, pp. 43–76. Springer (2012)
40. Plaza, L., Díaz, A., Gervás, P.: A semantic graph-based approach to biomedical summarisation. Artif. Intell. Med. **53**(1), 1–14 (2011)

41. Mallick, C., Das, A.K., Ding, W., Nayak, J.: Ensemble summarization of bio-medical articles integrating clustering and multi-objective evolutionary algorithms. Appl. Soft Comput. **106**, 107347 (2021)
42. Mallick, C., Das, A.K., Nayak, J., Pelusi, D., Vimal, S.: Evolutionary algorithm based ensemble extractive summarization for developing smart medical system. Interdisc. Sci. Comput. Life Sci. **13**(2), 229–259 (2021)
43. Unified medical language system (umls). https://www.nlm.nih.gov/research/umls/. Accessed 28 Feb 2019
44. Lee, J., Yoon, W., Kim, S., Kim, D., Kim, S., So, C.H., Kang, J.: Biobert: a pre-trained biomedical language representation model for biomedical text mining. Bioinformatics **36**(4), 1234–1240 (2020)
45. Afantenos, S., Karkaletsis, V., Stamatopoulos, P.: Summarization from medical documents: A survey. Artif. Intell. Med. **33**(2), 157–177 (2005)
46. Pubmed central. https://www.ncbi.nlm.nih.gov/pmc/. Accessed 28 Feb 2019
47. Savova, G.K., Masanz, J.J., Ogren, P.V., Zheng, J., Sohn, S., Kipper-Schuler, K.C., Chute, C.G.: Mayo clinical text analysis and knowledge extraction system (ctakes): architecture, component evaluation and applications. J. Am. Med. Inf. Assoc. **17**(5), 507–513 (2010)
48. Aronson, A.R., Lang, F.M.: An overview of metamap: Historical perspective and recent advances. J. Am. Med. Inf. Assoc. **17**(3), 229–236 (2010)
49. Rindflesch, T.C., Fiszman, M.: The interaction of domain knowledge and linguistic structure in natural language processing: interpreting hypernymic propositions in biomedical text. J. Biomed. Inf. **36**(6), 462–477 (2003)
50. Rush, A.M., Chopra, S., Weston, J.: A neural attention model for abstractive sentence summarization. Preprint at arXiv:1509.00685 (2015)
51. Nallapati, R., Zhou, B., Gulcehre, C., Xiang, B., et al.: Abstractive text summarization using sequence-to-sequence rnns and beyond. Preprint at arXiv:1602.06023 (2016)
52. Inza, I., Larrañaga, P., Saeys, Y.: A review of feature selection techniques in bioinformatics. Bioinformatics **23**(19), 2507–2517 (2007)
53. Mitra, P., Murthy, C.A., Pal, S.K.: Unsupervised feature selection using feature similarity. IEEE Trans. Pattern Anal. Mach. Intell. **24**(3), 301–312 (2002)
54. Song, L., Smola A., Gretton, A., Borgwardt, K.M., Bedo, J.: Supervised feature selection via dependence estimation. In: Proceedings of the 24th International Conference on Machine Learning, ICML '07, pp. 823–830. ACM, New York, NY, USA (2007)
55. Al-Radaideh, Q.A., Bataineh, D.Q.: A hybrid approach for arabic text summarization using domain knowledge and genetic algorithms. Cogn. Comput. **10**(4), 651–669 (2018)
56. Sakhare, D.Y., Kumar, R: Syntactic and sentence feature based hybrid approach for text summarization. Int. Inf. Technol. Comput. Sci. **2014**(3), 38–46 (2014)
57. Patil, M.S., Bewoor, M.S., Patil, S.H.: A hybrid approach for extractive document summarization using machine learning and clustering technique. Int. J. Comput. Sci. Inf. Technol. **5**(2), 1584–1586 (2014)
58. Grosan, C., Abraham, A.: Fuzzy expert systems. In: Intelligent Systems, pp. 219–260. Springer (2011)
59. Iezzi, D.F.: Centrality measures for text clustering. In: Communications in Statistics-Theory and Methods vol. 41(16–17), pp. 3179–3197 (2012)
60. Kozma, L.: k nearest neighbors algorithm (knn). Helsinki Univ. Technol. **32** (2008)
61. Li, H., Zhang, Q.: Multiobjective optimization problems with complicated pareto sets, MOEA/D and NSGA-II. IEEE Trans. Evol. Comput. **13**(2), 284–302 (2009)
62. Medline xml repository. https://www.nlm.nih.gov/databases/download/data_distrib_main.html. Accessed 28 Feb 2019
63. Pubmed open-access (oa) subset. https://www.ncbi.nlm.nih.gov/pmc/tools/ftp/. Accessed 28 Feb 2019
64. Mesh (medical subject headings). https://www.nlm.nih.gov/mesh/meshhome.html. Accessed 28 Feb 2019
65. Loper, E., Bird, S.: Nltk: The natural language toolkit. Preprint at arXiv:cs/0205028 (2002)

66. Umls metathesaurus metamap. https://www.nlm.nih.gov/research/umls/implementation_resources/metamap.html. Accessed 28 Feb 2019
67. 2018ab umls. https://www.nlm.nih.gov/research/umls/knowledge_sources/metathesaurus/release/abbreviations.html (2018). Accessed 28 Feb 2019
68. Sun, C., Qiu, X., Xu, Y., Huang, X.: How to fine-tune bert for text classification? In: China National Conference on Chinese Computational Linguistics, pp. 194–206. Springer (2019)
69. Steinbach, M., Tan, P.N.: knn: k-nearest neighbors. In: The Top Ten Algorithms in Data Mining, pp. 165–176. Chapman and Hall/CRC (2009)
70. Fonseca, C.M., Fleming, P.J.: An overview of evolutionary algorithms in multiobjective optimization. Evol. Comput. **3**(1), 1–16 (1995)
71. Zitzler, E., Laumanns, M., Thiele, L.: Spea2: Improving the strength pareto evolutionary algorithm. TIK-report 103 (2001)
72. Soumen Kumar Pati and Asit Kumar Das: Ensemble classifier design selecting important genes based on extracted features. Int. J. Data Min. Bioinform. **19**(2), 117–149 (2017)
73. Xia, X., Lo, D., Qiu, W., Wang, X., Zhou, B.: Automated configuration bug report prediction using text mining. In: 2014 IEEE 38th Annual Computer Software and Applications Conference, pp. 107–116. IEEE (2014)
74. Yang, Y., Pedersen, J.O.: A comparative study on feature selection in text categorization. In: Icml, vol. 97, p. 35 (1997)
75. Bird, S., Klein, E., Loper, E.: Natural Language Processing with Python. O'Reilly (2009)
76. Haque, M.M., Pervin, S., Begum, Z.: Enhancement of keyphrase-based approach of automatic bangla text summarization. In: 2016 IEEE Region 10 Conference (TENCON), pp. 42–46. IEEE (2016)
77. Mallick, C., Das, S., Das, A.K.: Evolutionary algorithm based summarization for analyzing covid-19 medical reports. In: Understanding COVID-19: The Role of Computational Intelligence, pp. 31–58. Springer (2022)
78. Reeve, L.H., Han, H., Brooks, A.: The use of domain-specific concepts in biomedical text summarization. Inf. Process. Manage. **43**, 1765–1776 (2007)
79. Erkan, G., Lexrank, D.R.R.: Graph-based lexical centrality as salience in text summarization. J. Artif. Intell. Res. **22**, 457–479 (2004)
80. Mihalcea, R., Tarau, P.: Textrank: Bringing order into text. In: Proceedings of the 2004 Conference on Empirical Methods in Natural Language Processing (2004)
81. Garg, N., Favre, B., Reidhammer, K., Hakkani-Tür, D.: Clusterrank: A graph based method for meeting summarization. In: Tenth Annual Conference of the International Speech Communication Association (2009)
82. Tixier, A., Skianis, K., Vazirgiannis, M.: Gowvis: A web application for graph-of-words-based text visualization and summarization. In: Proceedings of ACL-2016 System Demonstrations, pp. 151–156 (2016)
83. Luong, A.V., Tran, N.T., Ung, V.G., Nghiem, M.Q.: Word graph-based multi-sentence compression: Re-ranking candidates using frequent words. In: 2015 Seventh International Conference on Knowledge and Systems Engineering (KSE), pp. 55–60. IEEE (2015)
84. Nenkova, A., Vanderwende, L.: The impact of frequency on summarization. Microsoft Research, Redmond, Washington, Tech. Rep. MSR-TR-2005, 101 (2005)
85. Steinberger, J., Jezek, K.: Using latent semantic analysis in text summarization and summary evaluation. Proc. ISIM **4**, 93–100 (2004)

Chapter 8
An Optimistic Bayesian Optimization Based Extreme Learning Machine for Polycystic Ovary Syndrome Diagnosis

H. Swapnarekha, Pandit Byomakesha Dash, Janmenjoy Nayak, and Ashanta Ranjan Routray

Abstract The most prevalent endocrine disorder that exist in 5 to 10% of the women during their fertility period is the polycystic ovarian syndrome (PCOS). Women having PCOS problem are associated with serious consequences of health issues such as heart disease, obesity, infertility, ovarian cancer, type 2 diabetes and so on. To prevent the risks associated with PCOS, there is a need to develop prediction models for the accurate identification of PCOS at early stage. This chapter aims in developing prediction model based on ELM (Extreme learning machine) and Bayesian optimization algorithm for the detection of PCOS at early stage. The class imbalance problem has been overcome using a strategy known as random over-sampling. In this approach, Bayesian optimization is employed to choose the best hyperparameters of the models. The proposed architecture has been evaluated using PCOS dataset obtained from Kaggle. Further, the efficacy of the proposed ELM and Bayesian optimization algorithm has been compared with SVM, MLP, ELM and ELM and Genetic algorithm. The experimental results reveal that ELM and Bayesian optimization attained better performance of 99.31% accuracy when compared with other machine learning approaches.

Keywords Polycystic ovary syndrome · Extreme machine learning · Bayesian optimization · Healthcare · Machine learning

---

H. Swapnarekha · P. B. Dash (✉)
Department of Information Technology, Aditya Institute of Technology and Management, Tekkali 532201, India
e-mail: byomakeshdash2000@gmail.com

J. Nayak
Department of Computer Science, Maharaja Sriram Chandra Bhanja Deo (MSCBD) University, Mayurbhanj, Odisha 757003, India

A. R. Routray
Department of ICT, F. M. University, Balasore, Odisha, India

© The Author(s), under exclusive license to Springer Nature Switzerland AG 2023
J. Nayak et al. (eds.), *Nature-Inspired Optimization Methodologies in Biomedical and Healthcare*, Intelligent Systems Reference Library 233,
https://doi.org/10.1007/978-3-031-17544-2_8

8.1 Introduction

Polycystic ovarian syndrome (PCOS) also known as 'polycystic ovarian disease' is the most prevalent endocrine health problem in the fertility period of women [1]. In 1935, Stein and Leventhal originally defined the term Polycystic ovary syndrome [2]. It is basically represented by 12 or more follicles having diameter of 2-9 mm [3]. Approximately 5 to 10% of the women in their fertility period are affected with the PCOS [4]. It was reported that the predominance of PCOS in white women is 4.8% and 8% in African women [5, 6]. Women having PCOS suffer with problems of hormonal imbalance and metabolism that may impact the overall appearance and health of the women. PCOS is also considered as one of the frequent causes of infertility in women fertility period due to the inappropriate growth of follicles in the ovary at early stage [7]. In addition, women having PCOS disorder are inherent with high risk of type 2 diabetes mellitus, ovarian cancer, high blood pressure, cardiovascular disease and obesity [8–12]. Furthermore, several studies shows that women having PCOS are associated with the risk of miscarriage in first trimester of their pregnancy [13]. The following Figs. 8.1 and 8.2 represents the most prevalent risks and factors associated with PCOS. Therefore, it is necessary to detect the patients diagnosed with PCOS at early stage to avoid the risk factors associated with the disease.

Due to the advancement of technology, computing technology performs a crucial role in the diagnosis of disease in healthcare sector. In recent years, Machine learning (ML) algorithms have gained popularity in solving real life applications of distinct domains because of their ability to learn patterns from the observed data without being explicitly programmed. As machine learning approaches have been vastly used in the analysis of health data and efficient diagnosis, treatment and prevention of diseases, these techniques are gaining prominent importance in the biomedical and healthcare

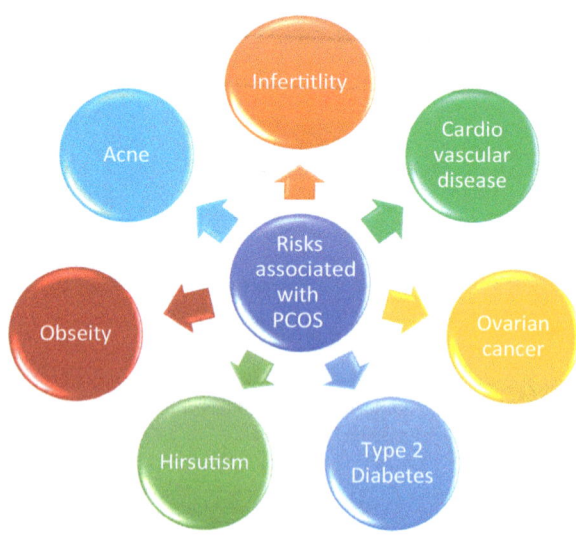

Fig. 8.1 Risks associated with PCOS

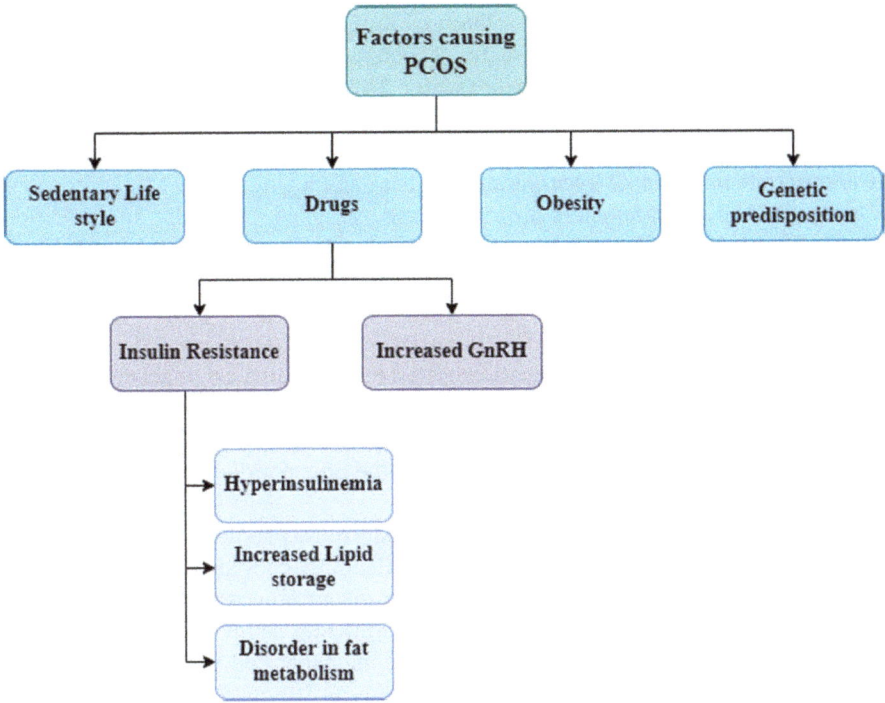

Fig. 8.2 Factors causing PCOS [14]

industry. Moreover, it also assists in successful decision-making process in the healthcare sector as it is capable of extracting hidden patterns in the database. Kumar et al. [15] have suggested a novel method that makes use of machine learning approaches for the efficient automatic diagnosis of disease. The suggested model is used for the efficient diagnosis of diabetes, cardiovascular and coronavirus disease. The proposed model collects the data through android app. Then logistic regression approach is used to perform the analysis of data for accurate prediction of disease. Finally, the model has been evaluated using COVID-19, diabetes and heart disease dataset and the results indicate logistic regression outperformed other machine learning approaches on three datasets in terms of accuracy and F1 measure.

Though machine learning approaches have been used in the efficient diagnosis and prediction of disease, they require more computational time. As artificial neural network depends on the principle of risk minimization, it also gets easily stuck into the local minima problem. To overcome these problems, a new algorithm known as ELM has been popularized by Huang [16] for SLFNs (single hidden layer feedforward neural networks). The weights of the output layer are decided by the ELM using MP (Moore–Penrose) generalized inverse by randomly choosing the weights of the input layer and hidden biases. ELM not only offers high performance with fast learning but also provides parameter tuning. Due to its advantages, ELM has been broadly used in diagnosis of various diseases [17–19]. Due to the availability of voluminous data from different data sources in health care sector, it becomes a challenging task to handle the prevalence information of the healthcare sector. This demands the need of developing more advanced machine learning approaches along with optimization techniques for the efficient handling of large volumes of data in healthcare industry [20]. Moreover, the appropriate selection of hyperparameters is a challenging task in ML approaches as most of the hyperparameters are continuous variables. Generally, the selection of hyper parameters is done on trial-and-error basis. However, such approach needs long time and sometimes it may not lead to optimized solutions. In recent years, Bayesian optimization has raised as an efficient approach for proper selection of hyperparameters in the models. The Bayesian optimization approach needs only less computational time for the selection of best hyperparameters when compared to other approaches. This strategy is particularly useful when the calculation of objective function is very costly. Therefore, the objective of proposed work is to make use of ELM and Bayesian optimization approach for the efficient diagnosis of polycystic ovarian syndrome at early stage.

The remaining sections of the paper is organized as follows. The analysis of works carried on the detection of PCOS using ML approaches have been represented in Sect. 8.2. Section 8.3 provides a description of the proposed methodology and dataset used in the experimentation. The experimental setup and analysis of the results has been described in Sect. 8.4. Finally, the paper end with conclusion and future scope in Sect. 8.5.

8.2 Related Work

PCOS is a condition that leads to hormonal disorder among women. It can lead to infertility problems in reproductive age group of women if not treated in early stage. This section represents a brief description of the several research works performed on diagnosis of PCOS using various machine learning approaches. Silva et al. [21] recommended a data driven approach for the efficient diagnosis of PCOS in women. The suggested approach makes use of CatBoost, voting soft and voting hard classifiers on the dataset consisting of PCOS data of 177 women. The dataset consists of 43 distinct characteristics for the identification of PCOS in women. Initially, the authors have identified the most relevant features of PCOS using feature elimination and univariate feature selection approaches for the accurate prediction of PCOS. Then the ratio of FSH (Follicle-stimulating hormone) to LH (Luteinizing hormone) is considered as the most significant character for the prediction of PCOS based on the ranking of the characteristics. The suggested approach has been evaluated on top most 13 significant features using cross validation method and the results indicate that soft voting attained better accuracy of 91.12% in the prediction of PCOS when compared with other ensemble classifiers.

To build a diagnostic model for PCOS based on the gene biomarkers, two ML approaches such as artificial neural network (ANN) and random forest (RF) has been suggested by Xie et al. [22]. The gene expression data has been collected from Geo (Gene Expression Omnibus) that consists of 76 samples of PCOS and 57 samples of normal. The suggested approach makes use of five different datasets (two datasets for training model, two datasets for testing model and one dataset for evaluating DEGs (differentially expressed genes)). Initially, 12 genes were identified as vital from 264 DEGs for classification of PCOS and normal shapes using RF. Then, the weight of these 12 vital genes were calculated by ANN using RNA-seq and microarray training dataset. Moreover, diagnostic models known as neuralPCOS have been constructed for these two datasets. Finally, the diagnostic models have been evaluated using testing datasets and the results reveal that the developed models attained better AUC of 0.7273 on microarray dataset and 0.6488 on RNA-seq dataset.

Gopalakrishnan. C & M. Iyapparaja [23] has suggested an efficient automatic computer-aided PCOS classification and detection system that is capable of analyzing unaffected and affected areas of PCOS from the ultrasound medical images. The suggested framework makes use of Gaussian low pass filter for pre-processing the input ultrasound images, multilevel thresholding approach for the segmentation of image and proposed GIST-MDR approach for the feature extraction. Moreover, it also makes use of supervised machine learning algorithms such as Support Vector Machine (SVM), RF, Naïve Bayes (NB) and Linear Discriminant analysis (LDA) for the categorization of PCOS. Finally, the model has been evaluated and the results indicate that the GIST-MDR attains an accuracy of 93.82, 89.7, 91.05 and 88.26% with SVM, RF, NB and LDA respectively.

For the classification of follicles that assist in the diagnosis of PCOS, a novel approach based on ANN and IFFOA (Improved Fruit Fly Optimization) has been recommended by Nilofer et al. [24]. Initially, the input images are resized and noise from the images has been removed to enhance the quality of image. Then the follicles segmentation is performed by applying adaptive k-means clustering algorithm. Moreover, the technique makes use of statistical GLCM approach for the extraction of features. Finally, IFFOA-ANN model is trained with obtained features to perform the classification of follicles. From the experimental outcomes, it is concluded that IFFOA-ANN attains an accuracy of 97.5% in the classification of follicles which further assist in the detection of PCOS effectively.

For the automatic detection of PCOS in early stage, a novel forecasting model based on SMOTE (Synthetic Minority Oversampling Technique) and machine learning approaches such as RF, Decision Tree (DT), SVM, K-Nearest Neighbour (KNN) and Logistic Regression (LR) has been developed by Dutta et al. [25]. Basically, the suggested framework consists of three layers. The responsibility of handling oversampling and missing values in the dataset is done by the first layer of framework. The second layer is responsible for finding most significant characters of the dataset using PCA (Principal component analysis) approach. Finally, the third layer is used for the deployment of the model. The model has been evaluated using PCOS dataset consisting of 541 instances and the results show that SMOTE based LR attained better performance in terms of 97.11% accuracy, 98% F1 score, 98% sensitivity,

98% precision and 95.6% AUROC (Area under Receiver Operating Characteristic). The following Table 8.1 provides an analysis of other literature works carried on the detection of PCOS using ML approaches.

Table 8.1 Analysis of other works performed on detection of PCOS using ML approaches

Author & Year	Approach	Dataset used	Results	Limitation	Ref
Zigarelli et al. [26]	CatBoost	Health information of 541 women obtained from 10 distinct hospitals in Kerala, India	Achieved prediction accuracy of 87.5% - 90.1% using both invasive and non-invasive predictor variables	Different diagnostic criteria have been used to diagnose PCOS patients	[22]
Rachana et al. [27]	Decision Tree, Naïve Bayes, SVM, KNN	50 ultrasound images of PCOS	Accuracy of KNN = 97%	Requires more computational time	[26]
Bharati et al. [28]	Gradient boosting, RF, RFLR (hybrid random forest and logistic regression) and LR	Dataset consist of 43 features of 541 instances of women out of which 177 instances of women are with PCOS disease	RFRL attains recall of 91.01% and accuracy of 91.01% using 40-fold cross validation	Different datasets have not been used for the validation of the model	[28]
Nandipati et al. [29]	KNN, SVM, RF, Adaboost, Bagging, Naïve bayes, Neural network	Dataset consisting of 541 instances with 42 attributes	Accuracy of RF using Rapidminer on complete dataset = 93.12%	Does not consider the nature of dataset	[29]
Prapty et al. [30]	KNN, SVM, RF and Naïve Bayes	Dataset consisting of 542 instances out of which 177 are instances of PCOS patients and remaining are normal instances	Accuracy of RF = 93.5%	Only considered 7 features out of 31 features	[30]

8.3 Proposed Work

In this segment, a detailed description of the proposed framework and the working of ELM and Bayesian optimization approaches has been presented.

8.3.1 Extreme Learning Machine

ELM is a kind of a SLFN resulting from the elimination of backpropagation in a multilayer perceptron [31]. It produces a nonlinear model with processing speed that is comparable to the processing speed of a linear model. In contrast to SLFN, ELM does not alter the weights by making use of back propagation or other iterative methods. There is no randomness in the weights, which are set analytically. Multi-hidden-layer networks are treated equally by ELM, unlike BP (Back Propagation) and SVM, which interpret them as a black box. ELM treats multi-hidden-layer networks as white boxes that are taught layer-by-layer. Unlike Deep Learning, which involves rigorous adjustments in hidden layers as well as in hidden neurons, hierarchical ELM does not require repeated tuning of all hidden neurons. ELM theories demonstrate that, while hidden neurons are essential (for both SLFNs and multi-hidden layer networks), they are not required to be tuned repeatedly for learning to occur [17]. Numerous domains [32–34] such as neurocomputing [35, 36], healthcare [37], energy estimate [38], cost forecasting [39], and others [40, 41] use ELM for a variety of purposes.

An ELM output function for a generalised SFLN with one output node can be described as in Eq. (8.1):

$$f_L(X) = \sum_{i=1}^{N} w_i h_i(X) = h(X)w \tag{8.1}$$

where $\omega = [\omega_1,\ldots, \omega_N]^T$, T is a vector containing the weights between the hidden layer of N nodes and the output node, and the hidden layer's output (row) vector is called $h(x) = [h1(X),\ldots, hL(X)]$. In reality, h(X) is a feature mapping since it transfers data from the d-dimensional input space to the N-dimensional hidden-layer of ELM feature space H. The decision function of the ELM for binary classification applications is shown in Eq. (8.2).

$$f_L(X) = sign(h(X)w) \tag{8.2}$$

ELM tends to attain the least norm of output layer weights in addition to the shortest training error, while conventional learning algorithms prefer to merely achieve the smallest training error. According to Bartlett's hypothesis, the lower the weight norms are for a feedforward neural network with a smaller training error, the better the networks' generalisation performance tends to be. We hypothesise that this may be true for generalised SLFNs in which the buried layer may not include identical neurons. ELM aims to minimise both the training error and the output weights' mean.

Minimize: $\|H\omega - T\|2$ and $\|\omega\|$

$$H = \begin{bmatrix} h(x_1) \\ \cdot \\ \cdot \\ \cdot \\ h(x_m) \end{bmatrix} = \begin{bmatrix} h_1(x_1) & \ldots & h_N(x_1) \\ \cdot & \ldots & \cdot \\ \cdot & \ldots & \cdot \\ \cdot & \ldots & \cdot \\ h_1(x_M) & \ldots & h_N(x_M) \end{bmatrix} \qquad (8.3)$$

where H is the hidden-layer output matrix represented in Eq. (8.3).

When seen from the point of view of $f_L(X)$, reducing the norm of the output weights means increasing the distance between the margins that define the two distinct classes in the ELM feature space: $2/\|\omega\|$. In the initial implementation of ELM [42], the minimum norm least square approach was used instead of the conventional optimisation method as shown in Eq. (8.4).

$$W = H^{\Psi}T \qquad (8.4)$$

8.3.2 Bayesian Optimization (BO)

Convex functions, which may be easily evaluated and have a well-established mathematical form, are often assumed in many optimization situations. To alter hyperparameters, the objective function is unknown and uses computationally expensive nonconvex function [43]. As a result, common optimization techniques like the Newton method and gradient descent are unsuccessful. In general, the goal of optimization is to discover a utmost value at the sampling point of an unknown function as shown in Eq. (8.5).

$$P^+ = argmax \vartheta(P) \qquad (8.5)$$

$$P \in \varnothing$$

where $\varnothing$ signifies the search space of P, and P+ indicates the location where ϑ, the unknown objective function is maximised. P represents a sample point.

This kind of optimization issue is well-suited to the use of BO [44]. With the use of the Bayesian formula, prior knowledge regarding unknown function ϑ is combined with sample points to provide posterior information about the function distribution. The global optimum value is then determined [45] based on this posterior knowledge.

8 An Optimistic Bayesian Optimization ...

BO has two primary responsibilities [46]. The Gaussian process (GP) is widely used for data fitting and function posterior distribution updates because of its high degree of flexibility and tractability. A multivariate Gaussian distribution on $\Re^z$ is implied by any finite set of Z points $p_z \in \varnothing{}^Z{}_{z=1}$. The marginals and conditionals are calculated using the assumption that the z-th point represents the value of the function $\vartheta(p_z)$. It is also possible to choose the next evaluation point based on the results of an acquisition function (AC). For simplicity, let's assume the function $\vartheta(p)$ is constructed from the posterior distribution of a GP function, and our observations are of the type $\xi n^Z{}_{z=1}$, where $\xi_z \sim N(\vartheta(p_z), \nu)$ is the z-th observed model performance and is the noise variance. Following this, the posterior function $\alpha(p)$ is used as a proxy optimization to determine which point it should be evaluated next, using $p_{next} = \text{argmax}_p \alpha(p)$. Model-dependent functions $\varpi(p)$ are used in this case to forecast the function's predictive mean and its predictive variance $\sigma^2(p)$.

A variety of methods, including the anticipated enhancement, probability of enhancement, and GP-UCB (GP upper confidence bound) [47], may be employed to solve AC. GP-UCB is used to assess whether the prevailing optimum value (corresponding to the high $\varpi(p)$) or additional low-confidence zones (corresponding to the high $\sigma(p)$ zone) that results in high performance in tuning of hyperparameters should be utilised for the next sample point. The choice of parameter k is based on these considerations. A formula for the function is as follows: Eq. (8.6).

$$\alpha_{UCB}(p) = \vec{\omega}(p) - k\sigma(p) \qquad (8.6)$$

Algorithm 1 [48] provides a description of the BO algorithm. Two components comprise the whole algorithm: updating the posterior distribution (Steps 3.3 and 3.4) and optimising the acquisition function (Step 3.1).

	Algorithm 1: Bayesian optimization algorithm
Step 1:	Randomly generate the initial population
Step 2:	Calculate the fitness of individuals

Step 3:	while (termination condition not satisfied) do
	Step 3.1: Find p_z by optimizing acquisition function $\alpha(p)$ over function ϑ
	$p_z = argmax_p \alpha(p \mid \varnothing_{1:z-1})$
	Step 3.2: Sample the objective function $\vartheta(p_z)$
	Step 3.3: Data is augmented using $\varnothing_{1:z} = \{\varnothing_{1:z-1}, (p_z, \vartheta(p_z))\}$
	Step 3.4: Update the posterior distribution of function ϑ
	End while

Step 4:	Report the best solution

8.3.3 Proposed ELM + BO Method

The ELM + BO model is put together by going through the first four phases outlined below. Also, the work flow diagram of proposed ELM + BO model is shown in Fig. 8.3.

Step 1—Finding suitable objective function is necessary for optimization. In order to develop the ELM model, initialization parameters are chosen in accordance with Eqs. (8.1) to (8.4). In addition, a five-fold cross-validation is performed to optimise hyperparameters using the BO approach. A root mean squared error with fivefold cross validation serves as the objective function.

Step 2—Establish the hyperparameters' search domain space. BO optimises the ELM parameters. n_hidden (p1), activation_func (p2), rbf_width (p3) and alpha (p4). One combination point of initialization hyperparameters is indicated as p = (p1, p2, p3, p4). The optimal ELM hyperparameters are determined within the following ranges:

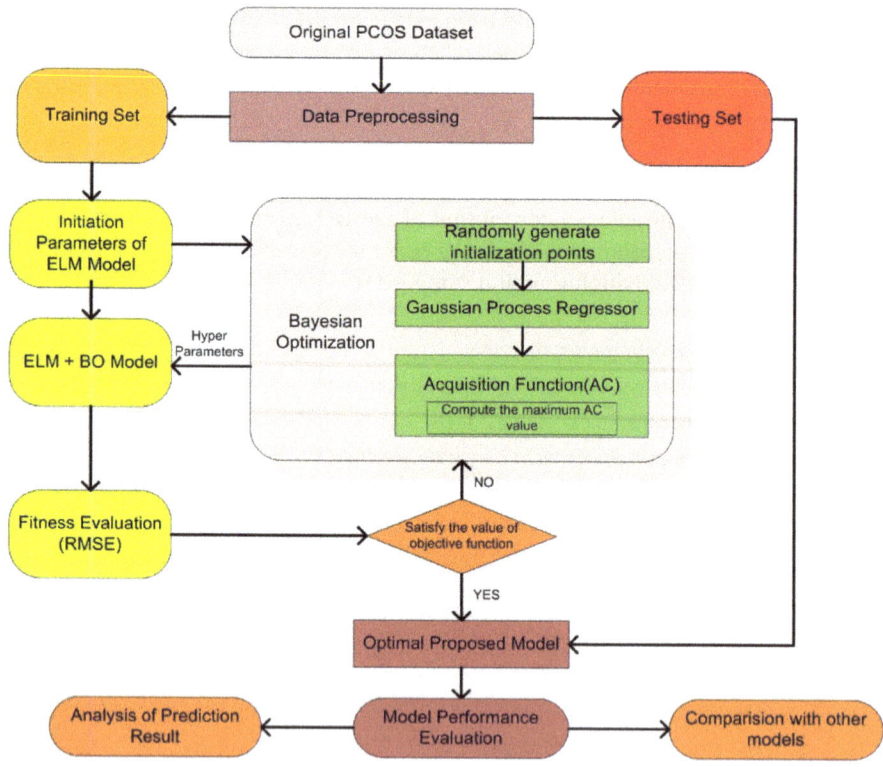

Fig. 8.3 Work flow of ELM + BO Model

- Number of hidden layer nodes - p1 = [20,40,60]
- Activation Function–p2 ['tanh', 'tribas', 'sigmoid', 'hardlim', 'softlim', 'sine', 'gaussian']
- rbf_width- p3 = [1.0,2.0,3.0,4.0,5.0,6.0,7.0]
- alpha – p4 = [0.5,0.1,0.2,0.3,0.4,0.6,0.7].

Step 3—Maximal optimization of hyperparameters. A probabilistic model is constructed using the Gaussian process, and the next set of hyperparameters are chosen by maximising an extraction function in order to evaluate the objective function. There is no limit to how many times a pattern may be repeated.

Step 4—keep a record of the iteration's output. In addition to hyperparameter values and ELM verification error, the results of each set of candidate hyperparameters are saved.

8.4 Discussion of Result Analysis and Simulation Setup

On the basis of an ensemble ELM with Bayesian optimization, this section describes the experimental setup and results of evaluating the suggested system.

8.4.1 Dataset Overview and Environmental Setup

The PCOS dataset that was used for the purpose of this investigation was obtained from the Kaggle repository [49]. The PCOS original dataset has 541 occurrences and 42 characteristics, one of which is file number of patient (not taken into consideration for data analysis). The last point to make is that there are a total of 41 characteristics, 40 of which are input attributes, and one of which is a class label called PCOS [Positive (Yes) and Negative (No)]. An Intel(R) Core (TM) i3-1115G4 @ 3.00 GHz in a 64-bit operating system, a CPU running at around 3.00 GHz, and 8 gigabytes of random access memory are used in the experiment, which is carried out on a machine that is operating on Windows 10 Pro. In order to carry out data preparation tasks and other classification strategies, such as machine learning and ensemble learning methods, amongst others, Sklearn and other Python programming frameworks are used. In order to finish the tasks involving data analysis, the frameworks numpy and pandas were used. The Matplotlib and seaborn frameworks were used in the creation of the data visualisation capabilities that are included in this module. By using a strategy known as random oversampling, Imblearn is able to resolve the problem of class imbalance that was previously present.

Table 8.2 Performance metrics of prediction models

Prediction models	Performance metrics				
	Precision	Recall	ROC-AUC	F1 Score	Accuracy
SVM	0.9264	0.9843	0.9616	0.9545	95.89
MLP	0.9402	0.9843	0.9677	0.9618	96.57
ELM	0.9411	1.0	0.9756	0.9696	97.26
ELM + Genetic Algorithm	0.9753	1.0	0.9850	0.9875	98.63
Proposed Model (ELM + Bayesian Optimization)	**0.9931**	**1.0**	**0.9934**	**0.9933**	**99.31**

8.4.2 Result Analysis

Experimentation has been conducted using a variety of learning strategies, including machine learning, ensemble learning, and others, with the goal of demonstrating that the technique that has been offered is successful. Moreover, the efficacy of the suggested method is tested by taking into account the k-fold cross-validation method. This method randomly splits the dataset into a certain number of folds, called k, and then compares the results of each fold to the original dataset. In this work, tenfold sampling with stratified sampling was used to keep error estimates as accurate as possible while also reducing bias and volatility. In addition, the performance of every strategy that has been examined, in addition to the performance of the approach that has been suggested, by employing evaluation measures such as precision, recall, F1 score, ROC-AUC, and accuracy. Table 8.2 displays a detailed relative analysis of the assessment criteria that were used in this work to analyse all of the different machine learning and ensemble ELM techniques, as well as the suggested method. The findings indicate that the performance of the suggested technique ELM + Bayesian Optimization in terms of precision, recall, F1 score, ROC-AUC values, and accuracy is better when contrasted with the other ML and ensemble ELM methods that were taken into consideration.

On data that has been stratified using tenfold cross-validation, the results of several ensemble methods, including ELM, ELM combined with GA, and ELM combined with Bayesian optimization, are summarised in Table 8.3. As a consequence of the empirical findings that are shown in Table 8.3, it has become apparent that the suggested ELM, in conjunction with Bayesian optimization, has outperformed the other two methods in virtually all of the folds of stratified tenfold cross verified data. On the basis of the categorization of the PCOS illness, Fig. 8.4a–e depicts the confusion matrix performance of all of the ML techniques that were contemplated in addition to the suggested model. Based on the findings presented in the figures, it has been observed that, with the exception of a select few strategies, such as SVM and MLP, the majority of the approaches, including ELM, ELM combined with the Genetic Algorithm (GA), and ELM in conjunction with Bayesian optimization, have

Table 8.3 Prediction results on stratified sampled cross-validated 10-Fold data

Stratified sampled cross-validated 10 Fold data	Accuracy		
	ELM	ELM + Genetic algorithm	ELM + Bayesian optimization
Fold 1	97.26	98.63	99.31
Fold 2	97.12	98.52	99.30
Fold 3	97.42	98.32	99.28
Fold 4	96.98	98.75	99.30
Fold 5	97.21	98.61	99.31
Fold 6	97.26	98.62	99.30
Fold 7	97.30	98.62	99.31
Fold 8	97.25	98.65	99.32
Fold 9	97.21	98.63	99.32
Fold 10	97.22	98.61	99.31

performed very well. It has also been observed that the suggested method excels all other methods that were taken into consideration by accomplishing the greatest projected outcomes in the best classification of PCOS illness categorization.

The findings of the area under the receiver operating characteristic curve (AUC-ROC) for the ELM, the ELM with the GA methodology, and the suggested ELM and Bayesian optimization strategy are displayed in Fig. 8.5a, b, and c respectively. It is clear from the visualisation data shown in Fig. 8.5c that ELM, in conjunction with Bayesian optimization, has consistently demonstrated its ability to forecast the PCOS illness categorization. A comparison of the accuracy of the suggested approach with that of many other methods that were taken into consideration is depicted in Fig. 8.6. The two models, ELM + GA and ELM + BO, both depict how the fitness of the individuals evolves over the course of numerous generations in Fig. 8.7.

8.5 Conclusion

PCOS which is considered as one of the most prevalent endocrine disorders is found in 5 to 10% of women during their fertility period. To prevent the serious health consequences associated with PCOS such as ovarian cancer, obesity, heart diseases, infertility, type 2 diabetes, a prediction model based on ELM approach and Bayesian optimization approaches has been developed in this paper. The recommended model has been evaluated on the PCOS dataset collected from Kaggle. The dataset consisting of 541 instances with 42 attributes out of which 177 instances are PCOS samples and remaining are normal samples. The class imbalance problem has been overcome using a strategy known as random oversampling. In this approach, Bayesian optimization is used to choose the best hyperparameters of the models. Finally, the model

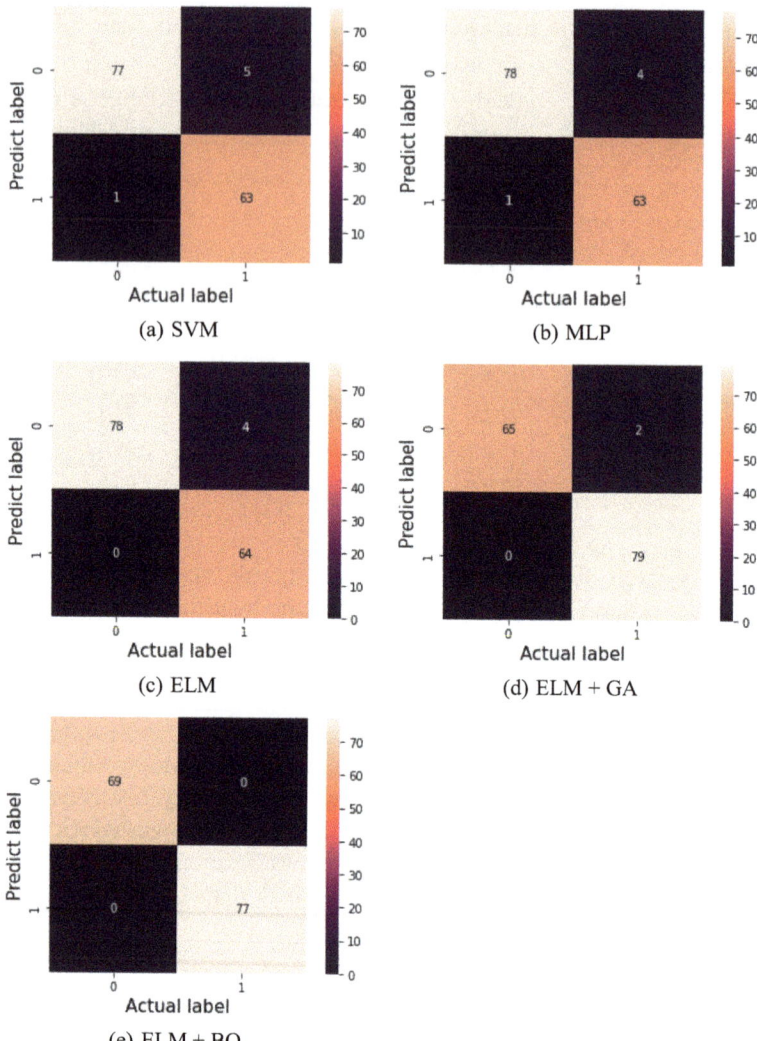

Fig. 8.4 Confusion matrix analysis of **a** SVM, **b** MLP **c** ELM **d** ELM + GA **e** ELM + BO

has been evaluated using tenfold cross validations and the results indicate ELM and Bayesian optimization approach acquired better performance of 99.31% accuracy in comparison with other ML approaches such as SVM, MLP, ELM and ELM and Genetic algorithm which attained an accuracy of 95.89, 96.57, 97.26 and 98.63% respectively.

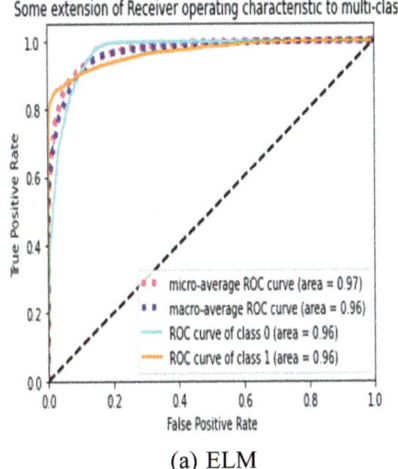
(a) ELM

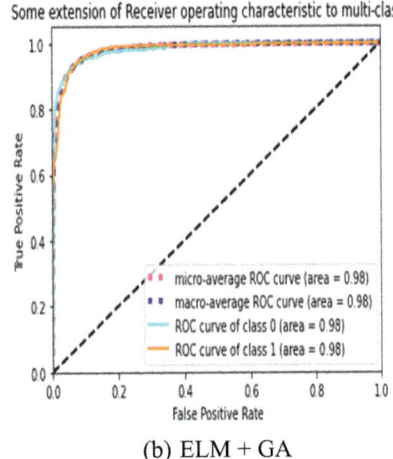
(b) ELM + GA

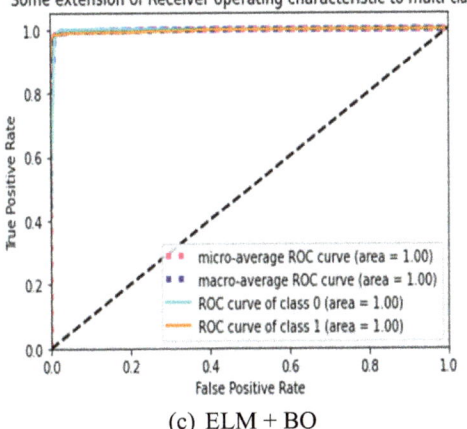
(c) ELM + BO

Fig. 8.5 ROC-AUC analysis of **a** ELM **b** ELM + GA and **c** ELM + BO

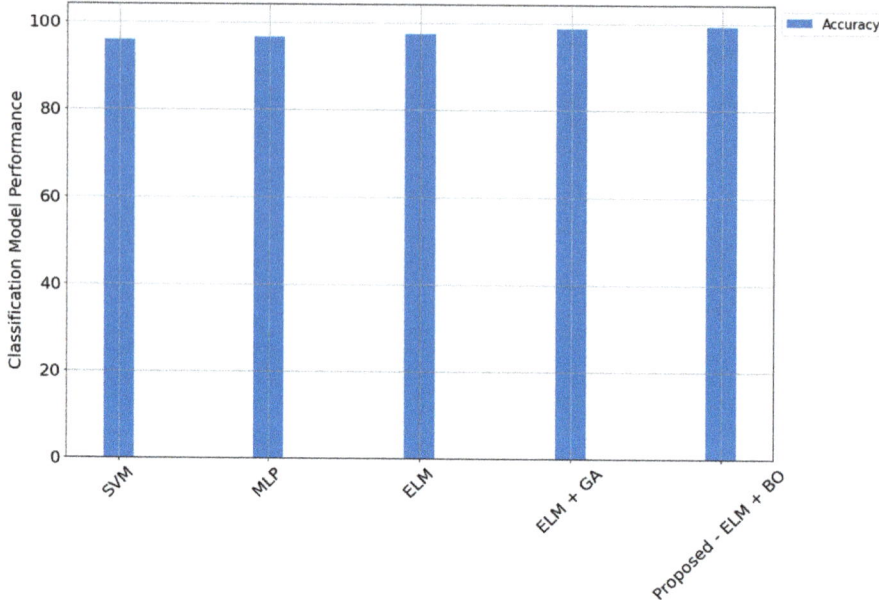

Fig. 8.6 Comparison analysis on different classification model

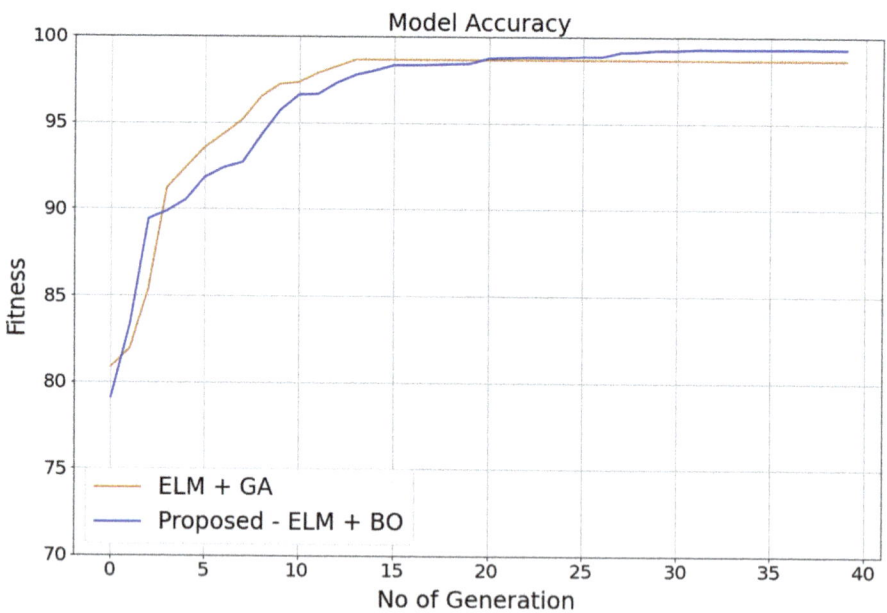

Fig. 8.7 Changes in fitness

References

1. Allahbadia, G.N., Merchant, R.: Polycystic ovary syndrome and impact on health. Middle East Fert. Soc. J. **16**(1), 19–37 (2011)
2. Stein, I.F.: Amenorrhea associated with bilateral polycystic ovaries. Am. J. Obstet. Gynecol. **29**, 181–191 (1935)
3. Saravanan, A., Sathiamoorthy, S.: Detection of polycystic ovarian syndrome: a literature Survey. Asian J. Eng. Appl. Technol. **7**(2), 46–51 (2018)
4. Franks, S.: Polycystic ovary syndrome. N. Engl. J. Med. **333**(13), 853–861 (1995)
5. Pasquali, R. et al.: PCOS Forum: research in polycystic ovary syndrome today and tomorrow. Clin. Endoc. **74.4**, 424–433 (2011)
6. Laganà, A.S. et al.: Current management of polycystic ovary syndrome: from bench to bedside. Intern. J. Endoc. 2018 (2018). doi:https://doi.org/10.1155/2018/7234543
7. Conway, G.S.: Polycystic ovary syndrome: clinical aspects. Baillieres Clin. Endocrinol. Metab. **10**(2), 263–279 (1996)
8. Rad, M.T.: BMI role in treatment of infertile patients with polycystic ovary syndrome. International Congress Series. Vol. 1271. Elsevier (2004)
9. Azziz, R., et al.: The prevalence and features of the polycystic ovary syndrome in an unselected population. J. Clin. Endoc. Metab. **89.6**, 2745–2749 (2004)
10. Ovalle, F., Azziz, R.: Insulin resistance, polycystic ovary syndrome, and type 2 diabetes mellitus. Fertil. Steril. **77**(6), 1095–1105 (2002)
11. Legro, R.S.: Polycystic ovary syndrome and cardiovascular disease: a premature association? Endocr. Rev. **24**(3), 302–312 (2003)
12. Hardiman, P., Pillay, O.S., Atiomo, W.: Polycystic ovary syndrome and endometrial carcinoma. The Lancet **361**(9371), 1810–1812 (2003)
13. Legro, R.S.: Polycystic ovary syndrome: the new millenium. Mol. Cell. Endocrinol. **184**(1–2), 87–93 (2001)
14. Legro, R. S. et al.: Diagnosis and treatment of polycystic ovary syndrome: an Endocrine Society clinical practice guideline. J. Clin. Endoc. Metab. **98.12**, 4565–4592 (2013)
15. Kumar, N., et al.: Efficient automated disease diagnosis using machine learning models. J. Healthcare Eng. 2021 (2021)
16. Huang, G.-B., Qin-Yu, Z., Chee-Kheong S.: Extreme learning machine: a new learning scheme of feedforward neural networks. 2004 IEEE international joint conference on neural networks (IEEE Cat. No. 04CH37541). Vol. 2. Ieee (2004)
17. Ismaeel, S., Ali, M., Dharmendra C.: Using the extreme learning machine (ELM) technique for heart disease diagnosis. 2015 IEEE Canada International Humanitarian Technology Conference (IHTC2015) IEEE (2015)
18. Chen, H.-L., et al.: An efficient hybrid kernel extreme learning machine approach for early diagnosis of Parkinson' s disease. Neurocomputing **184**, 131–144 (2016)
19. Li, L.-N., et al.: A computer aided diagnosis system for thyroid disease using extreme learning machine. J. Med. Syst. **36.5**, 3327–3337 (2012)
20. Asif, M.A.A.R., et al.: Performance evaluation and comparative analysis of different machine learning algorithms in predicting cardiovascular disease. Eng. Lett. **29**(2), 731–741 (2021)
21. Silva, I.S., et al.: Polycystic ovary syndrome: clinical and laboratory variables related to new phenotypes using machine-learning models. J. Endocrinol. Invest. **45**(3), 497–505 (2022)
22. Xie, N.-N., et al.: Establishment and analysis of a combined diagnostic model of polycystic ovary syndrome with random forest and artificial neural network. BioMed Research International 2020 (2020)
23. Gopalakrishnan, C., Iyapparaja, M.: Multilevel thresholding based follicle detection and classification of polycystic ovary syndrome from the ultrasound images using machine learning. Intern. J. Syst. Assur. Eng. Manag., 1–8 (2021)
24. Nilofer, N.S.: Follicles classification to detect polycystic ovary syndrome using Glcm and novel hybrid machine learning. Turkish J. Comp. Mathem. Educ. (TURCOMAT) **12**(7), 1062–1073 (2021)

25. Dutta, P., Shobhandeb, P., Madhurima, M.: An Efficient SMOTE Based Machine Learning classification for Prediction & Detection of PCOS (2021)
26. Zigarelli, A., Jia, Z., Lee, H.: Machine-aided self-diagnostic prediction models for polycystic ovary syndrome: observational study. JMIR Form. Res. **6**(3), e29967 (2022)
27. Rachana, B., et al.: Detection of polycystic ovarian syndrome using follicle recognition technique. Global Trans. Proc. **2**(2), 304–308 (2021)
28. Bharati, S., Prajoy, P., Rubaiyat Hossain Mondal, M.: Diagnosis of polycystic ovary syndrome using machine learning algorithms. 2020 IEEE Region 10 Symposium (TENSYMP). IEEE (2020)
29. Nandipati, S.C.R., Ying, C.X., Khaw Khai Wah.: Polycystic Ovarian Syndrome (PCOS) classification and feature selection by machine learning techniques. Appl. Math. Comput. Intell. **9**, 65–74 (2020)
30. Prapty, A.S., Tanzim T.S.: An efficient decision tree establishment and performance analysis with different machine learning approaches on Polycystic Ovary Syndrome. 2020 23rd International Conference on Computer and Information Technology (ICCIT). IEEE (2020)
31. Huang, G.B., Zhou, H., Ding, X., Zhang, R.: Extreme learning machine for regression and multiclass classification. IEEE Trans Syst Man Cybern Part B: Cybern **42**(2), 513–529 (2012)
32. Kariminia, S., Shamshirband, S., Motamedi, S., Hashim, R., Roy, C.: A systematic extreme learning machine approach to analyze visitors' thermal comfort at a public urban space. Renew Sustain. Energy Rev. **58**, 751–760 (2016)
33. Liu, X., Lin, S., Fang, J., Xu, Z.: Is extreme learning machine feasible? A theoretical assessment (Part I). IEEE Trans. Neural. Netw. Learn. Syst. **26**(1), 7–20 (2015)
34. Wong, P.K., Wong, K.I., Vong, C.M., Cheung, C.S.: Modeling and optimization of biodiesel engine performance using kernel-based extreme learning machine and cuckoo search. Renew. Energy **74**, 640–647 (2015)
35. Nianyin Z.H., Zhang, W., Liu, J., Liang, Alsaadi F.E.: A switching delayed PSO optimized extreme learning machine for short-term load forecasting. Neurocomputing (Elsevier) (2017)
36. Mao, W., Wang, J., He, L., Tian, Y.: Online sequential prediction of imbalance data with two-stage hybrid strategy by extreme learning machine. Neurocomputing (Elsevier) (2016)
37. Biredagn, N.K., Nehemiah, K.H., Kannan, A.: Hybrid approach using fuzzy sets and extreme learning machinefor classifying clinical datasets. Inform. Med. Unlocked (Elsevier) (2016)
38. Sánchez-Oro, J., Duarte, A., Salcedo-Sanz, S.: Robust total energy demand estimation with a hybrid Variable Neighborhood Search – Extreme Learning Machine algorithm. Energy Convers Manag (Elsevier) (2016)
39. Ou, T.-Y., Cheng, C.-Y., Chen, P.-J., Perng, C.: Dynamic cost forecasting model based on extreme learning machine – A case study in steel plant. Comput. Ind. Eng. (Elsevier) (2016)
40. Guo, P., Cheng, W., Wang, Y.: Hybrid evolutionary algorithm with extreme machine learning fitness function evaluation for two-stage capacitated facility location problems. Expert Syst. Appl. (Elsevier) (2016)
41. Al-Yaseen, W.L., Othman, Z.A., Nazri, M.Z.A.: Multi-level hybrid support vector machine and extreme learning machine based on modified K-means for intrusion detection system. Expert Syst. Appl. (Elsevier) (2016)
42. Huang, G.B., Zhu, Q.Y., Siew, C.K.: Extreme learning machine: theory and applications. Neurocomputing **70**(1), 489–501 (2006)
43. Zhou, J., Qiu, Y., Zhu, S., Armaghani, D.J., Khandelwal, M., Mohamad, E.T.: Estimation of the TBM advance rate under hard rock conditions using XGBoost and Bayesian optimization, Undergr. Sp. (2020). http://dx.doi.org/ https://doi.org/10.1016/j.undsp.2020.05.008.
44. Betrò, B.: Bayesian methods in global optimization. J. Global. Optim. **1**, 1–14 (1991). https://doi.org/10.1007/BF00120661
45. Wu, J., Chen, X.Y., Zhang, H., Xiong, L.D., Lei, H., Deng, S.H.: Hyperparameter optimization for machine learning models based on Bayesian optimization. J. Electron. Sci. Technol. **17**, 26–40 (2019). http://dx.doi.org/https://doi.org/10.11989/JEST. 1674–862X.80904120
46. Snoek, B.J., Larochelle, H., Adams, R.P.: Practical Bayesian optimization of machine learning algorithms, in: Proc. 25th Int. Conf. Neural Inf. Process. Syst., pp. 2951–2959 (2012)

47. Shahriari, B., Swersky, K., Wang, Z., Adams, R.P., De Freitas, N.: Taking the human out of the loop: A review of Bayesian optimization. Proc. IEEE **104**, 148–175 (2016). https://doi.org/10.1109/JPROC.2015.2494218
48. Brochu, E., Cora, V.M., de Freitas, N.: A tutorial on Bayesian optimization of expensive cost functions, with application to active user modeling and hierarchical reinforcement learning (2010). http://arxiv.org/abs/1012.2599
49. https://www.kaggle.com/datasets/shreyasvedpathak/pcos-dataset. Accessed on Feb 20, 2022

Chapter 9
Diabetes Twitter Classification Using Hybrid GSA

V. Diviya Prabha and R. Rathipriya

Abstract In today's world, it is important to understand individuals' health related opinions through sentiment analysis. Recently, many deep learning methods such as deep convolution neural network (CNN), Gated Recurrent Unit (GRU) and LSTM (Long short-term memory) are used to classify sentiments. This chapter focuses on diabetes tweet classification using the proposed Hybrid GSA, which is a combination of a Capsule Network (Deep Learning technique) and a Gravitational Search Algorithm. This approach is applied to perform sentiment classification such as positive, strong positive, negative, strong negative, and neutral using tweets on Twitter. It is observed from the results that the proposed approach produced better classification results compared to the existing approach. This work proved to be very effective in handling health tweets and accurate in classification.

Keywords Deep learning · Twitter · Sentimental analysis · Classification · GSA · Capsule network

9.1 Introduction

Machine Leanring (ML) techniques strongly rely on extracting useful features from healthcare data, which makes the classification task easier. This process becomes tedious to extract useful features from a huge amount of data and this decreases classification performance [1, 2]. However, healthcare depends on structured and unstructured data. This research tries to solve the problem by employing both data. ML techniques are difficult to analyze complex healthcare data. To overcome this problem, a branch of ML called Deep Learning (DL) techniques was introduced,

---

V. Diviya Prabha (✉)
Department of Computer Science, Sona College of Arts and Science, Salem, Tamil Nadu 636302, India
e-mail: diviyaprabha7@gmail.com

R. Rathipriya
Department of Computer Science, Periyar University, Salem, Tamil Nadu 636011, India
e-mail: rathipriyar@gmail.com

© The Author(s), under exclusive license to Springer Nature Switzerland AG 2023
J. Nayak et al. (eds.), *Nature-Inspired Optimization Methodologies in Biomedical and Healthcare*, Intelligent Systems Reference Library 233,
https://doi.org/10.1007/978-3-031-17544-2_9

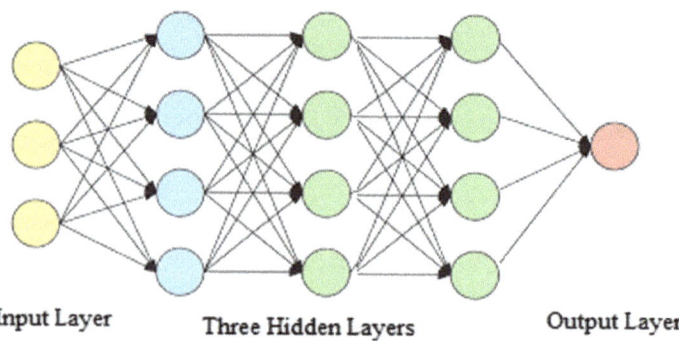

Fig. 9.1 Architecture of DL

which works on the concept of many layers connected to the NN (Neural Network) referred to as DL [3]. NN is an interconnection of neurons that consists of an input layer, a hidden layer and an output layer. Whereas, the main difference between NN and DL is the usage of many layers. DL also acts effectively to identify complex patterns from a huge amount of data. Therefore, successive layers consist of neurons that will inherit the more relevant features to improve the classification accuracy.

Figure 9.1 shows the structure of the DL consisting of one input layer, three hidden layers, and one output layer. The input layer contains structured or unstructured healthcare data which is transferred to three hidden layers. The result is passed on to the output layer in order to classify the diseases. The concept behind DL is that the raw input is given to the hidden layer and every hidden layer combines the values received from successive layers. Likewise, the model trains more complicated features from the dataset. The main advantage of using DL is to make the model learn feature stages, which will reduce human intervention [4].

DL is a leading Machine Learning technique that helps to frame healthcare analytics for data analysis. DL approaches are used to analyze patient data and prevent disorders like diabetes, cancer, heart attack, etc. It also acts as a mediator by developing efficient healthcare communication using clinical data. It has the potential to transform healthcare data into better clinical data by performing and modeling the complex hidden patterns in data. Its application is a great criterion in clinical data and provides guidance to personalized benefits for each individual. In recent years, multiple techniques have been integrated with DL for disease diagnosis and have helped to guide treatment plans in an efficient way. Classification using a single model for the same dataset with the same kind of parameter setting is suitable for only one dataset, while for different datasets, the existing model does not perform well. DL is a kind of neural network consisting of many hidden layers that has proved to be a better technique for handling huge amounts of data.

Text sentiment analysis [5] is a method for labeling information based on certain criteria. An ML study contains different types of methods for sentiment classification [5]. Obviously, some ML algorithms perform well on certain text datasets, but do not give better results on some large datasets.

To overcome this problem, instead of using a single classifier, it is better to combine optimization algorithm with classifier to improve the classification performance for all the datasets. This work proposes a Gravitational Search Algorithm (GSA) with capsule network. This will apparently increase the sentiment classification performance.

The contribution to this chapter is as followed

- To propose a better classification algorithm for twitter classification.
- To develop an optimization techniques which is a combination of GSA and capsule network.

This chapter is organized as follows: Sect. 9.2 discusses about related works. Section 9.3 explains in detail tweet extraction and also includes a study about the Twitter API that generates tokens. Section 9.4 defines the data collection with number of tweets collected. Section 9.5 describes the pre-processing of tweets and feature extraction techniques from text data. Section 9.6 explains the proposed work of the chapter and results obtained using the proposed work are tabulated. Finally, Sect. 9.7 concludes the chapter.

9.2 Related Works

This section provides a detailed description of ML techniques for unstructured data. These techniques are also used for solving text classification problems [6]. In recent years, social media data analysis has helped researchers to understand human behaviors consisting of a huge volume of unstructured data. One of the most developed social media platform is Twitter which helps people to communicate using small messages called tweets [7, 8]. It motivated people to share individual opinions on social media. However, social media is playing a vital role in improving the healthcare sector [9]. It gives more specific health related real-time opinions of each individual user and takes immediate actions in hospitals, at homes, etc. [10].

The survey stated that people searching for health related information [11] online is the third most popular online search activity. People rely on the web to find immediate health related information [12]. ML techniques are applied to social media text to understand users' opinions and interact with extremist users [13]. This paper analyzes 20,000 tweets collected from Twitter social media and achieves 93% accuracy using ML classification. Loyola et al. [14] were utilised to do sentiment analysis on tweets from six Mexican leaders.

The Naive Bayes classification model with an iterative approach provided good classification results for tweets collected regarding disasters [15]. Similarly, tweets based on topics are extracted to identify the relationship between them. Rehman et al. [16] proposed Hybrid CNN and LSTM for sentiment analysis using movies review dataset. Agarwal et al. [17] proposed a combination of feature set algorithm for tweets. Svm Classifier was applied by Zhang et al. [18] and Mohammad et al.

[19] to handle a text categorization issue better. The Naive Bayes classifier performed better for the Twitter sentiment classification task [20].

Multi-label classification was proposed using EL to classify drug side effects, which performed better in all aspects [21]. Chen et al. [22] proposed an ensemble mpdel which is a combination of CNN and RNN for text analysis. This approach showed that heterogeneous EL is better than the individual approach for multi-label text classification. Meanwhile, several combinations in DL are used for text analysis, which include CNN by RNN and hybridization of CNN with RNN [23, 24]. Table 9.1 represents other literature review for Text classification.

9.3 Tweets Extraction

Twitter provides an open environment for users to share their opinions in real-time that can be extracted by researchers. Tweets are extracted from Twitter using the Twitter API. Twitter helped to create an app that helps with the extraction of tweets. First, create a user login in the Twitter Health Related Record App. For each account, a unique key is generated representing the access key, access token, secret key and secret token. With the help of these keys, users can extract tweets one by one. Figure 9.2 shows the screenshot of the Health Related Records App that was used to extract tweets during the year 2020 about 'Diabetes'. Here, the keyword for diabetes tweets are 'Type 1 Diabetes', 'Type 2 Diabetes', 'Gestational Diabetes', and 'Young Diabetes'. Drugs related to diabetes keywords such as 'insulin', 'metformin' are used to extract tweets from Twitter.

9.4 Methodology

The main methods that are used in this chapter are discussed in this section. In recent days GSA proved to perform better to optimize better search space compared to other optimization algorithms. In the first section GSA optimization algorithm is discussed and in second section capsule network is discussed. Likewise, other DL methods that are used for text classification are discussed in detail.

9.4.1 GSA

Existing traditional algorithms do not work well to solve optimization problems in high-dimensional spaces. So, moving towards the better solution is needed. GSA is one of the important nature inspired algorithms that helps to solve many real-world problems [33]. It works on the concept of newton law of gravity. All these objects attract each other by the gravity force, and this force causes a global movement of all

Table 9.1 Literature review for text classification

Author and Refs.	Objective	Method	Pros	Cons
Jeow Li Huan et al. [25]	Emotionally charged text classification	It includes Naive Bayes, support vector machine, and stochastic gradient descent, k-nearest neighbour and ridge classifiers	1. Pre-trained GloVe vectors for LSTM 2. It is represented in multidimensional document	1. Semantic relationship between sentence and word are missing 2. While considering more number of documents in increases space there is no optimized word all words must considered for sentiment
Tai et al. [26]	To perform sentiment classification and predicting semantic of sentences	Tree-LSTM model, chain-structured LSTM	This methodology performs classification of sentiment and identify the semantic relatedness between two sentences	The methodology mainly focuses on the long-distance interaction in hierarchical model. Identifying certain words makes tedious in tree structure model
Basiri et al. [19]	Past and future context are considered for sentimental analysis	CNN-RNN deep learning model is proposed	The method is considered shot and long tweets	
Chauhan et al. [27]	To classify sentiments from the product reviews like amazon	The method follows to concentrate in adverbs, verbs and adjectives for the classification of sentiments to understand the polarity rate of the sentence	Considering adverbs in sentiments classification	Identifying adverbs are sometimes unstable several methods are used to identify and extract the adverbs properly. Extract adverbs are missing when moving to analyse large amount of tweets

(continued)

Table 9.1 (continued)

Author and Refs.	Objective	Method	Pros	Cons
Machova et al. [28]	To classify sentiments using machine learning and PSO	The method utilizes a particle swarm optimization algorithm and more precisely bare bone particle optimization algorithm	1. The methodology shows a simpler method to analyse the sentiments using the shift and switch method an effective lexicon based method is developed to improve the classification performance	1. Even though the methodology lands in great results it somehow falls in the accuracy bringing very low in accuracy
LV et al. [29]	To identify rumours based on the users opinion	The methodology utilizes an optimized LSTM model to improve the classification accuracy	1. Able to increases the accuracy 2. It doesn't require dimensionality reduction for the prediction of microarray data	The proposed methodology wasn't validated on consistency
Sanchez et al. [30]	To perform sentiment classification using hybrid model	The method used to classify labels at different levels using social context and community detection	1. The proposed approach is quite simple and time-efficient 2. The approach obtain high accuracy than existing model	The methodology even though its simple and fetches a great accuracy in this data, for a much larger dataset it crumbles. A better approach is needed to evaluate more number of dataset
Srinidhi [31]	To propose a hybrid model using LSTM and SVM for the sentiment classification	This methodology uses combination of model to improve the classification accuracy using two-word embedding vectors	Accuracy achieved is above which is greater than single model	Even though this approach works better for longer text for huge dataset it does not better which is the pitfall of the model

(continued)

Table 9.1 (continued)

Author and Refs.	Objective	Method	Pros	Cons
Zenun et al. [32]	To understand people opinion and thoughts in social media through sentiment analysis	The feature are extracted using attention mechanism, 1D-CNN, BiLSTM and hybrid model to understand the efficiency of feature and improve the performance of classification	The proposed methodology achieved an good classification accuracy to capture the semantic meaning of words	Very limited data are collected form Facebook in specific language. This may not suitable for all kids of sentiment classification of words. Since semantic meaning varies for every sentence collected from social media

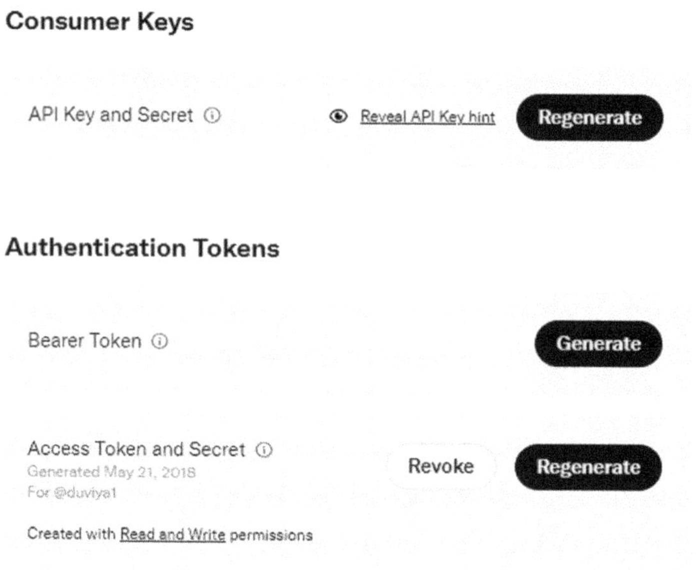

Consumer Keys

API Key and Secret ⓘ   ⊙ Reveal API Key hint   **Regenerate**

Authentication Tokens

Bearer Token ⓘ   **Generate**

Access Token and Secret ⓘ
Generated May 21, 2018   **Revoke**   **Regenerate**
For @duviya1

Created with Read and Write permissions

Fig. 9.2 Twitter health related records App

objects towards the objects with heavier masses. In GSA, the work on the concept of Kbest shows that choosing the right "K" values will make the algorithm work better. In an iteration, the best solutions are those that use gravitational force.

Pseudo Code for GSA
Step 1: Identify the search space t
Step 2: Randomly initialize the population X_i (i = 1, 2, ... N)
Step 3: Evaluate fitness of agents for each objects
Step 4: Update G(t), best(t), worst(t), Kbest
Step 5: Calculate acceleration and velocity of agent
Step 6: Update agent position
Step 7: Repeat step 3–6 until stopping condition is reached
Step 8: End.

9.4.2 CNN

CNN is used widely in image and text classification [34]. This method focuses on text, where the information in text data is stored and important features for classification are extracted. Therefore, CNN works better for text classification. Convolution layer is the most important part of CNN. The convolution layer works on the following concept: (i) Value containing input in matrix format, (ii) Filters are applied to input matrix and it becomes the final output, (iii) Convolution operation captures local dependencies existing in original data. The operation is denoted as follows:

$$I = V^{lw} \tag{9.1}$$

Equation (9.1), 'I' represents the input matrix, 'V' represents the vector matrix, 'l' represents the length and w represents the width of the input matrix. After the filtering process, the convolution operation is denoted as follows:

$$O_{p,q} = \sum_{l=1}^{N} \sum_{w=1}^{M} W_{lw} \otimes i_{p+l,q+w-1} \tag{9.2}$$

Equation (9.2) where 'O' is the output matrix, W_{lw} represents the weight of the matrix of length and width, and cross multiplication with the 'ith' element of the matrix.

9.4.3 GRU

The Gated Recurrent Unit (GRU) is similar to that of LSTM. They were developed mainly to overcome the memory problem in RNN. The model was proposed by [35] and it has a gating unit which helps with data flow within the limit without individual memory cells. It consists of two gates, namely the update and the reset gate. The task of both the gates is to determine the amount of information from previous layers to be moved either to the next layers or discarded. The formula for updating gate and resetting gate is represented in Eqs. (9.3) and (9.4).

$$U = S(W_U \cdot [h, x]) \tag{9.3}$$

$$R = S(W_R \cdot [h, x]) \tag{9.4}$$

Final equation is represented as

$$h = S(W_o \cdot [h, x]) * h + U * \tanh(W \cdot [R * h, x]) \tag{9.5}$$

From Eq. (9.5), 'W' represents the weight of the vector, 'S' denotes the sigmoid function and 'h' is the hidden unit of input 'x'.

9.4.4 LSTM

Long Short Term Memory (LSTM) is a type of RNN [36]. Here, a single layer LSTM is designed to contain 100 neurons. It contains memory cells to save the information. It is used to identify important features and to perform pre-calculation to produce the output. It consists of four gates: the input gate, the forget gate, the candidate gate and the output gate.

$$F_o = S(W_F \cdot [h, x]) + bw_F \tag{9.6}$$

$$C = \tanh(W_C \cdot [h, x]) + bw_F \tag{9.7}$$

$$I = S(W_F \cdot [h, x]) + bw_I \tag{9.8}$$

$$O = F_o * I + C * I \tag{9.9}$$

From Eqs. (9.6), (9.7) and (9.8) in which 'W' and 'bw' represents the weight of the vector gates. In Eq. (9.9), 'F' denotes the forget gate, 'C' denotes the candidate gate, 'I' represents the input gate and 'O' represents the output gate.

9.4.5 Embedding Layer

The embedding layer is the initial layer of all the three models, which helps to translate the tweets into vectors. Each word in the tweets is converted into numeric form and then represented as a word embedding. These vectors are given as the input to the next layer. Max_length is defined as 30, since, the tweets maximum character allowed by twitter is 280. The tweets consist of words w1, w2 ... wn and each word is assigned a numerical value vector. For this purpose, the size of the matrix is denoted as 300 multiplied by the embedding matrix size. For example, diabetes tweet's first word is represented as an embedding vector in the form of an 8×4 matrix. It is represented as (0.3, 0.4, 0.1, 0.5) with an index value of one.

9.4.6 Dropout Layer

A dropout layer is used to avoid over fitting of the value. It is set at 0.2 because the parameter ranges from 0 to 1 [37]. The process of the dropout layer is to deactivate the activated neurons. The network model is one of these three models, such as CNN, GRU or LSTM. The next layer in CNN is the pooling layer, and it is used to reduce the dimension. It is applied to each tweet in the dataset.

9.4.7 Maxpooling

Maxpooling has the efficiency to select the maximum value from tweets. The size of the window is set at 2 × 2. It extracts only the maximum elements from the window. After the process, a single element is selected. It chooses the largest values among all the values and then the output is produced at the Maxpooling layer. The next layer is the flatten. The main purpose of the layer is to convert the column vector value. It is fed as input into the layer and then passed into the neural network for classification. The flatten layer is used to transform the values into column vectors.

9.4.8 Output Layer

The output layer uses the softmax activation function to compute the five classes of output, such as strong positive, positive, negative, strong negative and neutral. The formula to calculating softmax function is

$$\sigma = \sum_{j}^{N} w_j i_j + bi \tag{9.10}$$

From Eq. (9.10), 'w' denotes the weight of the vectors, 'i' represent the input and the bias term 'bi'. The compile function represents the loss function, optimizers and metrics for accuracy. Furthermore, it requires the fitting of the model specifying the training and testing values with epoch value and batch size.

9.5 Data Collection

Diabetes [38] related 2,44,935 tweets are collected and labeled into 5 different classes which are described in Table 9.2. For example, diabetes drug related tweets are processed using keywords. 'Diabetes insulin', 'Diabetes metformin', etc.

9.6 Data Pre-processing

Data preprocessing is an important step for sentiment classification. This section explains some methods for text cleaning without losing the original meaning of the text. The following are certain pre-processing methods.

Table 9.2 Collected Twitter diabetes data

Diabetes dataset	Class	Tweets
Diabetes	5	105,811
Type 1 diabetes	5	14,157
Type 2 diabetes	5	10,259
Young diabetes	5	7886
Gestational diabetes	5	7600
Diabetes food	5	92,866
Diabetes drugs	5	6356

9.6.1 Conversion and Correction

Certain sentences in tweets consist of capital letters, which creates a problem while classifying a large number of tweets. Certain conversion methods [39] are used to change these letters to lower case. This method projects all kinds of words in tweets into feature space. Furthermore, it is challenging to handle misleading words. Some words are also represented in abbreviated form [40]. For example, COVID, which stands for Coronavirus Disease. This kind of word must be correctly identified and taken without losing original information.

9.6.2 Tokenization

Tokenization is an important step for pre-processing tweets. It breaks the sentence into words known as tokens [41, 42]. For text classification, tokens are important. For example,

Tweet: Covid19 is new while this one existed long years ago since 1978.

Tokens: 'Covid19', 'is', 'new', 'while', 'this', 'one', 'existed', 'long', 'years', 'ago', 'since', '1978'.

9.6.3 Stop Words

Tweets contain many words [20] that are not significant for sentiment classification. For example, {'for', 'above', 'this', 'that', 'before'…}. These words in tweets are difficult to identify the key concepts and will reduce the performance of classification. These words are manually assembled and removed from tweets.

9.6.4 Lemmatization

It is the process of removing the suffix of certain words to bring back the original meaning of the word. For example, 'move', 'moving', 'moved', 'moves'. These words represent a single form of 'move'. It is called a lemma. The process of dealing with these kinds of words is called lemmatization. The purpose of this method is to select the root.

9.6.5 Word Stemming

It is the method of analyzing tweets to produce morphological variants of the root words in tweets. These words can appear either in the singular or in the plural form. While the meaning of the word appears to be similar [43]. For example, consider the words 'playing' and 'play'. In tweets, one word can appear in different formats. Choosing an exact word improves the meaning of words.

9.6.6 Word Representation

This is a feature extraction technique used to represent the word without reducing the original meaning of the text. Words can be represented in numeric format by either randomly assigning vectors to text or adding weight as vectors. The Word Embedding method was proposed by [44]. It helps to map tokens to vectors, which makes the model easily understandable. The similarity between a single token and another token is considered in the vector space. If the words consist of similar meanings, these words appear closer in vector space; else the words appear far in vector space.

9.6.7 Bag of Word

This technique encodes each token into a vector. It consists of several methods, like 1-gram, 2-gram, 3-gram, and N-gram representations. It works on the concept of taking a single token and converting it to vector space, or taking a group of two tokens while mapping them to a vector. Similarly, it is considered for 3-gram and N-gram vector representations. The main drawback of this method is that semantic meaning between the words is missing.

An Example of a 2-Gram

    Tweet: basketball player David Edwards dies after battling COVID-19.
    Tokens: 'basketball player', 'David Edwards', 'dies after', 'battling COVID-19'.

An Example of a 3-Gram

Token: 'basketball player david', 'edwards dies after', 'battling COVID-19'.

9.6.8 TF-IDF

Term Frequency (TF) is an embedding method used to extract features from text. A certain scoring value is assigned to each token. The value is given based on the frequency of the token in the particular document.

$$\text{TF} = \frac{\text{No. of times token apppear in particular document}}{\text{Total no. of Tokens}} \quad (9.11)$$

In 1972, Spark Jones [45] developed a conjunction of TF which is called Inverse Document Frequency (IDF) represented in Eq. (9.11). It assigns higher weights to words based on the frequency of a word that appears in the document. TF-IDF is a multiplication of TF and IDF. It was developed to improve the performance of classification. It easily identifies common terms in the document.

9.6.9 Word2Vec

This approach is an enhanced word embedding method. Semantic meaning between tokens is acquired in this method. However, in previous methods, it was not possible. It can be implemented in two approaches, such as:

The first one is the Continuous Bag of Words method, which works by using multiple tokens as a target for a single word [44]. For example, 'patient' and 'doctor' are two tokens of the target word 'hospital'. It is mostly used for the unordered collection of tweets. It aims to segregate words from the collection corpus and identify the target token.

The second one is the Continuous Skip Gram Model. It helps to improve the classification of a token based on another token in the same tweet [44]. This model helps to maintain the semantic meaning of tweets.

9.7 Proposed Capsule Network with GSA

Proposed ensemble DL techniques perform better at extracting features from tweets. However, many hybrid models have been developed to extract the important features in a sentence, like C-LSTM [46]. Multi label text classification using Ensemble CNN-RNN is applied to understand the semantics of the text, thereby creating correlations between the information [22]. Zhu et al. [47] describes favorably characters in a document through hybrid techniques of CNN and RNN. This model provides better accuracy results when compared with existing word models. Several studies focused on hybrid models, but spatial information in the text is missing that leads to misclassification of the results. To address this problem, the Capsule Network (CapsNet) is used in the work [29, 48].

9.7.1 Capsule Network

The model works on the concept of capsules in which groups of neurons are represented in the form of parameters based on certain criteria. The capsule helps to select the most relevant features. The proposed algorithm consists of a convolution layer, GSA optimizer, primary capsule layer, and final capsule layer represented in Fig. 9.3.

The first layer is the convolution layer, which extracts features from input tweets using different filters. It extracts high-level features from tweets to form a sequence which is passed as an input to the GSA optimizer [49]. This layer works based on the function of gravity. Every element attracts other element by the function of gravity and mass. This optimizer is mainly used to reduce the parameters extracted from high-level features. This helps to minimize the value by choosing only the most suitable words to be passed as the input to the primary capsule layer.

Here, the maximization fitness function is used to engage relevant words for the labels. The next layer is the primary capsule layer. It accepts scalar inputs and it produces the output as vectors represented as capsules. When a certain number of capsules accept a specific capsule, then that capsule is activated to transmit from low-level to higher-level. The activated capsule formed a cluster to produce a high probability output. This kind of approach works better for low and high-dimensional data. CapsNet is designed with an Adam optimizer with a batch size as 40, and a learning rate is set between 0.0001 for 100 iterations. As a result, this approach is

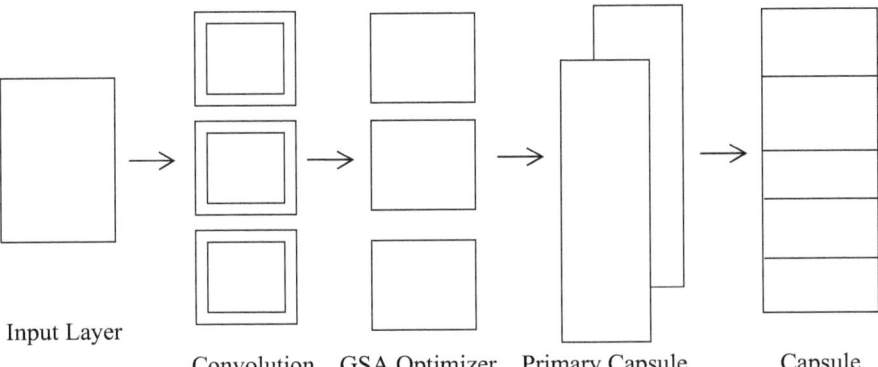

Fig. 9.3 Proposed CapsNet architecture

best suited for multi-label classification problems. The algorithm of the proposed work is represented as follows.

9.7.2 Capsule Network with GSA Algorithm

Step 1: Consider input tweets as Tw1, Tw2...Twn to be preprocessed as tokens (t1, t2...tm).

Step 2: Apply the convolution layer for the features.

$$f = \sum_{t}^{n} x_t + b \qquad (9.12)$$

Step 3: Important features are considered as agents in GSA. Each agents is attracted to other agents by force and mass. Agents = fi...fij.

Step 4: The total force that acts as an agent's ti can be weighed randomly.

$$TF = \sum_{i=1}^{n} \text{rand}(TF_i) \qquad (9.13)$$

Step 5: Find the best and worst value.

$$\text{fitness}_{\text{vlaue}(i)} = \text{Max (TF)} \qquad (9.14)$$

$$\text{Mass} = \frac{\text{fitness}_{\text{vlaue}(i)} - \text{worst}(i)}{\text{best}(i) - \text{worst}(i)} \qquad (9.15)$$

$$\widehat{M_{ij}} = W_{ij} * \text{Mass} \qquad (9.16)$$

Step 6: Apply capsule layer to change the scalar into vector transformation of capsule.

$$\widehat{u_{ij}} = W_i M_i \qquad (9.17)$$

Step 7: Apply squashing mass function to achieve the final capsule.

$$C_j = \frac{\left\|\widehat{M_{ij}}\right\|^2}{1 + \left\|\widehat{M_{ij}}\right\|^2} \frac{\widehat{M_{ij}}}{\left\|M_{ij}\right\|} \qquad (9.18)$$

Step 8: Apply the training model and compile it to evaluate the accuracy.

Step 1 describes the collection of input tweets it consists of tokens 't', the number of tokens 'n'. Step 2 represents the formula to calculate convolution layer where 'x' denotes the input vector with the bias term 'b in Eq. (9.12)'. Step 3 represents the extraction of important features as agents. Step 4 describes the calculation of total force and Eq. (9.13) denotes the formula for calculating the total force. The maximization fitness function is calculated in the next equation. Step 5 finds the best and worst value by calculating the fitness using Eq. (9.14). Mass calculation and weightes mass calculation is obtained by Eqs. (9.15) and (9.16). The Eq. (9.17) in step 6 represents the capsule layer. Finally, the most relevant features are extracted and are given as input to the capsule layer. $\widehat{u}_{ij}$ denotes the vector value multiplication of weight 'W' and mass function 'M'. The Squashing function is applied to the final capsule 'C' which is described in step 7 with Eq. (9.18). Finally, step 8 trains the model for compilation. This section discusses evaluation of the proposed work as shown in Fig. 9.4. The results are tabulated for 10 epochs of each dataset.

Table 9.3 describes the results of the proposed DL model for the Diabetes Twitter dataset. It calculates for 10 epochs. Finally, it received a classification accuracy of 95%. The loss function receives a minimum value of 29% during the final epoch.

The results of the proposed DL model for the Type 1 Diabetes Twitter dataset are presented in Table 9.4. It calculates for a total of ten epochs. Finally, it obtained a 94 percent categorization accuracy rating. In the last epoch, the loss function receives a minimum of 58%.

Table 9.5 displays the outcomes of the proposed DL model for the Type 2 Diabetes Twitter dataset. For a total of 10 epochs, it calculates. Finally, it received a 83% accuracy for classification. The loss function obtains a minimum of 29% in the most recent period.

Table 9.6 designates the result obtained for gestational diabetes dataset. Accuracy is increasing from the epoch 1 and at the end of epoch it receives 91% of accuracy. The loss function receives a minimum value of 0.02% during the final epoch.

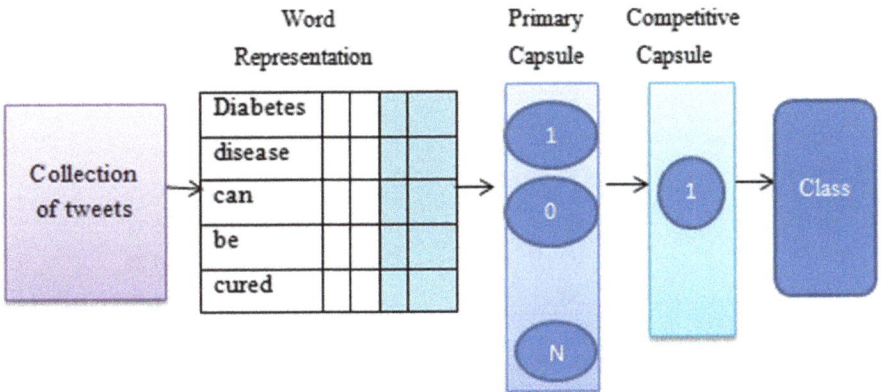

Fig. 9.4 Proposed work example

Table 9.3 Accuracy obtained using proposed model for diabetes Twitter dataset

Epochs	Accuracy	Loss
1	0.60	0.80
2	0.78	0.55
3	0.82	0.47
4	0.83	0.46
5	0.84	0.45
6	0.85	0.43
7	0.94	0.34
8	0.85	0.43
9	0.92	0.31
10	0.95	0.29

Table 9.4 Accuracy obtained using proposed model for type 1 diabetes dataset

Epoch	Accuracy	Loss
1	0.54	0.99
2	0.84	0.45
3	0.86	0.44
4	0.95	0.58
5	0.95	0.53
6	0.94	0.58
7	0.94	0.55
8	0.97	0.56
9	0.94	0.59
10	0.94	0.58

Table 9.5 Accuracy obtained using proposed model for type 2 diabetes dataset

Epoch	Accuracy	Loss
1	0.86	0.31
2	0.72	0.30
3	0.73	0.31
4	0.73	0.38
5	0.80	0.44
6	0.81	0.37
7	0.82	0.39
8	0.83	0.34
9	0.83	0.29
10	0.83	0.28

Table 9.6 Accuracy obtained using proposed model for gestational diabetes dataset

Epoch	Accuracy	Loss
1	0.36	1.14
2	0.55	0.77
3	0.74	0.49
4	0.83	0.25
5	0.89	0.06
6	0.90	0.09
7	0.91	0.06
8	0.91	0.04
9	0.91	0.03
10	0.91	0.02

Table 9.7 describes the results of the proposed DL model for the Young Diabetes Twitter dataset. It calculates for 10 epochs. Finally, it received a classification accuracy of 95%. The loss function receives a minimum value of 29% during the final epoch.

Table 9.8 describes the results of the proposed DL model for the Diabetes drug twitter dataset. For 10 epochs it receives an accuracy of 91% and loss function as 0.02.

Table 9.9 designates the results of the proposed model for diabetes food twitter dataset. It receives an accuracy of 93% of accuracy and loss 27%.

Table 9.10 describes the evaluation of the proposed work using different Twitter datasets. The proposed model outperforms better when compared with existing methods like GRU, LSTM, and CNN. Additionally, it overcomes the disadvantages of the Ensemble DL model. This model proved to be the most suitable for multi-label text classification of unstructured datasets.

Table 9.7 Accuracy obtained using proposed model for young diabetes dataset

Epoch	Accuracy	Loss
1	0.36	1.14
2	0.55	0.77
3	0.74	0.49
4	0.83	0.25
5	0.89	0.06
6	0.90	0.09
7	0.91	0.06
8	0.91	0.04
9	0.91	0.03
10	0.92	0.02

Table 9.8 Accuracy obtained using proposed model for diabetes drug dataset

Epoch	Accuracy	Loss
1	0.36	1.14
2	0.55	0.77
3	0.74	0.49
4	0.83	0.25
5	0.89	0.06
6	0.90	0.09
7	0.91	0.06
8	0.91	0.04
9	0.91	0.03
10	0.91	0.02

Table 9.9 Accuracy obtained using proposed model for diabetes food dataset

Epoch	Accuracy	Loss
1	0.75	0.47
2	0.80	0.43
3	0.84	0.39
4	0.85	0.36
5	0.86	0.37
6	0.87	0.35
7	0.91	0.29
8	0.89	0.31
9	0.90	0.30
10	0.93	0.27

Table 9.10 Accuracy obtained using proposed work for Twitter dataset

Dataset name	GRU	LSTM	CNN	Ensemble model	Proposed CapsNet with GSA
Diabetic	0.85	0.87	0.92	0.92	**0.94**
Type 1 diabetes	0.89	0.90	0.90	0.90	**0.95**
Type 2 diabetes	0.81	0.80	0.88	0.83	**0.96**
Gestational diabetes	0.89	0.90	0.92	0.91	**0.95**
Young diabetes	0.88	0.90	0.96	0.93	**0.98**
Diabetes drug	0.80	0.91	0.95	0.96	**0.97**
Diabetes food	0.87	0.92	0.95	0.93	**0.97**
COVID 19	0.92	0.95	0.93	0.93	**0.98**

Figure 9.5 shows the sentiment towards Diabetes and Type 1 Diabetes tweets were, SP represents strong positive, PS denotes positive, SN represents strong negative, NG represents negative and NT represents netural tweets classification. For Diabetes keyword nearly 60,000 tweets are strong positive sentiment, which is higher than other sentiments. For Type 1 Diabetes, the sentiment neutral is higher, which shows people's opinions are less aware of Type 1 Diabetes. Figure 9.6 illustrates Type 2 Diabetes and Gestational Diabetes. Nearly 4000 tweets are positive and negative sentiment is higher for Type 1 Diabetes. Above 2500 tweets are positive and above 2000 tweets are strongly positive and neutral tweets are high for Gestational Diabetes. For, Young diabetes and Diabetes Drug sentiment are illustrated in Fig. 9.7. Nearly 6000 tweets are positive for Young Diabetes and 3000 above tweets achieve positive sentiment for Diabetes Drug sentiment. Figure 9.8 explains sentiment towards Diabetes Food where positive sentiments are high compared to other sentiments.

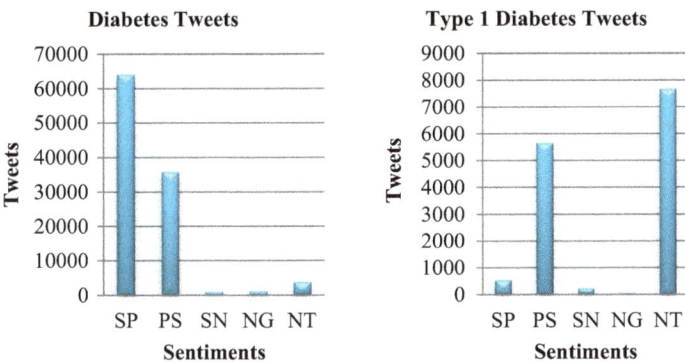

Fig. 9.5 Sentiments classification for diabetes and type 1 diabetes tweets

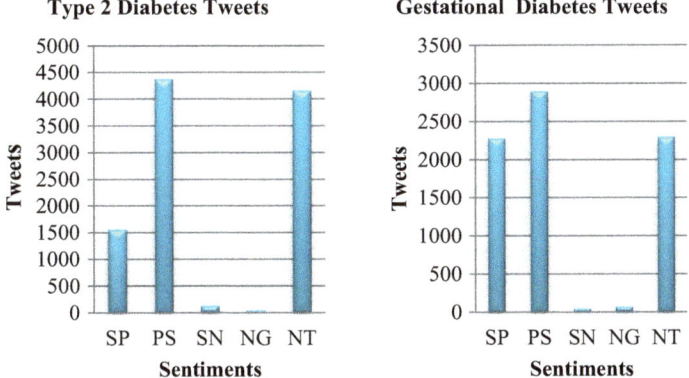

Fig. 9.6 Sentiments classification for type 2 diabetes and gestational diabetes tweets

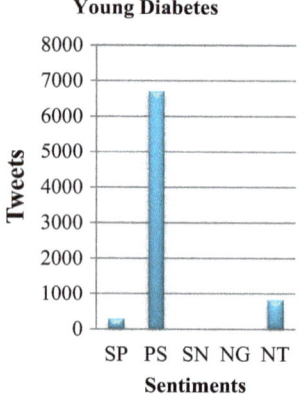 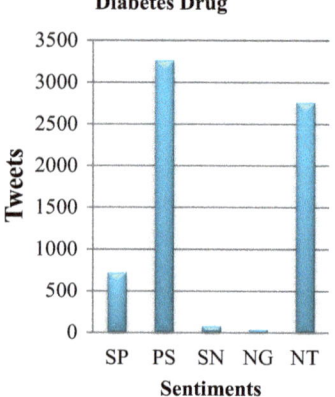

Fig. 9.7 Sentiments classification for young diabetes and diabetes drug tweets

Fig. 9.8 Sentiments classification for diabetes food and COVID-19 tweets

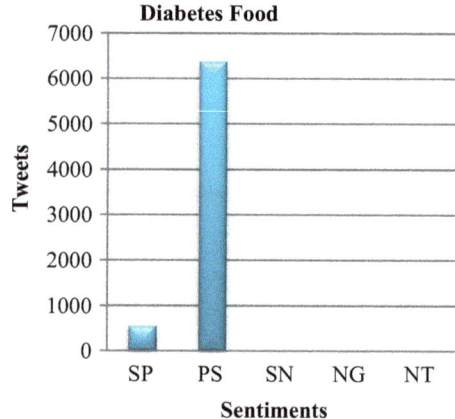

9.8 Conclusion

This chapter dealt with the proposed algorithm for twitter dataset. It showed that proposed hybrid GSA which is a combination of CapsNet and an GSA optimization algorithm. This algorithm performed better for Twitter sentiment analysis. In most cases, the proposed model showed superior performance compared with other standard models. In addition, the results in terms of accuracy are better for multi-label classification tasks.

This experiment reveal that the reliability of hybrid models outperformed well compared to existing models for sentiment analysis. Combining deep learning models with optimization techniques technique yields better results which is better than using an performance of individual model. In most of the twitter datasets, the consistency of hybrid models using optimization is higher than that of the ones not using it; however, better accuracy suggest for better classification of the model. It is also observed that the efficiency of the proposed algorithms depend mainly on the characteristics of datasets.

Twitter sentiment analysis has a large impact to understand people opinion. This chapter intended to study the performance of hybrid approaches for sentiment analysis on twitter datasets and helps in order to gain deeper insight in a specific topic in diabetes topic. From the opinion it is concluded that certain tweets obtain positive and negative sentiment.

References

1. Miotto, R., et al.: Deep learning for healthcare: review, opportunities and challenges. Brief. Bioinform. **19**(6), 1236–1246 (2017). https://doi.org/10.1093/bib/bbx044
2. Huan, J.L., Sekh, A.A., Quek, C., et al.: Emotionally charged text classification with deep learning and sentiment semantic. Neural Comput. Appl. **34**, 2341–2351 (2022). https://doi.org/10.1007/s00521-021-06542-1
3. Burt, J.R., et al.: Deep learning beyond cats and dogs: recent advances in diagnosing breast cancer with deep neural networks. Br. J. Radiol. 20170545 (2018). https://doi.org/10.1259/bjr.20170545
4. Bengio, Y.: Learning deep architectures for AI. Found. Trends Mach. Learn. **2**(1), 1–127 (2009). https://doi.org/10.1561/2200000006
5. Barbieri, F., et al.: Overview of the EVALITA 2016 sentiment polarity classification task. In: Evaluation of NLP and speech tools for Italian, pp. 146–155 (2016). https://doi.org/10.4000/books.aaccademia.1992
6. Aggarwal, C.C., Zhai, C.X.: A survey of text classification algorithms. In: Mining text data, pp. 163–222 (2012). https://doi.org/10.1007/978-1-4614-3223-4_6
7. Signorini, A., et al.: The use of Twitter to track levels of disease activity and public concern in the U.S. during the influenza A H1N1 pandemic. PLoS ONE **6**(5), (2011). https://doi.org/10.1371/journal.pone.0019467
8. Weiler, A., et al.: Editorial: survey and experimental analysis of event detection techniques for Twitter. Comput. J. (2016), https://doi.org/10.1093/comjnl/bxw056
9. Yonker, L.M., et al.: 'Friending' teens: systematic review of social media in adolescent and young adult health care. J. Med. Internet Res. **17**(1), 1–15 (2015). https://doi.org/10.2196/jmir.3692
10. Fox, S.: Health topics. In: MedlinePlus, U.S. National Library of Medicine (2017). https://medlineplus.gov/healthtopics.html. Accessed 15 Jan 2022
11. Krittanawong, C., et al.: Artificial intelligence in precision cardiovascular medicine. J. Am. Coll. Cardiol. **69**(21), 2657–2664 (2017). https://doi.org/10.1016/j.jacc.2017.03.571
12. Tan, S.S.-L., Goonawardene, N.: Internet health information seeking and the patient-physician relationship: a systematic review. J. Med. Internet Res. **19**(1), (2017). https://doi.org/10.2196/jmir.5729
13. Ferrara, E., et al.: Predicting online extremism, content adopters, and interaction reciprocity. In: Lecture Notes in Computer Science, pp. 22–39 (2016). https://doi.org/10.1007/978-3-319-47874-6_3
14. Loyola-González, O., et al.: Fusing pattern discovery and visual analytics approaches in tweet propagation. Inf. Fusion **46**, 91–101 (2019). https://doi.org/10.1016/j.inffus.2018.05.004
15. Li, H., et al.: Disaster response aided by tweet classification with a domain adaptation approach. J. Contingencies Cris. Manag. **26**(1), 16–27 (2017). https://doi.org/10.1111/1468-5973.12194

16. Rehman, A.U., Malik, A.K., Raza, B., Ali, W.: A hybrid CNN-LSTM model for improving accuracy of movie reviews sentiment analysis. Multimed. Tools Appl. **78**(18), 26597–26613 (2019)
17. Agarwal, A., et al.: Sentiment analysis of twitter data. In: Proceedings of the Workshop on Language in Social Media (LSM 2011), pp. 30–38 (2011)
18. Zhang, L., et al.: Combining lexicon-based and learning-based methods for Twitter sentiment analysis. In: HP Laboratories, Technical Report HPL-2011, vol. 89, pp. 1–8 (2011)
19. Basiri, M.E., Nemati, S., Abdar, M., Cambria, E., Rajendra Acharya, U.: ABCDM: an attention-based bidirectional CNN-RNN deep model for sentiment analysis. Future Gen. Comput. Syst. **115**(2020), 279–294 (2020)
20. Saif, H., et al.: "KDD'18." European Language Resources Association (ELRA). In: Proceedings of the Ninth International Conference on Language Resources and Evaluation (LREC'14), pp. 810–817 (2014)
21. Zhang, W., et al.: Predicting drug side effects by multi-label learning and ensemble learning. BMC Bioinform. **16**(1), 1–11 (2015). https://doi.org/10.1186/s12859-015-0774-y
22. Chen, G., et al.: Ensemble application of convolutional and recurrent neural networks for multi-label text categorization. In: 2017 International Joint Conference on Neural Networks (IJCNN) (2017). https://doi.org/10.1109/ijcnn.2017.7966144
23. Zhang, R., et al.: Dependency sensitive convolutional neural networks for modeling sentences and documents. In: Proceedings of the 2016 Conference of the North American Chapter of the Association for Computational Linguistics: Human Language Technologies (2016). https://doi.org/10.18653/v1/n16-1177
24. Lai, S., et al.: AAAI Press. In: AAAI'15: Proceedings of the Twenty-Ninth AAAI Conference on Artificial Intelligence, pp. 2267–2273 (2015)
25. Huan, J.L., Sekh, A.A., Quek, C., Prasad, D.K.: Emotionally charged text classification with deep learning and sentiment semantic. Neural Comput. Appl. (Springer) 2341–2351 (2022)
26. Tai, K.S., Socher, R., Manning, C.D.: Improved semantic representations from tree structure long short-term memory networks (2015). arXiv preprint arXiv:1503.00075
27. Chauhan, U.A., Afzal, M.T., Shahid, A., Abdar, M., Basiri, M.E., Zhou, X.: A comprehensive analysis of adverb types for mining user sentiments on amazon product reviews. World Wide Web **23**(3), 1811–1829 (2020). https://doi.org/10.1007/s11280-020-00785-z
28. Machova, K., Mikula, M., Gao, X., Mach, M.: Lexicon-based sentiment analysis using the particle swarm optimization. Electronics **9**, 1317 (2020)
29. Prabha, V.D., Rathipriya, R.: Sentimental analysis using capsule network with gravitational search algorithm. J. Web Eng. 762–778 (2020)
30. Sanchez-Rada, J.F., Iglesias, C.A.: CRANK: a hybrid model for user and content sentiment classification using social context and community detection. Appl. Sci. **10**(5), 1662 (2020)
31. Srinidhi, H., Siddesh, G., Srinivasa, K.: A hybrid model using MaLSTM based on recurrent neural networks with support vector machines for sentiment analysis. Eng. Appl. Sci. Res. **47**(3), 232–240 (2020)
32. Kastrati, Z., Ahmedi, L., Kurti, A., et al.: A deep learning sentiment analyser for social media comments in low-resource languages. Electronics **10**(10), 1133 (2021)
33. Mittal, H.: Chaotic Kbest Gravitational Search Algorithm (CKGSA) (2022). https://github.com/himanshuRepo/CKGSA).GitHub. Accessed 25 June 2022
34. Young, T., et al.: Recent trends in deep learning based natural language processing [Review Article]. IEEE Comput. Intell. Mag. **13**(3), 55–75 (2018). https://doi.org/10.1109/mci.2018.2840738
35. Choi, E., et al.: Doctor AI: predicting clinical events via recurrent neural networks. In: Machine Learning for Healthcare Conference. PMLR, pp. 301–308 (2016)
36. Hochreiter, S., Schmidhuber, J.: Long short-term memory. Neural Comput. **9**(8), 1735–1780 (1997). https://doi.org/10.1162/neco.1997.9.8.1735
37. Ahmad, S., et al.: Detection and classification of social media-based extremist affiliations using sentiment analysis techniques. Hum.-Centric Comput. Inf. Sci. **9**(1), (2019). https://doi.org/10.1186/s13673-019-0185-6

38. Diviya Prabha, V., Rathipriya, R.: Diabetes twitter analysis using improved ensemble machine learning techniques. Adv. Appl. Math. Sci. **21**(1), 241–250 (2021)
39. Dalal, M.K., Zaveri, M.A. Automatic text classification: a technical review. Int. J. Comput. Appl. **28**(2), 37–40 (2011). https://doi.org/10.5120/3358-4633
40. Whitney, D.L., Evans, B.W.: Abbreviations for names of rock-forming minerals. Am. Miner. **95**(1), 185–187 (2009). https://doi.org/10.2138/am.2010.3371
41. Gupta, G., Malhotra, S.: Text document tokenization for word frequency count using rapid miner (taking resume as an example). Int. J. Comput. Appl. 24–26 (2015)
42. Verma, T., et al.: Tokenization and filtering process in RapidMiner. Int. J. Appl. Inf. Syst. **7**(2), 16–18 (2014). https://doi.org/10.5120/ijais14-451139
43. Singh, J., Gupta, V.: Text stemming. ACM Comput. Surv. **49**(3), 1–46 (2016). https://doi.org/10.1145/2975608
44. Mikolov, T., et al.: Efficient estimation of word representations in vector space. arXiv preprint arXiv:1301.3781 (2013). https://doi.org/10.48550/arXiv.1301.3781
45. Jones, K.S.: A statistical interpretation of term specificity and its application in retrieval. J. Doc. (1972). https://doi.org/10.1108/eb026526
46. Zhou, C., et al.: A C-LSTM neural network for text classification. arXiv preprint arXiv:1511.08630 (2015). https://doi.org/10.48550/arXiv.1511.08630
47. Zhu, X., et al.: NRC-Canada-2014: recent improvements in the sentiment analysis of tweets. In: Proceedings of the 8th International Workshop on Semantic Evaluation (SemEval 2014) (2014). https://doi.org/10.3115/v1/s14-2077
48. Hinton, G.E., et al.: Transforming auto-encoders. In: Lecture Notes in Computer Science, pp. 44–51 (2011). https://doi.org/10.1007/978-3-642-21735-7_6
49. Prabha, V.D., Rathipriya R.: Clinical decision support systems. In: Handbook of research on disease prediction through data analytics and machine learning, pp. 268–280 (2021). https://doi.org/10.4018/978-1-7998-2742-9.ch014

Chapter 10
Advance Machine Learning and Nature-Inspired Optimization in Heart Failure Clinical Records Dataset

Dukka Karun Kumar Reddy, H. S. Behera, and Weiping Ding

Abstract ML is a subset of computing procedures that aims to imitate human astuteness by swotting from its surroundings. It has become a challenging task to diagnose the ailment and provide the appropriate treatment at the right time because of the increasing population and disease. The recent technological advancements have propelled the adoption of innovative functional biomedical solutions in the public health sector. Procedures based on traditional ML have been applied effectively in computational biology to biomedical and medical applications. Biomedical solutions entail a complex series of procedures ranging from consultation to treatment and beyond to ensure that patients react optimally. These are considered the working horse in the new era of the so-called big data. The process's complexity can vary and encompass multiple phases of nuanced human–machine interplay with decision-making, which certainly derive the application of ML algorithms to enhance and systematize the automate processes. A population-based Natured inspired swarm algorithms is proposed to extract the relevant parameters of Tree-based ML algorithms by using hyperparameter tuning. The proposed framework attains the desired performance by using "Heart failure clinical records dataset" prediction from the UCI ML data repository.

Keywords Nature-Inspired optimization · Clinical data · Hyperparameter tuning · Clinical dataset · Heart failure

---

D. K. K. Reddy (✉)
Department of Computer Science Engineering, Dr. L. Bullayya College of Engineering, Visakhapatnam, Andhra Pradesh 530013, India
e-mail: karun.redy@gmail.com

H. S. Behera
Department of Information Technology, Veer Surendra Sai University of Technology, Burla 768018, India
e-mail: hsbehera_india@yahoo.com

W. Ding
School of Information Science and Technology, Nantong University, Nantong, China

© The Author(s), under exclusive license to Springer Nature Switzerland AG 2023
J. Nayak et al. (eds.), *Nature-Inspired Optimization Methodologies in Biomedical and Healthcare*, Intelligent Systems Reference Library 233,
https://doi.org/10.1007/978-3-031-17544-2_10

10.1 Introduction

The rapid growth of biomedical data has encompassed several dimensions spanning from molecules to populations. It has increased the bandwidth, depth, and resolution of numerous entities in healthcare systems. These data prove to be a valuable resource for speeding up basic clinical science research and encouraging evidence-based medical treatments. Despite the fact that techniques for discovering data patterns have been around for decades, traditional analytical approaches still make it very difficult to convert enormous amounts of data into knowledge that can be applied. This drives the development of modern analytics methodologies, which use optimization and advanced ML techniques to discover helpful data representations or structures [1]. In Biomedical Informatics (BI), ML techniques and optimization are frequently used in two different groups of applications. One emphasis on knowledge acquisition and discovery by analysing historical data to explain what happened and why. Another focus is on prediction and decision-making applications that develop an extrapolative model and quantify it to generate predictions by means of unseen data utilizing a known dataset, including input data attributes and response values. The sheer quantity and complexity of data that we may easily gather nowadays in BI have been agreed upon as substantial hurdles to its translation into successful clinical interventions. As a result, there is a strong demand for advanced ML and NIO techniques, that address the unique problems of biomedical information and enable stakeholders and decision-makers to analyse and use the information [2]. ML has made strides in recent years when combined with sophisticated NIO approaches. BI data often contain rich contexts of characteristics with high dimensions and large volumes from heterogeneous sources. It is a challenging task to handle the pervasiveness existence of biomedical information with imbalanced classes, unstructured and weakly structured data, noise, incompleteness, and vague labelling. These rigorous characteristics are propelling the development of advanced ML algorithms in combination with NIO techniques [3]. NIO put into action what the healthcare sector has in spades. It has the power to make extraordinary improvements to the healthcare system by reducing subjectivity and variability in clinical diagnosis. NIO helps to leverage patient's health information to find correlations between various patient's symptoms with an assumed disease. These correlations with the mechanism of exploitation and exploration of NIO can help to forecast possible health outcomes before any health conditions occur and give doctors an understanding of underlying patterns of disease. In order to research and progress ML subjects and create influential tailored solutions for the newly emerging BI problems, NIO techniques scale up to the complexity of BI data with great attention. Besides the traditional ML methodological issues, advanced ML with optimization is much to practice for applications in the real world, in the context of the design framework, implementation, explication, and validation of these approaches. For the identification of superfluous information present in the biomedical dataset predictive analytics and predictive model building pacts with the problems allied with the dataset.

However, it is desirable to lessen the computational cost of the ML model and progress the model's performance. The performance of the ML model systems depends directly on the optimal features selection and with effective parameters selection, which leads to a simpler model, improved generalization, and better interpretation. The basic aim behind the use of the proposed optimization algorithms is that, they take on firm trade-off in choosing parameter by randomization and local search operation to deliver improved solution. The initialization of the parameters plays a foremost role in optimizing a Tree-based algorithms. These NIO algorithms can set the constraints of Tree-based algorithms by using various parameters. These constraints setting on Tree-based algorithms combat to improve predictive power of Tree-based algorithms. Optimizing the features and hyperparameters remains a substantial obstacle in designing ML models. The proposed work selects the NIO approaches for hyperparameter selection that have not been extensively exploited for this task. NIO approaches usually involve minimizing a specific predictive error measure and overfitting of ML models that may fit the noise rather than the signal of interest for different data subsets.

10.1.1 Cardiovascular Disease (CVD)

Heart disease is one of the primary factors in morbidity and mortality among people worldwide. 17.9 million people globally died from CVDs in 2019, making up 32% of all fatalities. 85% of the deaths were caused by heart attacks and strokes. Around three-quarters of Mortality rates occurs in low- and middle-income countries. CVDs were associated for 38% of the 17 million premature deaths caused by noncommunicable diseases in 2019 (before the age of 70) [4]. Heart and blood vessel illnesses collectively are referred to as CVDs, which are classified into six types as mentioned in Fig. 10.1. CVDs are conditions characterised by blocked or narrowed blood arteries, which can result in an angina or heart attack. Heart disease also includes additional cardiac conditions that damage the heart's muscle, valves, or rhythm. The vast percentage of heart attacks transpire because of a blockage in the blood vessels that supply blood to the heart. This happens because of a sticky substance (plaque) that can build inside the arteries. Atherosclerosis is the name for this build-up. Plaque deposits inside the coronary arteries can sometimes break open or rupture, causing a blood clot to form where the rupture occurs. If the clot blocks the artery, the heart muscle will be deprived of blood, resulting in a heart attack.

The lifestyle choices are also influencing factors of having a heart attack. Heart attack risk is increased by the following lifestyle factors like Insufficient physical activity, a high intake fat diet & sugar, smoking, overindulging in alcoholic beverages, and abuse of drugs. Additionally, diabetes, obesity, high blood pressure, abnormal pulse rate, high cholesterol, and eating disorders, and many other factors can increase the risk of heart attack [5, 6]. However, due of the aforementioned contributory risk factors, it is difficult to detect cardiac disease. This leads the cardiac disease a key

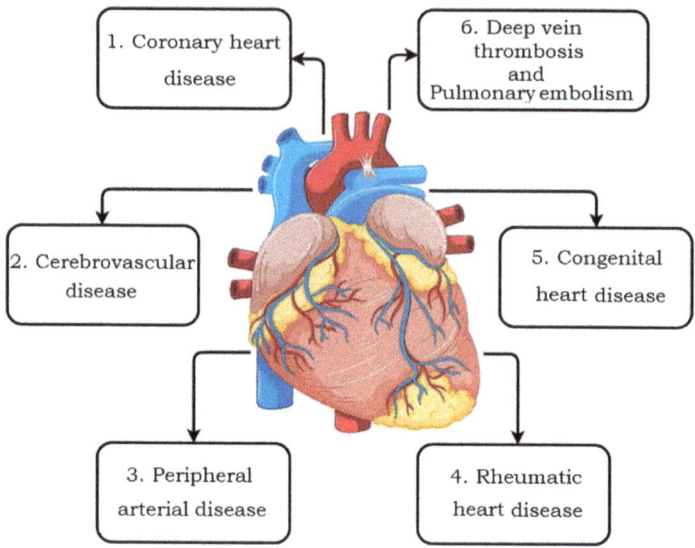

Fig. 10.1 CVDs of the heart and blood vessels

concern to be dealt with. Due to such constraints, researchers have focused towards modern ML approaches for predicting the cardiac disease.

The use of ML with NIO has proven to be beneficial in supporting decision-making and forecasting from the vast amounts of data generated by the healthcare industry. The aim of this chapter is to present unconventional ML with optimization techniques to address BI's practical problems. This chapter, deals with applying ML and optimization methods for categorizing whether a person is suffering from CVD or not. The sooner if we able to detect CVD, the easier it is to treat. A novel "heart failure clinical records data set" is taken into account in the study from the UCI repository.

The objective of the research reported in this chapter is

i. To investigate and evaluate the heart failure dataset's influencing factors in order to pinpoint the likely effects and improve its capacity for correctly diagnosing heart illness.
ii. Making use of Tree-based ML algorithms under different NIO based hyperparameters tuning to differentiate between the person who is prone to heart failure and no chance of heart failure.
iii. Precision, recall, F1-score, and accuracy metrics are employed to evaluate the effectiveness of the suggested algorithms.

The proposed method has a long-term effect on the heart failure dataset in comparison to existing supervised ML classifiers. The structure of the chapter is as follows: Sect. 10.2 covers some of the most significant related research in this area. Sections 10.3 and 10.4 describes the classification models used in the experiments and NIO technique used for hyperparameter tuning. Section 10.5 gives a brief basic preliminaries of optimization techniques. Section 10.6 gives a concise description of the datasets. Section 10.7 describes the experimental design and outcomes analysis, and Sect. 10.8 concludes the chapter.

10.2 Related Works

One of the most life-threatening issues in the biomedical field that demands rapid attention is CVDs. A number of researchers have been working toward the most advanced clinical diagnostic and early treatment possible. This section provides a synopsis of each researcher's work, the results of their analysis on the heart failure clinical records data set, and some quick facts about CVD detection. The majority of prior work on the UCI dataset has shown useful findings, and many improvements in classification algorithms are still being developed to improve forecast accuracy. However, throughout our survey, we discovered a dataset titled "Heart Failure Dataset" on which no major research has been done earlier. So, the goal of this study is to use ML methods to build an accurate and effective heart disease diagnosis on the "Heart Failure Dataset" with NIO by hyperparameter tuning.

Sai Krishna Reddy et al. [7] proposed the study to predict CVD with improved accuracy by proposing Decision Tree (DT), Gaussian Naïve Bayes (GNB) classifiers. The foremost objective of this research paper provides an insight of prediction models for Heart Failure Dataset. The classifiers GNB and DT were recorded with accuracies of 86.0 and 82.0% respectively. The proposed ML classification techniques are employed with 299 instances, where 200 instances are considered as training data and 99 instances as test data. The confusion matrix for DT shows that 64 and 18 are precisely classified with the target classes values respectively, and 18 instances values are incorrectly classified. Similarly, for GNB, 86 instances are precisely classified with the target classes and 14 instances are incorrectly classified.

Chicco and Jurman [8] proposed survival ML prediction on all the clinical characteristics employed by various ML algorithms to envisage the patients' ability to survive. Where each ML algorithm is applied hundred times and derived the mean result score with randomly selected data instances. The k-Nearest Neighbours (k-NN), Support Vector Machine (SVM), and Artificial neural network (ANN), the dataset is split into 60% for the training (179 patients' instances), 20% for the validation (60 patients' instances), and 20% for the testing (60 patients' instances). The hyperparameter optimization with grid search is performed on these ML methods based on highest Matthew's correlation coefficient. For the RF, One Rule, Linear Regression (LR), Naïve Bayes (NB), and DT ML methods the dataset is split into 80% for the training (239 patients' instances), and 20% for the testing (60 patients' instances). The DT obtained the top results with sensitivity of 0.532 and F1 score of 0.554, and able to predict precisely the majority of patients with deceased. The prediction results shows that RF outdid by obtaining the top MCC of + 0.384, and ROC AUC of 0.8, and accuracy of 74%.

Ishaq et al. [9] proposed to predict patient's survival with effective Synthetic Minority Oversampling Technique (SMOTE) technique and highest ranked features selected by RF to boost the performance of cardiovascular patient's survivor prediction model. The author employed Gradient Boosting, DT, AdaBoost, LR, RF, ETC, GNB, Stochastic Gradient and SVM classifier. The results are compared with ML classifiers using total features. The experimental outcome determines that ETC overtopped and achieved an accuracy of 92.62% with SMOTE.

10.3 Tree Based Algorithms

One of the finest and most widely used supervised learning approaches is Tree-based algorithms. Tree-based algorithms provide great accuracy, stability, and interpretability to prediction models. They map non-linear interactions relatively well, unlike linear models. They are adaptable at solving classification or regression problem. A Tree-based model requires essentially two fundamental components: determining which features to split on by minimizing entropy and maximizing information gain, and then deciding when to stop splitting. To stop splitting, the model will split until each final node has a small number of data points, but this will almost certainly lead to "overfitting". This classic problem in ML model will have enormously high accuracy with nonsensical outputs but fail to generalize when exposed to a new data, because as it has learned from the noises. To combat this a technique is referred called as "tree pruning". Where the model can set constraints on Tree-based algorithms by using various parameters like limit the maximum depth, maximum features, estimators, the number of leaf nodes in the tree etc. These Constraints Setting on Tree-based algorithms combat to improve predictive power [10]. For the study three Tree-based supervised ML algorithms DT, RF and Extra Trees classifier (ETC) are taken into consideration.

10.4 Natured Inspired Optimization (NIO)

A mathematical model with many parameters that must be learned from data is known as an ML model. When developing an ML model, the model architecture can be specified in a number of different ways. It is never easy to determine the ideal parameters for a particular model design because it calls for a careful analysis of many different possibilities. An internal model configuration called swarm-based parameter tweaking has a fitness function that can be learned or inferred during training. The agents, which are independent of the model are calculated from the data, by carry out the exploration. These swarms automatically choose the best parameters for a ML model based on assessing the fitness function. One always applies numerous pertinent algorithms based on the problem and chooses the best model, based on the models' top performance indicators. The ML model has both parameters and hyperparameters, although they have different functions. The variables known as parameters are those that the ML algorithm employs to forecast outcomes based on the input of past data. Hyperparameters are variables that the user specifies throughout the ML model construction process. In order to assess the ideal model parameters, hyperparameters are used. The performance of a model can be enhanced by using hyperparameters. Thus, locating the proper hyperparameters will help us develop the model that performs the best. The manual search method uses a hit-and-trial approach to find the best hyperparameters by spending a lot of time on a single model. A model's hyperparameters can be chosen using a variety of methods, including grid search, random search, manual search, Bayesian optimization etc., depending on how many hyperparameters are involved, and these solutions add time and expense to processing. NatureInspiredSearchCV is discussed in the study, which uses the to explore the best hyperparameters to up the performance of the model. The Bat algorithm (BA) [11], Hybrid Bat algorithm (HBA) [12], Hybrid Self Adaptive Bat algorithm (HSABA) [13], Firefly algorithm (FF) [14], and Grey Wolf Optimizer (GWO) [15] are considered in the investigation of Tree-based ML hyperparameter adjustment. A basic explanation of how nature-inspired search functions is shown in the following Algorithm 1 and the Fig. 10.2 shows the detail workflow that is used in this chapter.

Algorithm 1: Hyperparameter tuning by NatureInspiredSearchCV	
Step 1:	Initialize with randomly defined parameters of ML algorithm
Step 2:	Generate initial population of hyperparameters with size of solutions: $X = \{x_i\}_i^n$ at maximum number of generations uniformly
Step 3:	Partition the training dataset into folds
Step 4:	The number of candidate solutions generated depends upon the initial population size, maximum number of generations, and training dataset folds
Step 5:	While (until candidate solutions criteria not reached) **Step 5.1** Every individual is a parameter combination trained during the optimization run. The optimization run computes the fitness function (F1-score) $f(X_{(t)})$ for each individual of the population with dataset folds **Step 5.2** Select a proportion of the best optimized solution $B_{(t)}$ parameters, from the population of a certain size for a certain number of generations **Step 5.3** Build a ML model $ML_{(t)}$ based on $B_{(t)}$ **Step 5.4** The ML model is updated by sampling $ML_{(t)}$ to generate new solutions $X'_{(t)}$ and substituting $X'_{(t)}$ in $X_{(t)}$ **Step 5.5** The parameter combinations are being cached with optimization runs
Step 6:	Finally, output the best parameter combination solution for selected ML model

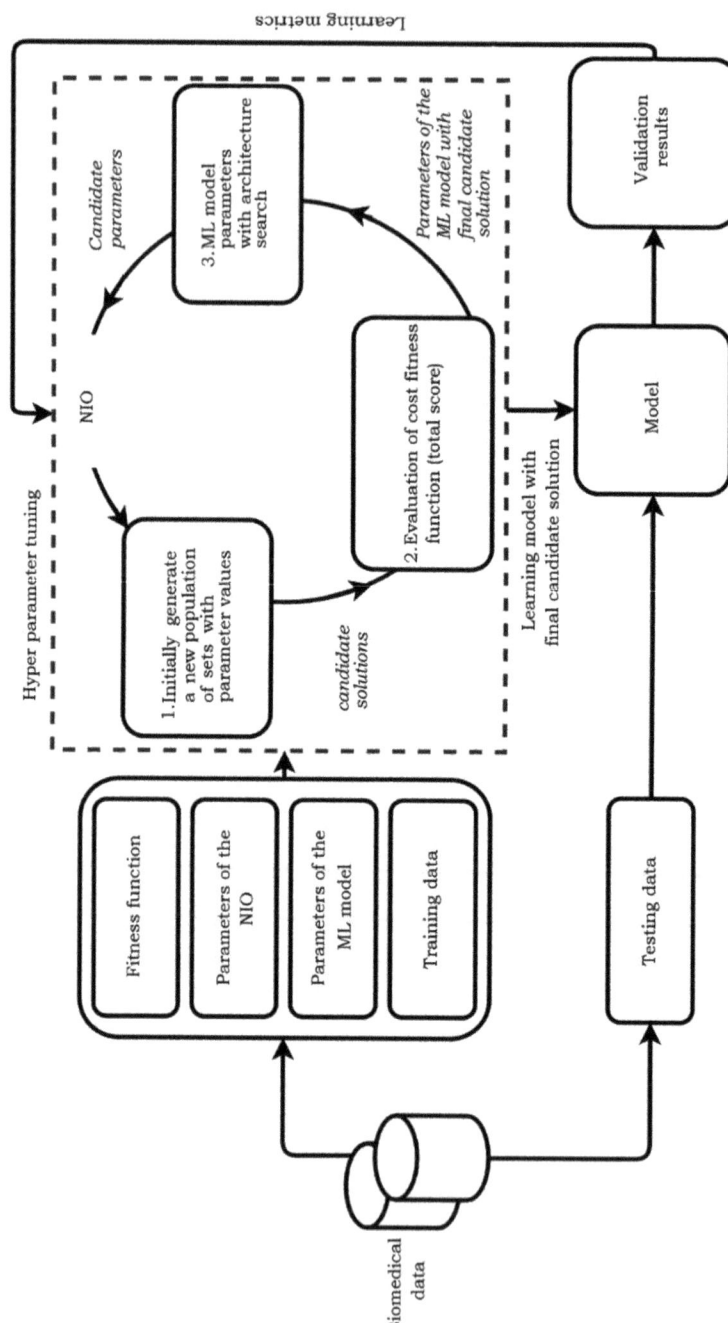

Fig. 10.2 Proposed framework

10.5 Basic Preliminaries of Optimization Techniques

The demand for optimization is universal, Optimization is a mathematical study that seeks out the optimal answer from a plethora of possibilities, whether in engineering, health, economics, or any other discipline. The foundation of mathematical NIO technique is to construct an objective function that must be maximised or minimised depending on the situation at hand, and to take numerous parameters as input. Then a search will be conducted to determine which set of parameters provides the best value. Typically, optimization algorithms attempt to intelligently steer the solution to global optimums while avoiding being locked in local optimum regions.

In general, too much exploitation will result in a local optimum, whereas too much exploration will result in the inability to locate the best solution. Mother nature has stepped in to help us find better solutions to real-world challenges with her intelligent solutions. Furthermore, these nature-inspired algorithms properly balance the processes of exploration, which is a departure from normal space in search of new, unknown regions and expanding the solution space, and exploitation, which is a search for a potential solution by utilising information from existing solutions in the search space, ultimately leading to an optimum solution. Some of the problem-solving methodologies and a set of novel approaches derived from natural processes of Nature-inspired algorithms are taken into consideration for the study.

10.5.1 Bat Algorithm

Bat algorithm was developed by Xin-She Yang [11] and is a population-based metaheuristic technique based on bat hunting behaviour. The idealized rules for developing program for the BAT algorithm are as follows.

1. By using echolocation, all bats can recognize and locate their prey.
2. Bats fly at a velocity v_i at point x_i can alter the wavelength (λ) and loudness A_0 of their produced pulses to fly randomly in search of prey. They vary their frequency based on the proximity of their target while keeping the minimum set frequency f_{min}.
3. The bat's loudness has a maximum value of A_0 and a minimum value of A_{min}. The volume levels range from A_0 to A_{min}.

The core operations of BA are encapsulated in the block diagram of Fig. 10.2 based on the initial assumptions. Equation (10.1) defines the initial location of all bats in the BA algorithm. The pseudo-random number generated by the uniform distribution is called rand. The *low* and *up* are the bottom and upper limits of boundary conditions, respectively. The *low* and *up* are both row vectors. Equations (10.2) and (10.3) are used to calculate each bat's pulse frequency and velocity. Where x^* is the current global best solution and a random vector (β) is created by uniform distribution. The exploitation is controlled by the parameter r and exploration by the parameter A.

Similarly, the minimum and maximum pulse frequencies are denoted by f_{min} and f_{max}, respectively. Equation (10.4) is used to calculate each bat's next location. The Bat pseudo code procedure is presented in Algorithm 2.

$$x_{ij} = rand(up_j - low_j) + low_j \tag{10.1}$$

$$f_i = \beta(f_{max} - f_{min}) + f_{min} \tag{10.2}$$

$$v_i^t = v_i^{t-1} + (x_i^t - x^*)f_i \tag{10.3}$$

$$x_i^t = x_i^{t-1} + v_i^t \tag{10.4}$$

Algorithm 2: BA optimization technique	
Step 1:	Initialize the fitness function $f(x)$, $x = (x_1, ..., x_d)^T$
Step 2:	Initialize the bat population x_i and v_i for $i = 1...n$
Step 3:	Define pulse frequency $Q_i \in [Q_{min}, Q_{max}]$
Step 4:	Initialize pulse rates r_i and the loudness A_i
Step 5:	While ($t < T_{max}$)
	Step 5.1: Generate new solutions by adjusting frequency
	Step 5.2: Update velocities and locations using Eq. (10.1-10.3)
	Step 5.3: $if(rand(0, 1) > r_i)$
	Step 5.3.1: Select a solution among the best solutions
	Step 5.3.2: Generate a local solution around the best solution
	Step 5.4: Generate a new solution by randomly flying
	Step 5.5: $if(rand(0, 1) < A_i$ and $f(x_i) < f(x^*))$
	Step 5.5.1: Accept the new solutions
	Step 5.5.2: Reduce A_i and increase r_i
	Step 5.6: Rank the bat population and find the current best

10.5.2 Hybrid Bat Algorithm

Fister I, D. Fister, and X. S. Yang [12] proposed a novel BA by employing Differential Evolution (DE) methods to hybridize the original BA and propose a new BA, called HBA. DE optimizes a problem by retaining a population of candidate solutions and creating new candidate solutions by merging the existing ones using simple equations, and then keeping the candidate solution with the best score or fitness on the optimization problem. DE supports a differential mutation, a differential crossover and a differential selection. DE can be accomplished in a variety of ways in terms of mutation, crossover, and differential selection. Algorithm 3 gives a pseudo code for HBA.

Algorithm 3: HBA optimization technique	
Step 1:	Initialize the fitness function $f(x)$, $x = (x1, ..., xd)^T$
Step 2:	Initialize the bat population x_i and v_i for $i = 1...n$
Step 3:	Define pulse frequency $Q_i \in [Q_{min}, Q_{max}]$
Step 4:	Initialize pulse rates r_i and the loudness A_i
Step 5:	While $(t < T_{max})$
	Step 5.1: Generate new solutions by adjusting frequency
	Step 5.2: Update velocities and locations using Eq. (10.1-10.3)
	Step 5.3: if $(rand(0, 1) > r_i)$
	Step 5.3.1: Modify the solution using $DE/rand/1/bin$
	Step 5.4: Generate a new solution by randomly flying
	Step 5.5: if $(rand(0, 1) < A_i$ and $f(x_i) < f(x^*))$
	Step 5.5.1: Accept the new solutions
	Step 5.5.2: Reduce A_i and increase r_i
	Step 5.6: Rank the bat population and find the current best

10.5.3 Hybrid Self Adaptive Bat Algorithm

Applying the Self-Adaptive Bat Approach (SABA) to a population-based algorithm has two distinct advantages: (i) There is no need to establish control parameters prior to the algorithm's execution. (ii) Throughout the run, the control parameters are modified to account for the fitness landscape, which is determined by the locations of potential solutions inside the search space and their corresponding fitness values. Although the SABA method surpassed the original BA algorithm by a large margin, it suffered from a lack of domain-specific understanding of the problem to be solved. So, hybridising the SABA, derives to a new local search heuristic that better harnesses the algorithm's self-adaptation mechanism. The local search is initiated when the self-adapted pulse rate r_i reaches a certain threshold. On average, every 10th virtual bat modifies this parameter. The local search is a DE-inspired implementation of the crossover and mutation operators. To begin, the four virtual bats are chosen at random from the bat population, and a random position within the virtual bat is chosen at random. The trial solution is modified as follows by the appropriate DE strategy as given in Eq. (10.5). Where the DE Strategy is implemented based on the probability of crossover (CR). The term $n = D$ assures that the trial solution is subjected to almost one modification. Where dimension of the problem is determined by D and the population size is determined by N_p. The different strategies used in DE for

Table 10.1 DE strategies

Strategies	Functions
$DE/rand/1/bin$	$y_j = x_{r1,j} + F.(x_{r2,j} - x_{r3,j})$
$DE/randToBest/1/bin$	$y_j = x_{i,j} + F.(best_j - x_{i,j}) - F.(x_{r1,j} - x_{r2,j})$
$DE/best/2/bin$	$y_j = best_j + F.(x_{r1,j} + x_{r2,j} - x_{r3,j} - x_{r4,j})$
$DE/best/1/bin$	$y_j = best_j + F.(x_{r1,j} - x_{r2,j})$

HSABA algorithm is mentioned in Table 10.1 and Algorithm 4 shows the HSABA pseudo code.

$$y_n = \begin{cases} DE_{starategy}, & if\ Rand(0,1) \leq CR \vee n = D, \\ x_i, & otherwise \end{cases} \quad (10.5)$$

Algorithm 4: HSABA optimization technique	
Step 1:	*Initialize the fitness function $f(x)$, $x = (x1, ..., xd)^T$*
Step 2:	*Initialize the bat population x_i and v_i for $i = 1...n$*
Step 3:	*Define pulse frequency $Q_i \in [Q_{min}, Q_{max}]$*
Step 4:	*Initialize pulse rates r_i and the loudness A_i*
Step 5:	$While(t < T_{max})$
	Step 5.1: *Generate new solutions by adjusting frequency*
	Step 5.2: *update velocities and locations using Eq. (10.1-10.3)*
	Step 5.3: $if(rand(0,1) > r_i)$
	Step 5.3.1: $r_{i=1,...,4} = \lfloor rand(0,1) * Np + 1 \rfloor \wedge r_1 \neq r_2 \neq r_3 \neq r_4$
	Step 5.3.2: $n = rand(1, D)$
	Step 5.3.3: $for\ i \leftarrow 1\ to\ D\ w.r.t\ to\ DE\ Strategies$
	Step 5.3.3.1: $if((rand(0,1) < CR) \| (n == D))$
	Step 5.3.3.1.1: $y_n = DE_{Strategy}(n, i, r1, r2, r3, r4)$
	Step 5.3.3.2: $n = (n+1)\%(D+1);$
	Step 5.4: *Generate a new solution by randomly flying*
	Step 5.5: $if(rand(0,1) < A_i\ and\ f(x_i) < f(x^*))$
	Step 5.5.1: *Accept the new solutions*
	Step 5.5.2: *Reduce A_i and increase r_i*
	Step 5.6: *Rank the bat population and find the current best*

10.5.4 Firefly Algorithm

Different animals communicate with one another through diverse techniques of communication. FA are winged beetles or insects that produce light and blinking at night. Inspired by the flashing characteristics of the fireflies, Yang [16] discovers how to use the qualities of firefly activity to solve real-life challenges. Fireflies use their flashing property to communicate. There are three important assumptions (i) FA are unisex and will be attracted to each other, (ii) brightness plays a vital role in attracting others, and (iii) FA will move randomly when their brightness is the same. Where α determines the maximum radius of the random step, β determines the step size towards an optimum solution, I is the intensity, d observer distance from the source, n determines the population size, γ determines light absorption coefficient, $\mathcal{E}$ is a random vector with values ranging from 0 to 1 drawn from a uniform distribution, and max_t determines maximum iterations. The position of individual fireflies is updated with position i.e., move firefly i towards firefly j by Eq. (10.6), and firefly move randomly in case, not any brighter one is recognized by Eq. (10.7). The FA pseudo code is presented in Algorithm 5.

$$x_i(t+1) = x_i(t) + \beta e^{\gamma r_{ij}^2}(x_j^t - x_i^t) + \alpha_t \epsilon_i^t \qquad (10.6)$$

$$x_i(t+1) = x_i(t) + \alpha \varepsilon_i \qquad (10.7)$$

Algorithm 5: FA optimization technique	
Step 1:	$Initialize\ n, \beta, \alpha, d, max_t\ parameters$
Step 2:	$Randomly\ generate\ N\ initial\ solutions$
Step 3:	$While\ t \leftarrow 1\ to\ max_t$
	Step 3.1 $Calculate\ the\ fitness\ value\ (light\ intensity)\ for\ each\ firefly\ i.e,\ I_i$ at x_i is computed by the objective function $F(x_i)$
	Step 3.2 $for\ i \leftarrow 1\ to\ n-1$
	Step 3.2.1 $for\ j \leftarrow i+1\ to\ n$
	Step 3.2.1.1 $if\ I_i > I_j$
	Step 3.2.1.1.1 $Update\ position\ i.e.,$ $move\ firefly\ i\ towards\ firefly\ j\ as$ $given\ in\ Eq.\ (10.6).$
	Step 3.3 $Move\ firefly\ randomly\ in\ case,\ not\ any\ brighter\ as\ give\ in$ $Eq.(10.7).$
Step 4:	$Report\ the\ best\ solution$

10.5.5 Grey Wolf Algorithm

The behaviour of the grey wolf, which hunts huge prey in packs and relies on cooperation among individual wolves, is the inspiration for this algorithm. There are two features of this behaviour that are worth noting i.e., social hierarchy, and hunting mechanism. Because the grey wolf is a highly gregarious species, it has a complicated social hierarchy. The term "dominance hierarchies" refers to a hierarchical system in which wolves are graded according to their strength and power. As a result, alphas, betas, deltas, and omegas exist. Applying the described skills to solve the optimization problem, the three best answers are indicated by alpha, beta, and delta, at each stage. Mathematically GWO examines two points in an n-dimensional space and updates the location of one of them based on that of another as given in Eqs. (10.8–10.11). where $X(t+1)$ is the next location, $X(t)$ is current location of the wolf, and $r_1 \& r_2$ is a vector for randomly generated numbers in the interval [0,1]. The A and D indicates the coefficient matrix and vector that is dependent on the prey's location X_p. X_p is dependent on the three best solutions to identify the real position of the optimal solution, and the formulas for updating each of the wolves are as given in Eqs. (10.12–10.13). The GWO pseudo code is presented in Algorithm 6.

$$X(t+1) = X(t) - A.D \qquad (10.8)$$

$$A = 2a.r_1 - a \qquad (10.9)$$

$$D = |C.X_p(t) - X(t)| \qquad (10.10)$$

$$C = 2.r_2 \qquad (10.11)$$

D_α, D_β and D_δ are calculated using Eq. (10.12).

$$\begin{aligned} D_\alpha &= |C_1.X_\alpha - X| \\ D_\beta &= |C_2.X_\beta - X| \\ D_\delta &= |C_3.X_\delta - X| \end{aligned} \qquad (10.12)$$

where X_1 and X_2 and X_3 are calculated with Eq. (10.13)

$$\begin{aligned} X_1 &= X_\alpha(t) - A_1.D_\alpha \\ X_2 &= X_\beta(t) - A_2.D_\beta \end{aligned} \qquad (10.13)$$

$$X_3 = X_\delta(t) - A_3.D_\delta$$

The Eq. (10.14) indicates that the position of the wolf will be updated accordingly to the best three wolves from the previous iteration as given in Eq. (10.13)

$$X(t+1) = \frac{X_1 + X_2 + X_3}{3} \qquad (10.14)$$

Algorithm 6: GWO technique	
Step 1:	Initialize the grey wolf population $X_i, i = 1\ldots n$
Step 2:	Initialize a, A, and C
Step 3:	Calculate the fitness of best search agent (X_α), second best search (X_β) agent and third best search agent (X_δ)
Step 4:	While $t \leftarrow 1$ to max_t
	Step 4.1: for *each search wolves* do
	Step 4.1.1: Randomly initialize r_1 and r_2
	Step 4.1.1: Update the position of the current search agent by the Eq.(10.14)
	Step 4.2: Update a, A, and C
	Step 4.3: Calculate the fitness of all search agents
	Step 4.4: Update X_α, X_β, and X_δ
Step 5:	Report the best solution

10.6 Experiment Setup and Datasets Descriptions

The system environment and the dataset utilised are briefly described in this section.

10.6.1 System Environment

Google Colab Notebook was used to conduct the experiment. Data pre-processing was done using the NumPy framework, Tree-based ML algorithms are executed using the Scikit-Learn framework, and hyperparameter optimization was done using the NatureInspiredSearchCV framework.

Table 10.2 The comprehensive description of the dataset

Attributes	Measurement	Range
Age	years	(40 to 95)
Anaemia	boolean	(0,1)
High blood pressure	boolean	(0,1)
Creatinine phosphokinase	mcg/L	(23 to 7861)
Diabetes	boolean	(0,1)
Ejection fraction	percentage	(14 to 80)
Platelets	kiloplatelets/mL	(25.01 to 850.00)
Sex	binary	(0,1)
Serum creatinine	mg/dL	(0.50 to 9.40)
Serum sodium	mEq/L	(114 to 148)
Smoking	boolean	(0,1)
Time	days	(4 to 285)
Death event	boolean	(0,1)

10.6.2 Heart Failure Clinical Records Data Set

The "Heart Failure Clinical Records Dataset" is a multivariate numerical dataset composed of 13 clinical features. The dataset comprises of 299 patients' medical records who had deceased with heart failure. The key tasks of this dataset are to predict heart failure based on the given characteristics of the patients. The experimental objective is to diagnose and extract numerous insights from this dataset which could aid in comprehending the problem whether or not that a particular person is at risk of developing heart failure. The dataset is collected from UCI ML repository [8]. The Table 10.2, briefly describes about the dataset through clinical report and lifestyle information with various attributes, their description, their measurement, and range. Additionally, the quantitative characteristics of the dataset are given in Table 10.3.

10.7 Results

It is crucial to test the process to make sure that the dataset's visualisation and study analysis are suitable. So, a fivefold cross validation process with binary classification is performed for the study. The simulation work's results based on the existing dataset discloses the cases that were undetected. The outcomes of the suggested Tree-based ML algorithms with NIO are outlined in this section. The assessment measures that are taken into the study are TPR, FPR, F1-score, precision, and accuracy are used to validate the performance of our suggested techniques. Precision and recall are less comprehensible measurements when used alone, hence the chosen hyperparameters are tuned using swarm optimization with F1-score as the fitness function. For data

Table 10.3 The outlined category features description

Category feature	Total patients		Survived patients		Dead patients	
	No. of patients	% of patients	No. of patients	% of patients	No. of patients	% of patients
Sex (1: man)	194	64.88	132	65.02	62	64.58
Sex (0: woman)	105	35.12	71	34.98	34	35.42
Anaemia (1: true)	129	43.14	3	40.89	46	47.92
Anaemia (0: false)	170	56.86	120	59.11	50	52.08
Smoking (1: true)	96	32.11	66	32.51	30	31.25
Smoking (0: false)	203	67.89	137	67.49	66	68.75
Diabetes (1: true)	125	41.81	85	41.87	40	41.67
Diabetes (0: false)	174	58.19	118	58.13	56	58.33
High blood pressure (1: true)	105	35.12	66	32.51	39	40.62
High blood pressure (0: false)	194	64.88	137	67.49	57	59.38
Death event (1: true)	–	–	–	–	96	32.1
Death event (0: false)	–	–	203	67.89	–	–

with imbalanced classes, the F1-score is a more accurate evaluation metric and is easier to interpret when looking for data distribution between precision and recall. Table 10.4 shows the classifiers with optimized hyperparameters for "Heart Failure Dataset". The precision, recall, and F1-Macro avg score of proposed algorithms without optimization are given in Table 10.5 and Fig. 10.9 shows the proposed approach accuracies. Tables 10.6, 10.7, 10.8, 10.9 and 10.10 shows the proposed approach with false positive rate (FPR), area under ROC curve, and error rate of individual class metrics. It is referred that for HSABA with RF showed the least FPR of zero for Class 1, on the other hand DT for Class 0 gained the highest FPR. The ROC expectancy of ETC showed 0.84 maximization for both the classes, and produced a minimum error rate of 0.083 for both RF and ETC. However, hyperparameter optimization of GWO with ETC improved and derived the least FPR of zero for Class 1, on the other hand DT for Class 1 gained the highest FPR with 0.28. All the Tree-based ML algorithms are likewise well functioning for the ROC and error rate. The HBA algorithm with RF obtained the least FPR for Class 0 when compared to other algorithms. The ROC and error rate of ETC have achieved the majority of correctly deceased patients and next RF, but a poor score compared of error rate of DT compared to other Tree-based algorithms. The BA optimization with RF showed outcomes, validated with minimum error rate of 0.06 and high ROC area of 0.88 compared algorithm outcomes. The results from the tested data of Tree-based algorithms with FA showed a likewise functioning for the ROC and error rate. But for class 1 ETC showed a minimum FPR and highest for class 0. The simulation work result analysis discloses the incidences of heart failure that went unnoticed on the dataset. The Figs. 10.3, 10.4, 10.5, 10.6 and 10.7 depicts the classification report of the proposed work with Tree-based classification approach with the quantitative characteristics of the dataset. The Fig. 10.8 illustrates the fitness function(F1-score) score of the optimization techniques with respect to Tree-based algorithms. ETC fared well among all Tree-based ML techniques with an accuracy of 95% using GWO and a fitness function score of 0.9242. And for all other optimization techniques, the ETC derived a consistent accuracy of 91.66%, with a fitness function sore of 0.8737 and 0.8664. The RF fits with a highest accuracy of 93.33% for BA technique and a low accuracy of 90% for HBA. Where the fitness value of BA is 0.9018 and for HBA is 0.8527. Similarly, the DT produced a highest accuracy of 88.33% with HSABA technique and a lowest accuracy of 85% for FA technique. Where the fitness value of HSABA is 0.8117 and for FA is 0.8043. We compared the suggested work with other researchers work in order to determine the significance of our research. The Table 10.11, shows the proposed system proved comparatively better in predicting the results.

10.8 Conclusion and Future Work

The aim of this chapter is to examine and find the suitable techniques for developing the model for predicting heart failure. NIO algorithms with clinical data leads to identify CVD and validate the possibility to predict heart failure. NIO solves problems iteratively in an effort to enhance a potential solution with respect to a specified fitness function quality metric. In this work, we examined how well tree-based ML classification tasks performed with respect to NIO techniques. This chapter presents an interplay between sensitivity, precision of the correct instance's prediction and also the cost of missed and erroneous instances prediction of heart failure. The suggested work successfully illustrated its sturdiness using the heart failure dataset. The empirical study demonstrates that hyper parameter tuning with optimization approaches can greatly enhance the overall performance of the clinical datasets. The chapter main contribution is a comprehensive assessment of heart failure data set features with Tree-based ML algorithms and hyperparameter tuning. The proposed algorithm outperformed well in categorizing no chance of heart failure and person

Table 10.4 Tree-based ML algorithms with optimized hyperparameters by NIO

Tree-based ML algorithms	Hyperparameters	Optimized hyperparameters				
		FA	BA	HBA	GWO	HSABA
DT	max_features = (auto, sqrt, log2), splitter = (best, random), max_depth = range (5, 30), criterion = (gini, entropy)	max_features = log2, splitter = best, max_depth = 5, criterion = entropy	max_features = auto, splitter = best, max_depth = 5, criterion = gini	max_features = log2, splitter = best, max_depth = 5, criterion = entropy	max_features = log2, splitter = best, max_depth = 5, criterion = entropy	max_features = sqrt, splitter = random, max_depth = 5, criterion = entropy
ETC	max_features = (auto, sqrt, log2), n_estimators = range (10, 100), max_depth = range (5,30), criterion = (gini, entropy)	max_features = sqrt, n_estimators = 30, max_depth = 10, criterion = entropy	max_features = log2, n_estimators = 10, max_depth = 20, criterion = gini	max_features = auto, n_estimators = 30, max_depth = 20, criterion = entropy	max_features = log2, n_estimators = 30, max_depth = 25, criterion = gini	max_features = auto, n_estimators = 40, max_depth = 10, criterion = gini
RF	max_features = (auto, sqrt, log2), n_estimators = range (10, 100), max_depth = range (5, 30), criterion = (gini, entropy)	max_features = log2, n_estimators = 30, max_depth = 5, criterion = gini,	max_features = log2, n_estimators = 40, max_depth = 5, criterion = gini	max_features = log2, n_estimators = 10, max_depth = 25, criterion = gini	max_features = auto, n_estimators = 10, max_depth = 5, criterion = gini	max_features = sqrt, n_estimators = 10, max_depth = 5, criterion = entropy

Table 10.5 Evaluation metrics of ML algorithms

Tree-based ML algorithms	Without optimization			
	Precision	Recall	F1-score	Accuracy (%)
DT	0.737	0.795	0.753	80%
RF	0.86	0.86	0.86	90%
ETC	0.877	0.896	0.886	91.66%

Table 10.6 The FPR, ROC, and Error rate of Tree-based alg. using HSABA

Metrics	RF		ETC		DT	
	Class 0	Class 1	Class 0	Class 1	Class 0	Class 1
FPR	0.357	0	0.28	0.02	0.42	0.02
Area under ROC	0.82	0.82	0.84	0.84	0.77	0.77
Error rate	0.083	0.083	0.083	0.083	0.11	0.11

Table 10.7 The FPR, ROC, and Error rate of Tree-based alg. using GWO

Metrics	RF		ETC		DT	
	Class 0	Class 1	Class 0	Class 1	Class 0	Class 1
FPR	0.21	0.04	0.21	0	0.28	0.08
Area under ROC	0.87	0.87	0.89	0.89	0.81	0.81
Error rate	0.083	0.083	0.05	0.05	0.13	0.13

Table 10.8 The FPR, ROC, and Error rate of Tree-based alg. using HBA

Metrics	RF		ETC		DT	
	Class 0	Class 1	Class 0	Class 1	Class 0	Class 1
FPR	0.28	0.04	0.35	0	0.42	0.04
Area under ROC	0.83	0.83	0.82	0.82	0.76	0.76
Error rate	0.09	0.09	0.08	0.08	0.13	0.13

Table 10.9 The FPR, ROC, and Error rate of Tree-based alg. using BA a>

Metrics	RF		ETC		DT	
	Class 0	Class 1	Class 0	Class 1	Class 0	Class 1
FPR	0.21	0.021	0.35	0	0.28	0.08
Area under ROC	0.88	0.88	0.82	0.82	0.81	0.81
Error rate	0.06	0.06	0.08	0.08	0.13	0.13

Table 10.10 The FPR, ROC, and Error rate of Tree-based alg. using FA

Metrics	RF		ETC		DT	
	Class 0	Class 1	Class 0	Class 1	Class 0	Class 1
FPR	0.28	0.02	0.35	0	0.21	0.13
Area under ROC	0.84	0.84	0.82	0.82	0.82	0.82
Error rate	0.08	0.08	0.08	0.08	0.15	0.15

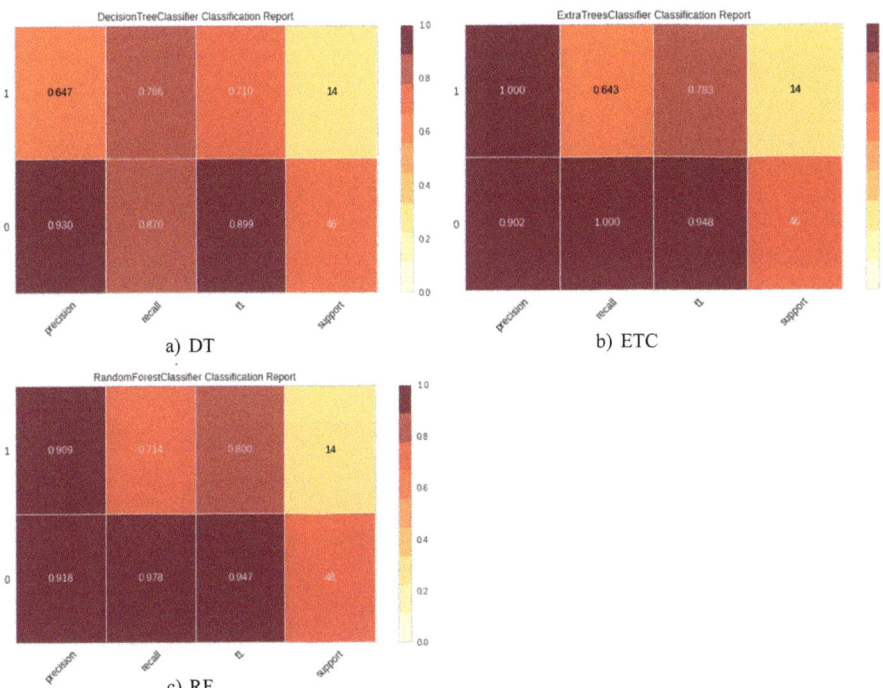

Fig. 10.3 Classification report with FA optimization

who is prone to heart failure activities with 95% of accuracy. The future research work would be concentrated on iterative improvement and discovering a newly optimum value set of parameters using different swarm intelligence approaches on various benchmark datasets.

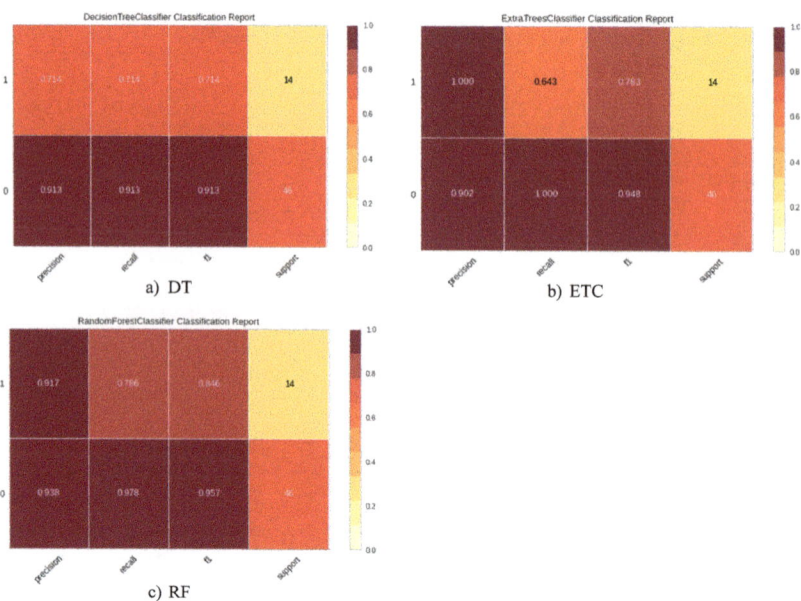

Fig. 10.4 Classification report with BA optimization

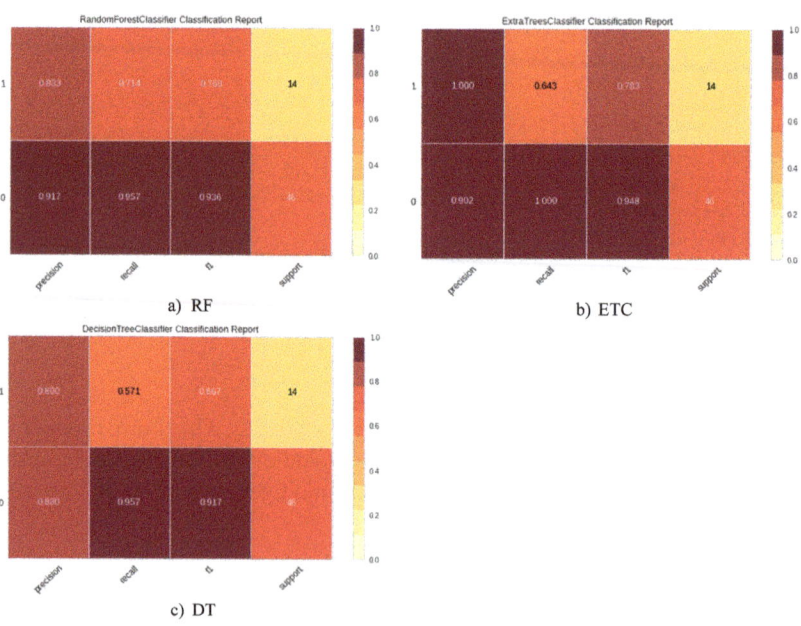

Fig. 10.5 Classification report with HBA optimization

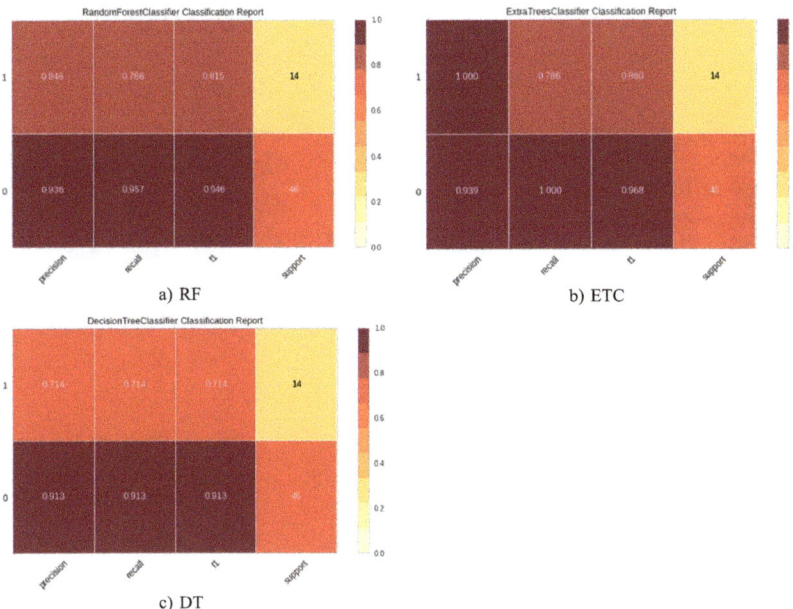

Fig. 10.6 Classification report with GWO

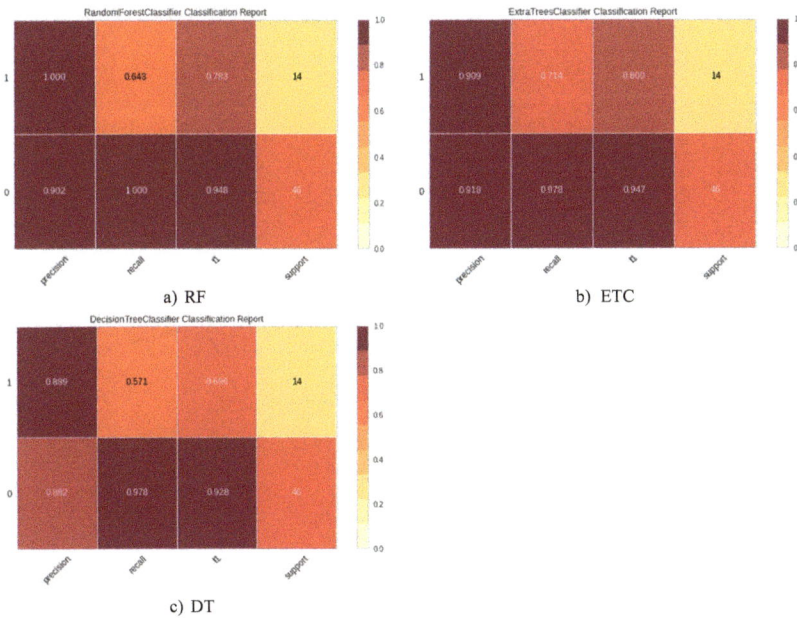

Fig. 10.7 Classification report with HSABA optimization

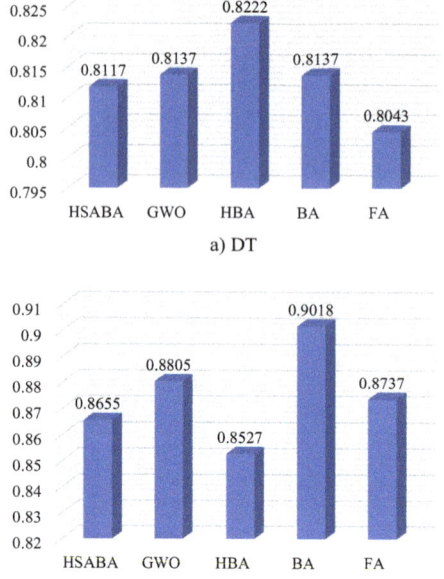

Fig. 10.8 The F1-Score of NIO for Tree-based ML algorithms

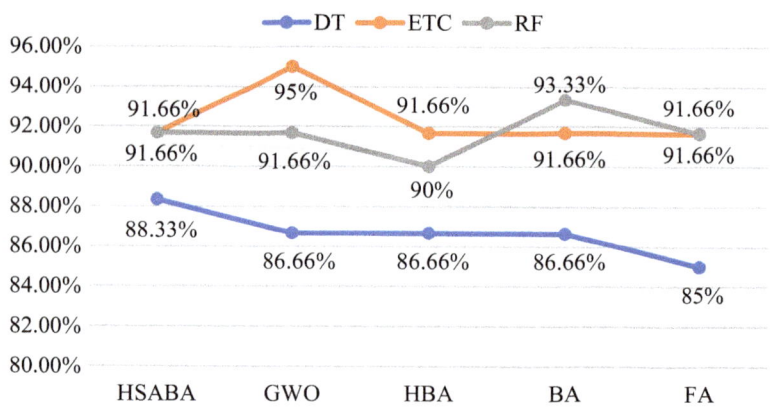

Fig. 10.9 Proposed model accuracies

Table 10.11 Comparative study for heart failure dataset

Various researchers work	Proposed model	Metrics
Sai Krishna Reddy et al. [7]	GNB	Accuracy = 86%
	DT	Accuracy = 82%
Chicco and Jurman [8]	ANN	Accuracy = 68%, F1-score = 0.483
	SVM	Accuracy = 69%, F1-score = 0.182
	k-NN	Accuracy = 62%, F1-score = 0.148
	RF	Accuracy = 74%, F1-score = 0.547
	One rule	Accuracy = 72.9%, F1-score = 0.465
	LR	Accuracy = 73%, F1-score = 0.475
	NB	Accuracy = 69.6%, F1-score = 0.364
	DT	Accuracy = 73%, F1-score = 0.554
	Gradient boosting	Accuracy = 73.8%, F1-score = 0.527
Ishaq et al. [9]	ETC with nine significant features and SMOTE	Accuracy = 92.62%, F1-score = 0.93, Precision = 0.93, Recall = 0.93
Proposed work	ETC with GWO	Accuracy = 95%, F1-score = 0.9242, Precision = 0.96, Recall = 0.89

References

1. Ghosh, P., et al.: Efficient prediction of cardiovascular disease using machine learning algorithms with relief and LASSO feature selection techniques. IEEE Access **9**, 19304–19326 (2021). https://doi.org/10.1109/ACCESS.2021.3053759
2. Asif, M.A.A.R., et al.: Performance evaluation and comparative analysis of different machine learning algorithms in predicting cardiovascular disease. Eng. Lett. **29**(2), 731–741 (2021)
3. Sree Sandhya, N., Beena Bethel, G.N.: Impact of Bio-inspired Algorithms to Predict Heart Diseases. Smart Computing Techniques and Applications. Springer, Singapore, pp. 121–127 (2021)
4. World Health Organization: Cardiovascular diseases. https://www.who.int/news-room/fact-sheets/detail/cardiovascular-diseases-(cvds). Accessed on May 6, 2022
5. Joshi, A., Rienks, M., Theofilatos, K., Mayr, M.: Systems biology in cardiovascular disease: a multiomics approach. Nat. Rev. Cardiol. **18**(5), 313–330 (2021). https://doi.org/10.1038/s41569-020-00477-1

6. Reddy, D.K.K., et al.: A Fog-Based Intelligent Secured IoMT Framework for Early Diabetes Prediction. Intelligent Internet of Things for Healthcare and Industry. Springer, Cham, pp. 199–218 (2022)
7. Sai Krishna Reddy, V., Meghana, P., Subba Reddy, N.V., Ashwath Rao, B.: Prediction on Cardiovascular disease using Decision tree and Naïve Bayes classifiers. J. Phys. Conf. Ser. **2161**(1), 012015 (2022). doi:https://doi.org/10.1088/1742-6596/2161/1/012015
8. Chicco, D., Jurman, G.: Machine learning can predict survival of patients with heart failure from serum creatinine and ejection fraction alone. BMC Med. Inform. Decis. Mak. **20**(1), 1–16 (2020). https://doi.org/10.1186/s12911-020-1023-5
9. Ishaq, A., et al.: Improving the prediction of heart failure patients' survival using SMOTE and effective data mining techniques. IEEE Access **9**, 39707–39716 (2021). https://doi.org/10.1109/ACCESS.2021.3064084
10. Huang, Y., Talwar, A., Chatterjee, S., Aparasu, R.R.: Application of machine learning in predicting hospital readmissions: a scoping review of the literature. BMC Med. Res. Methodol. **21**(1), 1–14 (2021). https://doi.org/10.1186/s12874-021-01284-z
11. Yang, X.S., He, X.: Bat algorithm: literature review and applications. Int. J. Bio-Inspired Comput. **5**(3), 141 (2013). https://doi.org/10.1504/IJBIC.2013.055093
12. Fister, I., Fister, D., Yang, X.S.: A hybrid bat algorithm. Elektroteh. Vestnik/Electrotechnical Rev. **80**(1–2), 1–7 (2013)
13. Fister, I., Fong, S., Brest, J., Fister, I.: A novel hybrid self-adaptive bat algorithm. Sci. World J. **2014**(i), 1–12 (2014). doi:https://doi.org/10.1155/2014/709738
14. Yang, X. S.: Firefly algorithms for multimodal optimization. *Lect. Notes Comput. Sci. (including Subser. Lect. Notes Artif. Intell. Lect. Notes Bioinformatics)*, vol. 5792 LNCS, pp. 169–178 (2009). doi:https://doi.org/10.1007/978-3-642-04944-6_14
15. Mirjalili, S., Mirjalili, S.M., Lewis, A.: Grey wolf optimizer. Adv. Eng. Softw. **69**, 46–61 (2014). https://doi.org/10.1016/j.advengsoft.2013.12.007
16. Yang, X.-S., Karamanoglu, M.: Nature-inspired computation and swarm intelligence: a state-of-the-art overview, in *Nature-Inspired Computation and Swarm Intelligence*, vol. 927, Elsevier, pp. 3–18 (2020)

Chapter 11
Early Detection of Chronic Obstructive Pulmonary Disease Using LSTM-Firefly Based Deep Learning Model

P. Suresh Kumar, Pandit Byomakesha Dash, B. Kameswara Rao, S. Vimal, and Khan Muhammad

Abstract Identifying Chronic Obstructive Pulmonary Disease (COPD) is essential for reducing mortality and cost burden. However, the population suffers from an underdiagnosis of chronic obstructive pulmonary disease. This chapter aims to create COPD detection models and assess the relative effectiveness of several modeling paradigms to discover the optimal model for the task on the dataset of 563 hospital or emergency ward visits in China-Japan Friendship Hospital performed between February 2011 and March 2017. We investigated the use of a Long Short Term Memory Network (LSTM), a kind of deep learning, for the automated identification of COPD, with the model hyperparameters modified using the firefly algorithm. Three optimization variations have been used to optimize the hyperparameters of the proposed LSTM Model: random search, hyperband, and firefly algorithm. Firefly algorithm with LSTM obtained superior results than the LSTM-Random Search and LSTM-Hyperband. Therefore, the adoption of LSTM-Firefly is beneficial in terms of COPD detection and diagnosis with clinically acceptable performance compared to LSTM—Random Search, LSTM—Hyperband, LSTM, and other machine learning algorithms such as LR, KNN, NB, DT, and RF.

P. S. Kumar (✉)
Department of Computer Scinece and Engineering, Aditya Institute of Technology and Management, Tekkali 532201, India
e-mail: reshu.suri@gmail.com

P. B. Dash
Department of Information Technology, Aditya Institute of Technology and Management, Tekkali 532201, India

B. K. Rao
Department of Computer Science and Engineering, Gandhi Institute of Technology and Management (Deemed to be University), Visakhapatnam 530045, India

S. Vimal
Department of AI & DS, Ramco Institute of Technology, Tamil Nadu, Rajapalayam 626117, India

K. Muhammad
Department of Applied Artificial Intelligence, School of Convergence, College of Computing and Informatics, Sungkyunkwan University, Seoul 03063, Republic of Korea

© The Author(s), under exclusive license to Springer Nature Switzerland AG 2023
J. Nayak et al. (eds.), *Nature-Inspired Optimization Methodologies in Biomedical and Healthcare*, Intelligent Systems Reference Library 233,
https://doi.org/10.1007/978-3-031-17544-2_11

Keywords Chronic obstructive pulmonary disease · LSTM · Machine learning · Firefly

11.1 Introduction

COPD is a public health issue that health care systems are increasingly concerned about, and it is on track to be the world's third-biggest cause of death in the near future. According to the Global Burden of disease survey, COPD killed over 3 million people in 2010, and there were 251 million cases of COPD worldwide in 2016 [1]. It is a broad phrase that encompasses disorders such as chronic bronchitis, emphysema, and refractory asthma. According to the World Health Organization, around 3.17 million individuals have died as a result of such life-threatening diseases [2]. Figure 11.1 depicted the top 10 nations afflicted by COPD from 2001 to 2010. According to the National Vital Statistics system, the mortality rates of the United States population are shown in Fig. 11.2. COPD is identified by an irreversible chronic airflow limitation induced by sustained exposure to toxic particles or gases. As the disease advances, patients often encounter acute exacerbations characterized by sudden cough, the onset of dyspnea, sputum production, and hastened lung function decrease. The intensity of airway obstruction must be assessed in order to determine the chance of potential symptoms and to guide treatment. Spirometry is often used to accomplish this assessment; nevertheless, spirometry requires a significant amount of effort and support from patients. Elderly individuals, those who cannot comprehend, and those who have significant medical disorders often have trouble passing this test [3]. COPD is often connected with hospitalizations and readmissions, and substantial mortality. Diagnosing CPOD is quite expensive from a financial aspect. Costs associated with the condition are projected to rise in tandem with its frequency in the future years. These expenditures tend to increase as the severity of COPD worsens, mainly owing to the hospitalization of COPD patients. As a result, COPD is marked by a high prevalence, death rate, high health-care expenses, primarily due to hospitalization, and a severe decline in the quality of life of those afflicted.

COPD is an obstructive sort of lung disease. COPD illness has a notably negative influence on our respiratory. This illness generally involves an airflow impairment that is not totally reversible. COPD is a common lung disease that results in persons suffering from chronic bronchitis as well as emphysema. In emphysema, the alveoli at the end of the bronchioles (the tiny air passageways of the lungs) are damaged, often as a result of smoking. An accurate diagnosis of COPD is crucial for the prompt commencement of medications that lower the likelihood of future exacerbations and hospitalizations, postpone disease progression, and improve patients' overall prognosis [4]. Without a doubt, early detection of COPDs is essential for decreasing the associated mortality and cost burden. Clinical notes contain essential facts about illness development that aren't accessible anywhere else in a patient's electronic health record, but they're difficult to access for medical researchers. These difficulties prompted the development of illness progression modeling techniques. The

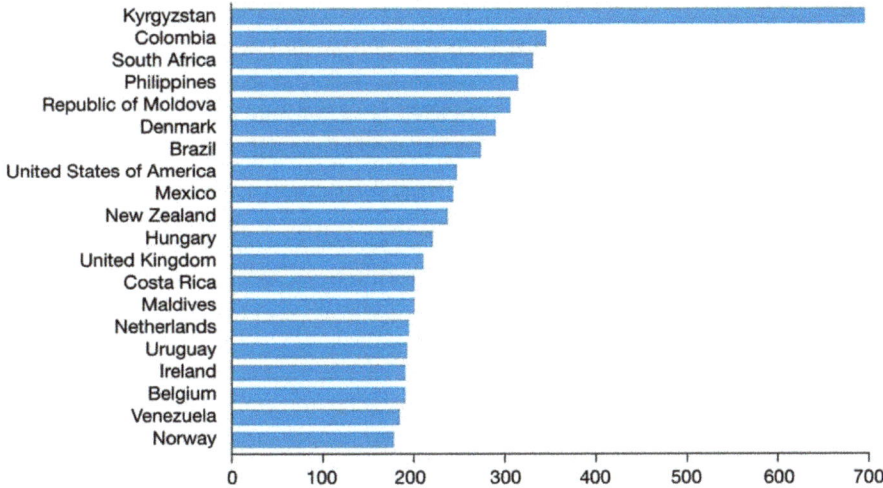

Fig. 11.1 Top 20 nations with the most COPD fatalities per million per year between 2001 and 2010. *Source* https://statistics.blf.org.uk/copd

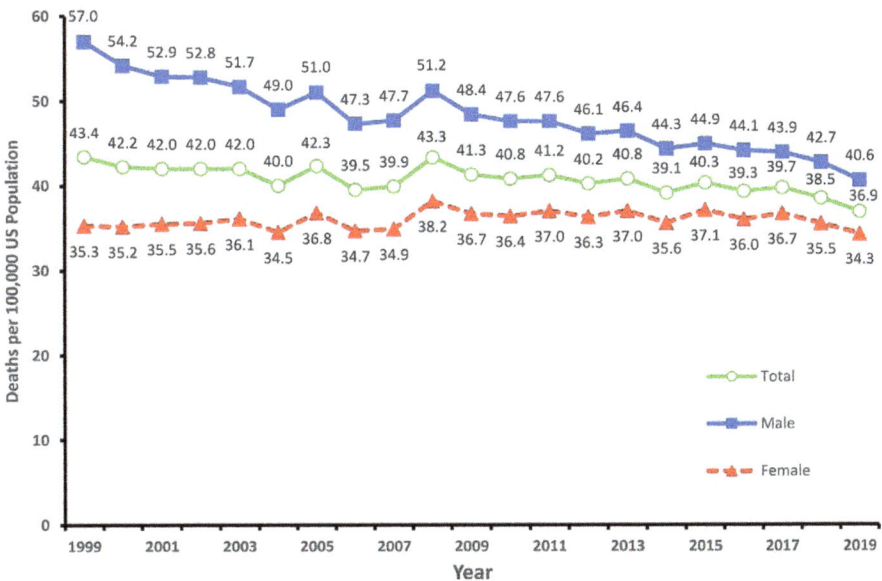

Fig. 11.2 COPD death rates in US from 1999–2019. *Source* National Vital Statistics System detailed mortality data at http://wonder.cdc.gov, https://www.cdc.gov/copd/data.html

spirometry pulmonary function test is the most basic and well-organized primary care strategy for COPD diagnosis among the current analysis and discovery tools. Patients' lung capacity is assessed during in–out breathing cycles as part of this examination. The morbidity and death associated with COPD are often underdiagnosed because of the spirometry test's low sensitivity of 64.5%. As a result, a proper machine learning technique with high clinical reliability is essential for diagnosing, treating, and self-management of COPD. Machine learning (ML) is a powerful approach for predicting medical diseases and allowing caregivers to make accurate medical choices.

Despite the fact that machine learning algorithms are strong at prediction, they have several drawbacks compared to deep learning. When the data amount is high, Deep Learning outperforms conventional approaches. On the other hand, traditional machine learning techniques are preferred when dealing with tiny amounts of data. Deep learning provides several benefits, including automated feature development, managing unstructured data, self-learning capabilities, scalability, and cost-efficiency. However, effective hyper-parameter optimization is critical for controlling the learning process in deep learning approaches. The appropriate selection of hyper-parameters increases the model's overall performance compared to any single solution. Furthermore, hyperparameters can effectively explore the space, making it more straightforward to manage many experiments [4]. In this chapter, we present a deep learning model based on the Long Short Term Memory Network (LSTM), and the hyperparameters of the proposed methodology are optimized using a swarm-inspired firefly method.

The following are the primary contributions of this chapter:

1. Deep learning approach Long Short-Term Memory Network, has been presented to address the early diagnosis of Chronic Obstructive Pulmonary Disease.
2. The Firefly approach is presented to regulate the learning process and improve overall model performance by tuning the hyper-parameters of LSTM.
3. The proposed model's efficiency is demonstrated by comparing existing state-of-the-art machine learning techniques.

The following is how the rest of the article is organized: The literature on COPD is briefly discussed in Sect. 11.2. In Sect. 11.3, the proposed framework, which incorporates firefly, LSTM, and LSTM plus Firefly technique, is thoroughly discussed. Section 11.4 discusses the experimental setup, including a description of the dataset, the simulation environment, and performance metrics. The experimental findings and the method's efficacy are discussed in Sect. 11.5. Section 11.6 concludes with a discussion of the chapter's future scope.

11.2 Literature Study

Chenshuo Wang et al. [3] aim to create acute exacerbations in chronic obstructive pulmonary disease (AECOPD) detection models and assess the relative performance of several modelling paradigms to discover the optimal model. They examined the data in the form of electro medical records from COPD patients hospitalized in China-Japan Friendship Hospital between February 2011 and March 2017. They selected features by combining information gain and hypothesis test; they evaluated them using support vector machine (SVM), random forest (RF), K-nearest neighbor (KNN), logistic regression (LR), and naïve Bayes (NB) machine learning techniques. The findings concluded that the proposed model based on the support vector machine with the feature selection is powerful in identifying AECOPDs patients. Haider et al. 2019 [2] employed machine learning techniques to investigate the classification of COPD and normal individuals based on respiratory sound analysis. Several parametric and non-parametric tests have been used to extract the features, such as the Mann–Whitney U-test, t-test, spearman's rank correlation coefficient, correlation analysis, ANOVA, etc. Various ML models have been used, and it has been concluded that the SVM and LR are the two best classifiers for COPD classification. In Table 11.1, we've included a few more studies focused on COPD identification.

11.3 Proposed Method

The suggested model is known as the Firefly-based optimized Long Short-Term Memory Network (LSTM + firefly) model because it combines two algorithms, namely the firefly optimization method and LSTM approaches. The firefly-based method has been used to discover architectural LSTM's hyperparameter factors. Therefore, compared to traditional machine learning approaches, the classification of early detection of COPD illness using the LSTM + firefly model is enhanced efficiently.

11.3.1 Firefly Optimization Algorithm

A firefly optimization method is a meta-heuristic algorithm inspired by firefly behaviour. A firefly's natural habit is to produce periodic and shorter blazes caused by a bioluminescence mechanism that follows the inverse square law. Fireflies use their bursts of light for hunting, communicating, and warning their predators. Consider the light power (I) at a specific distance (R), where the light power decreases as the distance between the fireflies increases. In addition, as distance increases, the light and its power are reduced due to air absorption, making it more vulnerable. As a result, most fireflies communicate within a hundred meters, which was originally

Table 11.1 Literature on COPD

Intelligent method	Compared methods	Data source	Evaluation factors	Performance	Ref
KNN, RF	KNN, RF, SVML, and SVMR	FOT Parameters from 128 volunteers	AUC	AUC ≥ 0.9	Amaral et al. [5]
Deep Residual Network	–	2153 CT scans acquired from a separate cohort of individuals	AUC, PPV, NPV, f1-macro, Precision-macro, Recall-macro	AUC = 0.889	Tang et al. [6]
C5.0	Neural networks and Support vector machine	414 patients' psychological parameters derived from pulmonary function tests	Sensitivity, Specificity, and Accuracy	Sensitivity = 98.39, Specificity = 96.2, and Accuracy = 97.4	Iadanza et al. [1]
LS-SVM		128 individuals from First Affiliated Hospital of Wenzhou Medical University	Accuracy, and AUC	Accuracy = 84.62, and AUC = 0.90	Zheng et al. [7]
LightGBM-RFE (feature eliminations) Genetic algorithm Grid search (Optimization) Multistage ensemble voting classifier (Classification)		Exasens	Accuracy, Precision, Recall, f1-measure, AUC	Accuracy = 0.9820, Precision = 0.9800, Recall = 0.9600, f1-measure = 0.9667, AUC = 0.9912	Dhar [8]

(continued)

Table 11.1 (continued)

Intelligent method	Compared methods	Data source	Evaluation factors	Performance	Ref
RBF, K-means, PNN		16 COPD patient's questionnaire during 6 months	Accuracy, Sensitivity, Specificity	Accuracy = 89.3, Sensitivity = 84.1, Specificity = 92.5	Vicente et al. [9]
XGBoost	KNN, LR, SVM, DT, MLP	633 subjects from China collected during jan-dec 2017	AU-ROC, AU-PRC, Accuracy, Precision, Recall, F1-Score	AU-ROC = 0.94, AU-PRC = 0.97, Accuracy = 0.91, Precision = 0.95, Recall = 0.93, F1-Score = 0.94	Ma et al. [10]
Logistic regression with lasso regularization		44,929 hospitalized individuals from nationwide administrative database in Japan	Sensitivity, Specificity	Sensitivity = 0.67, Specificity = 0.50	Goto et al. [11]
DT, LR	KNN, Naïve Bayes, Ada-Boost	101 COPD patients from Bangladesh	Recall, Precision, F1Score, Accuracy	Recall = 100, Precision = 88.89, F1Score = 94.12, Accuracy = 95.24	Das Joshe et al. [12]
MLNN, SVm, XGBoost		MaPCReN	Sensitivity, Specificity, Accuracy	Sensitivity = 0.82, Specificity = 0.84, Accuracy = 0.83	Zafari et al. [13]

the distance limit. As a result, the goal function is a blazing light from which a population-based firefly algorithm has been formed.

The inverse square law may be used to calculate the light power I(R) at a distance of R from a light source (L$_S$) as shown in Eq. (11.1).

$$L(R) = LS/R2 \tag{11.1}$$

The light is submerged in the air with a constant light absorption coefficient ($\gamma \in (0, \infty)$). As a result, the gaussian equation is produced, and the Eq. (11.2) is presented below

$$B(R) = B_0 e^{-\gamma R^2} \tag{11.2}$$

where (R) represents the attractiveness of fireflies at a distance of R, and B$_0$ is the attractiveness of fireflies when R = 0.

Consider the position of two fireflies, i and j, respectively X$_i$ (x$_i$, y$_i$) and X$_j$ (x$_j$, y$_j$). R$_{ij}$ is the distance between two fireflies, and the formula is euclidean, as given in Eq. (11.3)

$$R_{ij} = \|X_i - X_j\| = \sqrt{(x_i - x_j)^2 - (y_i - y_j)^2} \tag{11.3}$$

The following Eq. (11.4) is the new position and movement (j) of the brighter firefly.

$$X_i = X_i + B_0 e^{-\gamma R^2}(X_j - X_i) + a\epsilon_i \tag{11.4}$$

where ϵ_i is random vector variables and also the parameter of randomness (α) $\in$ [0,1].

11.3.2 Long Short-Term Memory (LSTM)

In LSTM, the activation function is replaced with a "gating" function that maintains track of the input and, if it is remembered, sends it on to the next hidden node or layer. Because the network is trained on the network's combination of gates, as long as the network's gates are all 1, the network can recall early input values and identify how they affect expected output. A standard LSTM architecture was used, with each block including gates that determine if an input is relevant, whether it should be remembered or forgotten, and when it should be outputted. The method is then fine-tuned by adding a dense layer on top of the LSTM, with the number of hidden nodes acting as the major tuning parameter. A sigmoid activation function translates the dense layer's values into real numbers between 0 and 1 once they've been formed. After that, a binary detection decision (0 or 1) is made based on a

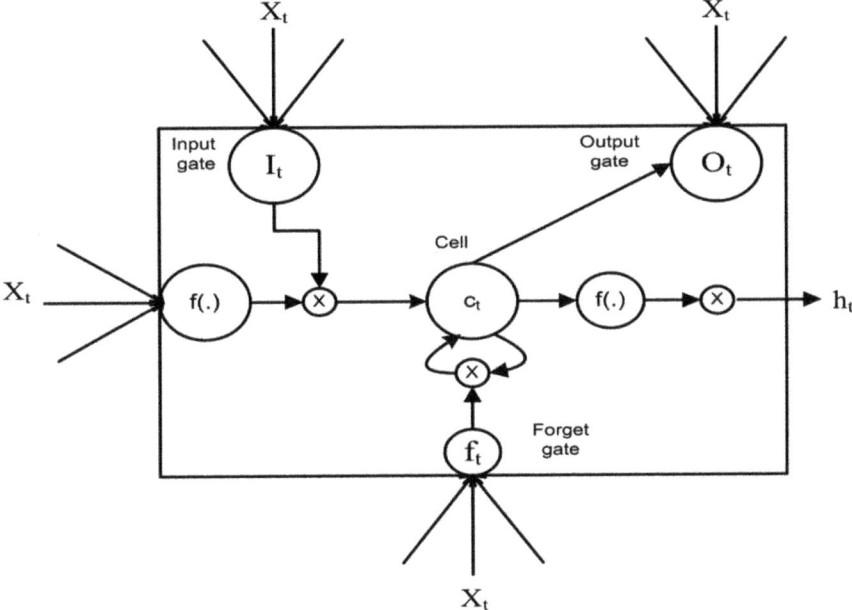

Fig. 11.3 Architecture of LSTM cell

predefined threshold. This threshold determines whether a COPD disease has been detected and if it is exceeded, COPD disease has been found. The LSTM cell structure is shown in Fig. 11.3.

Three gates are available in LSTM and they are responsible for the cell state protection and control. The following Eqs. (11.5) to (11.9) are implemented for LSTM.

$$I_t = \sigma\left(W_i[h_{t-1}, x_t] + b_i\right) \tag{11.5}$$

$$f_t = \sigma\left(W_f[h_{t-1}, x_t] + b_f\right) \tag{11.6}$$

$$c_t = \tanh(W_c[h_{t-1}, x_t] + b_c) \tag{11.7}$$

$$O_t = \sigma(W_o[h_{t-1}, x_t] + b_o) \tag{11.8}$$

$$h_t = O_t \tanh(c_t) \tag{11.9}$$

σ is the logistic sigmoid function, and i, f, o, and c are respectively the input gate, forget gate, output gate, and cell activation vectors, all of which are the same size as the hidden vectors h Where W_f, W_i and W_c are weights, and b_i, b_f and b_c are bias.

The weight matrices from the cell to gate vectors are diagonal, so element m in each gate vector-only receives input from element *m* of the cell vector.

11.3.3 LSTM + Firefly Methodology

In general, LSTM makes use of earlier data throughout the learning process, and choosing the right time frame is crucial for achieving consistent results. The suggested prediction consists of two stages: appropriate hyperparameter selection and analysis of LSTM architectural factors using the Firefly optimization method. The Firefly method examines the ideal number of hidden neurons in each hidden layer, as well as the dropout rate, optimizer learning rate, and hidden layer activation function. The network's primary weights are set to random values, and the network's weight is fine-tuned via a gradient-based "Adam" optimizer. The LSTM + firefly framework is shown in Fig. 11.4.

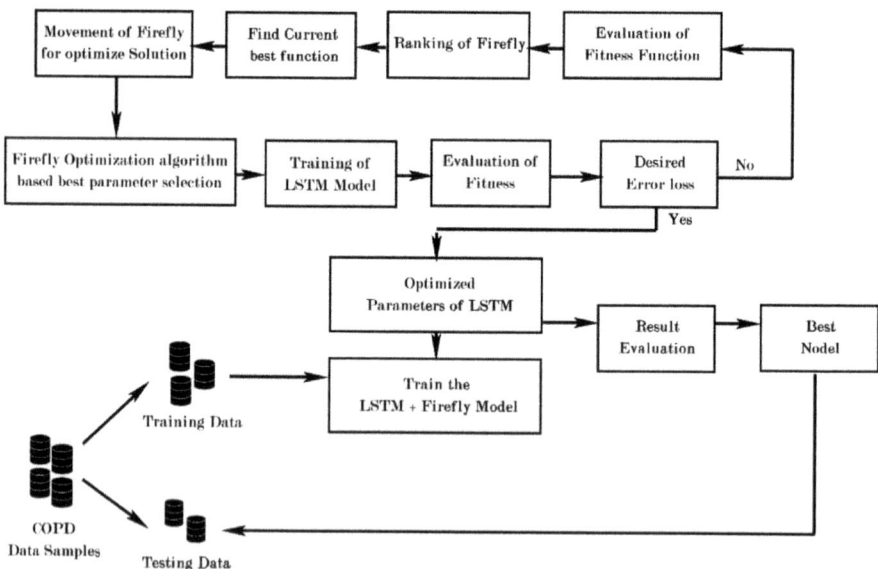

Fig. 11.4 The framework of the proposed method

Algorithm 1: optimized parameters using LSTM + Firefly Methodology
1. Initialize the current position of the firefly and the LSTM hyperparameters to be tuned by estimating the upper and lower limits
2. Replace the LSTM hyperparameters that correspond to each firefly position
3. By updating current data, divide the dataset into train-set and test-set, and then forecast the train-set next Sequence
4. Compare the predicted value with the test-set data
5. Calculate the difference between the expected value and the test-set values
6. Evaluating the fitness function by brightening flashes of a firefly and every change in firefly position using Eq. (11.4)
7. Steps 3–6 should be repeated until satisfied
8. The hyperparameter value of the firefly using LSTM is the result of optimal prediction

11.4 Experimental Setup

This section contains the dataset and features, data preparation process, parameters, and performance measurements of the proposed and comparable machine learning approaches.

11.4.1 Dataset

The data includes electronic medical reports from 563 COPD patients admitted to the China-Japan friendship hospital between February 2011 and March 2017. Each patient's EMR contains various clinical data, including demographics, hospital information, biomedical tests, vital signs, diagnosis, medication, etc. Exclusion and inclusion criteria have been used to identify the obtained EMRs. The following were the study's exclusion criteria: (i) a Patient who has asthma, (ii) A patient with eight or more comorbidities (iii) A diagnosis of COPD is either ambiguous or absent. (iv) More than 30% of an exciting feature gets missed. The following have been the criteria for inclusion: (i) After treatment, the patient is discharged from the hospital (ii) Aged 36 to 80 years (iii) The patient has been diagnosed with COPD.

The EMRs obtained 33 input parameters and one output feature extensively described in Table 11.2. Before building the identification model, the categorical features were encoded using the one-hot encoding approach. We used the following imputation approach to cope with missing data management: (i) if the categorical data is missing, we replaced it with the most common category associated with that feature. (ii) if the continuous data is missing, the relevant feature's average was used to replace it. Then, all features were normalized to prevent within-subject variations in amplitude and variance across features.

Table 11.2 An overview of the features that have been extracted

Feature	Units	Type
Patient profile		
Age	Years	Continuous
Gender	Female/Male	Categorical
Smoking history	No/Yes	Categorical
History of alcohol use	No/Yes	Categorical
COPD/AECOPD	No COPD/AECOPD	Categorical
Timespan	Days	Continuous
Vital signs		
Respiratory rate	BPM	Continuous
Pulse rate	BPM	Continuous
Diastolic blood pressure	mm Hg	Continuous
Systolic blood pressure	mm Hg	Continuous
Potential of hydrogen	N/A	Continuous
PaCO2	mm Hg	Continuous
PO2	mm Hg	Continuous
FEV1/FVC	%	Continuous
FEV1/FEV1predicted	%	Continuous
Comorbidities		
Diabetes	No/Yes	Categorical
Hyperlipidemia	No/Yes	Categorical
Hypertension	No/Yes	Categorical
Heart disease	No/Yes	Categorical
Symptoms		
Cold	No/Yes	Categorical
Fever	No/Yes	Categorical
Cough	No/Yes	Categorical
Dyspnea	No/Yes	Categorical
Wheezing	No/Yes	Categorical
Sputum	No/Yes	Categorical
Sputum volume	There are a few things that aren't covered in EMR	Categorical
Difficulty of cough	Easy EMR Tough does not mention this	Categorical
Sleep quality	Bad EMR Normal does not mention this	Categorical
Chest tightness	No/Yes	Categorical
Shortness of breath	No/Yes	Categorical
Chest pain	No/Yes	Categorical
Supine position	No/Yes	Categorical

(continued)

Table 11.2 (continued)

Feature	Units	Type
Activity capability	"At least one symptom becomes worse after walking about 100 yards" is preferable to "After walking approximately 100 yards, at least one symptom gets worse." EMR does not mention it	Categorical

11.4.2 Simulation Environment

We commenced using Google Colab's python notebook on GPU servers with Tensor Flow's Keras and Tensor Flow frameworks to perform our study. For this experiment, we used an Intel Core i7 CPU 2.20 GHz, 16 GB RAM, Windows 10 (64-bit), and an NVIDIA GeForce GTX 1050. Various PYTHON library software packages, such as Pandas, Imblearn, and Numpy framework, are utilized to evaluate the data further. In addition, other frameworks are used to visualize the data, such as Matplotlib and Mlxtend, while sklearn is used to analyze the data. We have used Keras and Tensorflow libraries, where Keras is a neural network library. In contrast, TensorFlow is an open-source machine learning framework that may be used for various applications.

11.4.3 Performance Measures

The experiment is performed on the proposed approach and various existing machine learning classifiers. Accuracy, Precision, Recall, f1 score, f2-score, and ROC-AUC are used to verify the suggested technique and other machine learning classifier methods [14]. The calculation of the above performance measures has been obtained using the Eqs. (11.10) to (11.15) presented in Table 11.3.

Table 11.3 Performance measures and their equations

Performance measure	Equation	Equation no
Accuracy	$(TP + TN)/(TP + TN + FP + FN)$	(11.10)
Precision	$(TP)/(TP + FP)$	(11.11)
TPR / Recall/ Sensitivity	$(TP)/(TP + FN)$	(11.12)
FPR	$(FP)/(TN + FP)$	(11.13)
TNR	$(TN)/(TN + FP)$	(11.14)
f-measure	$2 \times \frac{Precision \times Sensitivity}{Precision + Sensitivity}$	(11.15)

11.5 Result Analysis

In this research work, we have examined the overall performance of the selected models, beginning with an analysis of Machine Learning metrics and concluding with an explanation of the deep learning LSTM model's performance. Various measurement metrics (e.g., accuracy, precision, recall, F1-score, F2-score, and ROC-AUC) are utilized to demonstrate the findings, with the achieved accuracy demonstrating the suggested model's overall performance. Furthermore, we have emphasized the F1-Score measure of all approaches since it supports achieving a balanced precision-recall ratio. The distribution of class labels is non-uniform and extremely imbalanced in this study, F1-Score is a valuable measure for accurately evaluating performance. We used a wide variety of cases in our investigation, each with its own set of characteristics. For this purpose, we perform experiments using hidden layer units, dropout rates, a variety of hidden layer activation functions, and different learning rates in optimizers. These important parameters have a big impact on how the performance metrics for the Deep learning-based LSTM model are calculated. The values examined in each of the scenarios are presented in Table 11.4 as part of the optimization of many hyperparameters of the LSTM technique and also presented the parameters of various compared machine learning models.

Several machine learning techniques, including LSTM with random search and LSTM with hyperband, have been compared with the suggested approach We utilized

Table 11.4 Optimized parameters of all investigated models

Models	Optimized parameters
LSTM + Random Search	dropout = 0.1, dense_units = 320, dense_activation = 'sigmoid', learning_rate = 0.0006
LSTM + Hyperband	dropout = 0.25, dense_units = 352, dense_activation = 'relu', learning_rate = 0.0001
Proposed approach (LSTM + Firefly)	dropout = 0.1, dense_units = 32, dense_activation = 'tanh', learning_rate = 0.001
LR	penalty = 'l2', tol = 0.0001, C = 1.0, fit_intercept = True, intercept_scaling = 1, solver = 'lbfgs', max_iter = 100, multi_class = 'auto',
NB	var_smoothing = 1e-09
KNN	n_neighbors = 5, weights = 'uniform', algorithm = 'auto', leaf_size = 30, p = 2, metric = 'minkowski'
DT	criterion = 'gini', splitter = 'best', min_samples_split = 2, min_samples_leaf = 1
RF	n_estimators = 100, criterion = 'gini', min_samples_split = 2, min_samples_leaf = 1,
LSTM	Dropout = 0.3, num_hidden_layer = 300, number_neurons = 256, Learning_rate = 0.1, activation_fun_hidden layer = 'relu'

Table 11.5 Results of ML models vs. suggested model

Prediction models	Precision	Recall	F1 Score	F2 Score	ROC-AUC	Accuracy
LR	0.8787	0.8357	0.8566	0.8574	0.9215	86.18
NB	0.6297	0.7432	0.7476	0.7440	0.8281	79.00
KNN	0.9004	0.9038	0.9021	0.9035	0.9531	90.31
DT	0.8354	0.6149	0.7084	0.7012	0.8283	75.00
RF	0.8846	0.7980	0.8391	0.8345	0.9082	84.88
LSTM	0.9440	0.9467	0.9454	0.9446	0.9860	94.42
LSTM + Random Search	0.9639	0.9671	0.9645	0.9643	0.9926	96.55
LSTM + Hyperband	0.9443	0.9456	0.9446	0.9438	0.9865	94.43
Proposed LSTM + Firefly	0.9717	0.9721	0.9718	0.9713	0.9959	97.41

Keras-tuner for hyperband implementation. Deep learning methods can be implemented using the Keras Python package. LSTM model hyper-parameter selection is done via hyperband in Keras-tuner. Three factors are taken into account: the range of hyper-parameters, the number of trials (max_trial), and the number of executions per trial (exes _per_trial). The algorithm's goal is to reduce the amount of data that is invalidated. Our chosen hyper-parameters include, for example, the number of layers, the number of hidden units, the dropout layer percentage, the activation function, and the learning rate of the model. Table 11.4 lists the hyperparameters and their respective optimal values.

Table 11.5 shows a comparison of ML approaches such as linear regression (LR), Naive Bayes (NB), K-Nearest Neighbors (KNN), Decision Tree (DT), Random Forest, and the proposed LSTM + Firefly based on deep learning neural network. KNN outperforms other ML algorithms and has the greatest F1-Score of 0.9021, whereas NB has a poor F1-Score. Similarly, LSTM, LSTM + Random Search, LSTM + Hyperband, and LSTM + Firefly models have been studied. The proposed LSTM + Firefly model has the greatest accuracy of 97.41%, the precision of 0.9717, recall of 0.9721, F1-score of 0.9718, F2-score of 0.9713, and ROC AUC of 0.9959.

Figure 11.5 depicts the AUC-ROC analysis for all machine learning and deep learning approaches. Here in this study, deep learning approaches are extremely dominating ML methods; AUC-ROC analysis is displayed between all ML methods and the deep learning methods, as it was in all prior performance analyses. The suggested LSTM + Firefly method is proven to be superior to previous comparison strategies in terms of the coverage area for all classes.

Figure 11.6 illustrates a comparison of the selected deep learning models' performance accuracy measures (LSTM, LSTM + RS, LSTM + Hyperband, and LSTM + Firefly). For our analysis, we used 50 epochs. In the validation phase, the suggested LSTM + Firefly achieves the best accuracy score. The accuracy of the suggested model improves significantly in epoch 5 and progressively advances to a value of 97.41% at epoch 50. Also, a comparison of the loss performance metrics of the selected deep learning models is shown in Fig. 11.7.

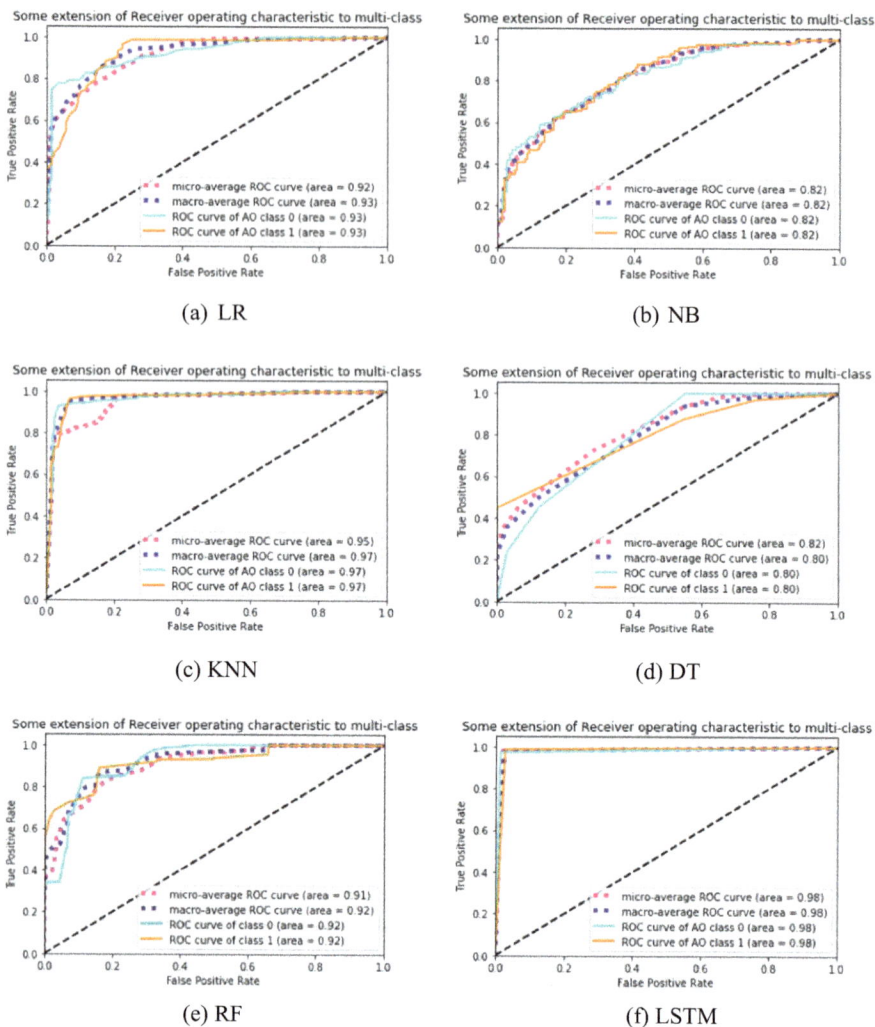

Fig. 11.5 ROC-AUC Curve for **a** LR **b** NB **c** KNN **d** DT **e** RF **f** LSTM **g** LSTM + Random Search **h** LSTM + Hyperband **i** Proposed LSTM + Firefly

In Fig. 11.8, a comparison of the examined Machine Learning and Deep Learning-based approaches is made using the accuracy metric. Precision, recall, F1 score, and F2 score are depicted in Fig. 11.9. In contrast to existing approaches, the suggested LSTM + Firefly method outperforms them and is determined to be an effective classifier.

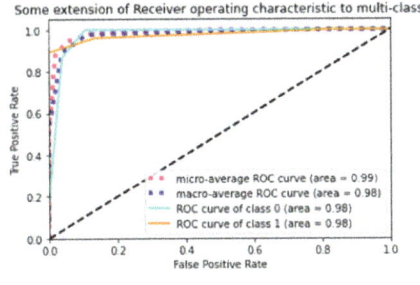
(g) LSTM + Random Search

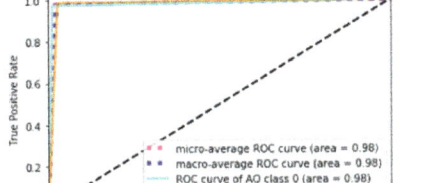
(h) LSTM + Hyperband

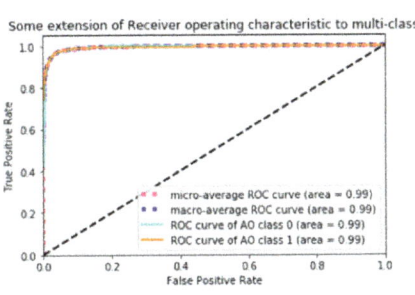
(i) Proposed LSTM + Firefly

Fig. 11.5 (continued)

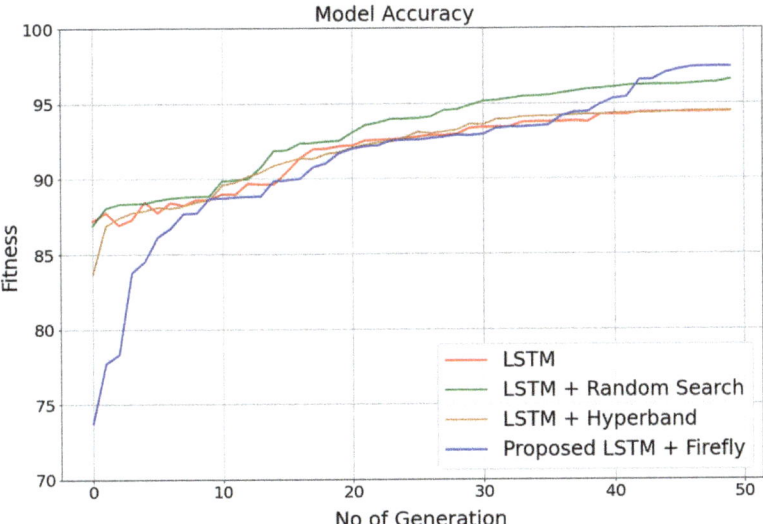

Fig. 11.6 Comparisons of the Accuracy performance metrics of the selected deep learning models

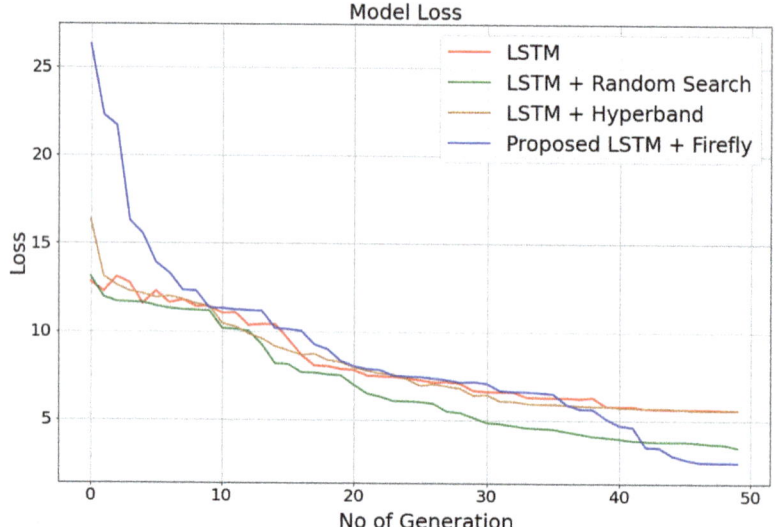

Fig. 11.7 Comparisons of the loss performance metrics of the selected deep learning models

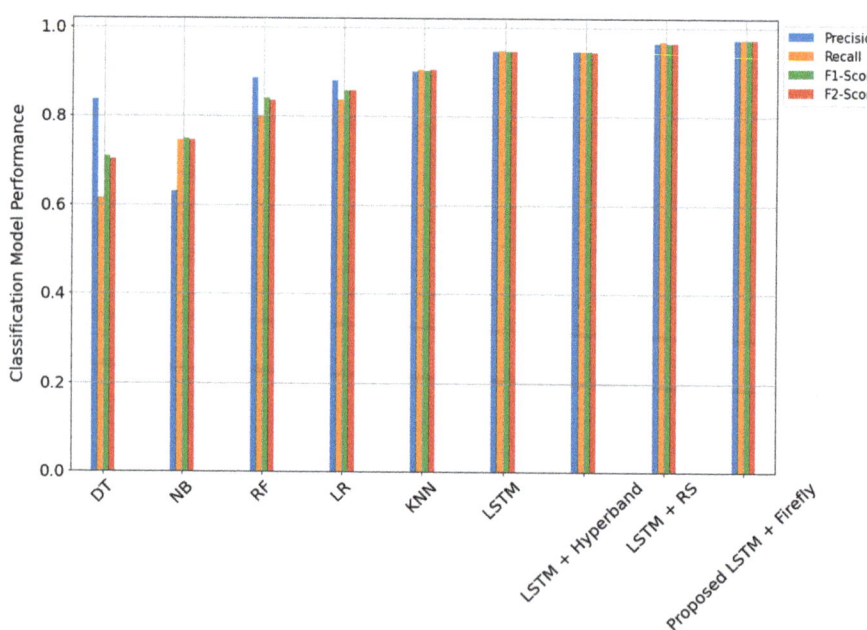

Fig. 11.8 Comparison of Precision, Recall, F1 score, and F2 score for examined models

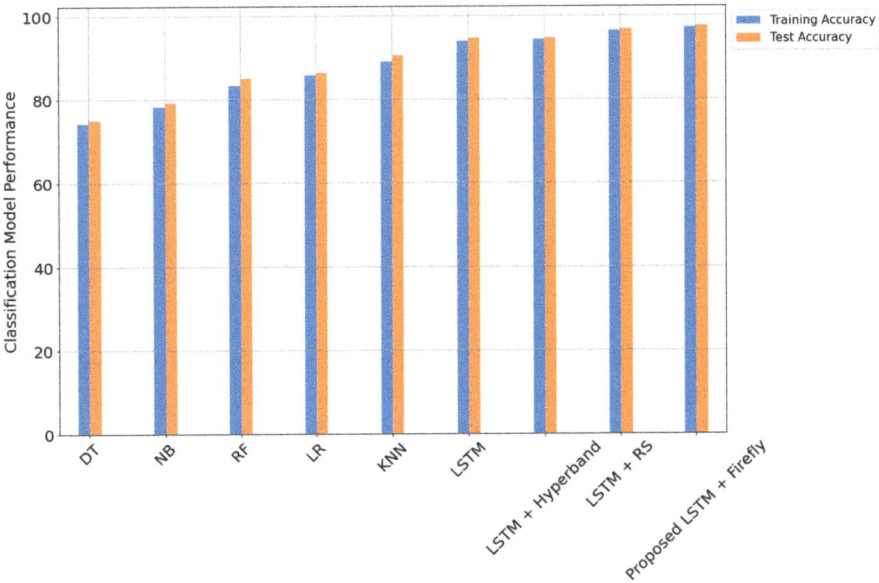

Fig. 11.9 Comparison of Accuracy Score for examined models

11.6 Critical Discussion

Throughout evolution, a variety of solutions, ranging from traditional models to models at the forefront of technology, such as neural networks (NN), have been presented to solve this problem. Long Short Term Memory (LSTM) is a form of RNN, and it incorporates numerous hyper-parameters to get the ideal model by reducing the training loss. LSTM was developed by Google. The Firefly algorithm was utilized in this study to choose an ideal configuration of hyper-parameters, and that model was subsequently applied for COPD illness identification. The performance of the many prior studies on COPD has been described in the literature section. Apart from them Table 11.6 gives the earlier research findings on the same dataset selected for experimentation. It is evident from previous research that the performance of different classification measures spans between 0.8 and 0.9, but our suggested technique yielded results in the range 0.97 to 0.99. Therefore, it can be inferred that the proposed approach outperformed the prior research and approaches that were compared.

11.7 Conclusion

We developed a clinical decision support system for COPD patients by designing and evaluating multiple classifier algorithms. The use of hyperparameter tuning will

Table 11.6 Performance comparision of the proposed method with the previous studies

Technique	Sensitivity	Specificity	AUC	Reference
LR	0.83	0.79	0.9	Wang et al. [3]
NB	0.85	0.65	0.85	
KNN	0.71	0.8	0.83	
SVM	0.8	0.83	0.9	
RF	0.83	0.71	0.8	
Proposed method	0.9721	–	0.9959	

influence the effectiveness of the classification model; we have used random search, hyperband, and firefly algorithms to acquire the hyperparameters that are appropriate for the suggested classification model LSTM for the considered data. Apart from these, numerous machine learning methods, including DT, NB, RF, LR, and KNN, were assessed to validate the suggested method's performance. The most appropriate are LSTM—Random search, LSTM—Hyperband, and notably LSTM—Firefly, which attains values that allow for a highly accurate clinical diagnosis. The suggested LSTM-Firefly achieved 97.14 percent accuracy, 0.9717 precision, 0.9721 recall, 0.9718 f1-score, 0.9713 f2-score, and ROC-AUC is 0.9959. Future work will be done on a dataset with more instances and specific inclusion criteria.

References

1. Iadanza, E., Mudura, V., Melillo, P., Gherardelli, M.: An automatic system supporting clinical decision for chronic obstructive pulmonary disease. Health Technol. (Berl) **10**(2), 487–498 (2020). https://doi.org/10.1007/s12553-019-00312-9
2. Haider, N.S., Singh, B.K., Periyasamy, R., Behera, A.K.: Respiratory sound based classification of chronic obstructive pulmonary disease: a risk stratification approach in machine learning paradigm. J. Med. Syst. **43**(8), 255 (2019). https://doi.org/10.1007/s10916-019-1388-0
3. Wang, C., Chen, X., Du, L., Zhan, Q., Yang, T., Fang, Z.: Comparison of machine learning algorithms for the identification of acute exacerbations in chronic obstructive pulmonary disease. Comput. Methods Programs Biomed. **188**, 105267 (2020). https://doi.org/10.1016/j.cmpb.2019.105267
4. Fister, I., Yang, X.-S., Fister, I., Brest, J.: Memetic firefly algorithm for combinatorial optimization. Proc. 5th Int. Conf. Bioinspired Optim. Methods their Appl. BIOMA 2012, pp. 75–86 (2012), [Online]. Available: http://arxiv.org/abs/1204.5165
5. Amaral, J.L.M., Lopes, A.J., Faria, A.C.D., Melo, P.L.: Machine learning algorithms and forced oscillation measurements to categorise the airway obstruction severity in chronic obstructive pulmonary disease. Comput. Methods Programs Biomed. **118**(2), 186–197 (2015). https://doi.org/10.1016/j.cmpb.2014.11.002
6. Tang, L.Y.W., Coxson, H.O., Lam, S., Leipsic, J., Tam, R.C., Sin, D.D.: Towards large-scale case-finding: training and validation of residual networks for detection of chronic obstructive pulmonary disease using low-dose CT. Lancet Digit. Heal. **2**(5), e259–e267 (2020). https://doi.org/10.1016/S2589-7500(20)30064-9

7. Zheng, H., et al.: Predictive diagnosis of chronic obstructive pulmonary disease using serum metabolic biomarkers and least-squares support vector machine. J. Clin. Lab. Anal. **35**(2), 1–8 (2021). https://doi.org/10.1002/jcla.23641
8. Dhar, J.: Multistage ensemble learning model with weighted voting and genetic algorithm optimization strategy for detecting chronic obstructive pulmonary disease. IEEE Access **9**, 48640–48657 (2021). https://doi.org/10.1109/ACCESS.2021.3067949
9. Vicente, J.M.F., Álvarez-Sánchez, J.R., De La Paz López, F., Toledo-Moreo, F.J., Adeli, H.: Artificial Computation in Biology and Medicine: International Work-Conference on the Interplay Between Natural and Artificial Computation, IWINAC 2015 Elche, Spain, June 1–5, 2015 Proceedings, Part I. Lect. Notes Comput. Sci. (including Subser. Lect. Notes Artif. Intell. Lect. Notes Bioinformatics) **9107**, 305–311 (2015). doi:https://doi.org/10.1007/978-3-319-18914-7
10. Ma, X., et al.: Comparison and development of machine learning tools for the prediction of chronic obstructive pulmonary disease in the Chinese population. J. Transl. Med. **18**(1), 1–14 (2020). https://doi.org/10.1186/s12967-020-02312-0
11. Goto, T., Jo, T., Matsui, H., Fushimi, K., Hayashi, H., Yasunaga, H.: Machine learning-based prediction models for 30-day readmission after hospitalization for chronic obstructive pulmonary disease. COPD J. Chronic Obstr. Pulm. Dis. **16**(5–6), 338–343 (2019). https://doi.org/10.1080/15412555.2019.1688278
12. Das Joshe, M., Emon, N.H., Islam, M., Ria, N.J., Masum, A.K.M., Noori, S.R.H.: Symptoms Analysis Based Chronic Obstructive Pulmonary Disease Prediction In Bangladesh Using Machine Learning Approach, no. December, pp. 1–5 (2021). doi:https://doi.org/10.1109/icccnt51525.2021.9580078
13. Zafari, H., Langlois, S., Zulkernine, F., Kosowan, L., Singer, A.: Predicting chronic obstructive pulmonary disease from EMR data. 2020 IEEE Conf. Comput. Intell. Bioinforma. Comput. Biol. CIBCB 2020 (2020). doi:https://doi.org/10.1109/CIBCB48159.2020.9277712
14. Suresh Kumar, P., Behera, H.S., Nayak, J., Naik, B.: Bootstrap aggregation ensemble learning-based reliable approach for software defect prediction by using characterized code feature. Innov. Syst. Softw. Eng. (September 2019), 1–22 (2021). doi:https://doi.org/10.1007/s11334-021-00399-2

Chapter 12
GACO: A Genetic Algorithm with Ant Colony Optimization—Based Feature Selection for Breast Cancer Diagnosis

Satyajit Panigrahi, H. Swapnarekha, and Sharmila Subudhi

Abstract Breast cancer is the most prevalent cancer diagnosed and the basis of mortality among women worldwide. However, the early prognosis and treatment can avoid the death rate of the patients. Since the traditional method of detecting cancer is error-prone, machine learning has shown significant promise in aiding the accurate diagnosis. Moreover, using a minimal number of features is highly pertinent in decision-making. Therefore, this chapter proposes a novel evolutionary algorithm-based feature selection method to identify the most appropriate attributes. The suggested model fuses the Genetic Algorithm with Ant Colony Optimization to increase the search operation in the global search space. Finally, the Random Forest classifier is employed on the reduced attribute subset to examine and determine the nature of breast tumors. The developed system is evaluated on the Wisconsin Diagnostic Breast Cancer dataset. The experimental outcomes demonstrate the efficiency of the proposed method over other popular single algorithms and ensemble learners.

Keywords Breast cancer · Genetic algorithm · Ant colony optimization · Random forest

12.1 Introduction

Breast cancer is the most frequently occurring malignancy in women and is the second leading source of mortality cancer among women. Generally, breast cancer

---

S. Panigrahi
Department of Computer Science and Engineering, Institute for Technical Education and Research, Siksha 'O' Anusandhan Deemed to be University, Bhubaneswar, Odisha 751030, India

H. Swapnarekha
Department of Information Technology, Aditya Institute of Technology and Management, Tekkali, Andhra Pradesh 532210, India

S. Subudhi (✉)
Department of Computer Science, Maharaja Sriram Chandra Bhanja Deo University, Mayurbhanj, Odisha 757003, India
e-mail: sharmilasubudhi1@gmail.com; sharmilasubudhi@ieee.org

© The Author(s), under exclusive license to Springer Nature Switzerland AG 2023
J. Nayak et al. (eds.), *Nature-Inspired Optimization Methodologies in Biomedical and Healthcare*, Intelligent Systems Reference Library 233,
https://doi.org/10.1007/978-3-031-17544-2_12

appears in the epithelium of the ducts or the lobules of the breast glandular tissue when cancerous lumps start to raise from the breast cells. According to World Health Organization (WHO), more than 2.3 million women were identified with breast cancer, and approximately 6,85,000 deaths occurred due to breast cancer worldwide in 2020 [1]. Figures 12.1 and 12.2 show the statistics of the percent of cases and 5 year survival rate of breast cancer by stage [2]. The severity of breast cancer refers to the extent the cancer cell grows in the body, which can be used to determine the treatment and survival rate. If the cancer is observed in the body part where it has begun, it signifies a localized stage or stage 1. If it extends to distinct parts of the body, then it is referred to as regional or distant.

The figures prove that if breast cancer is identified in the earlier stage, the survival rate of the person from cancer can be improved with appropriate treatment. The tumor in the breast can be detected by self-examining the individual by touching it after the size increases to lemon size shape. Generally, the cancer is seen at a very late stage using self-examination [3]. Therefore, mammography is used for the early

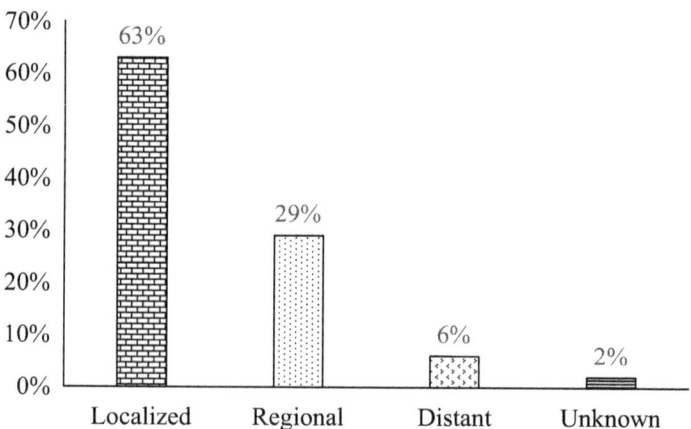

Fig. 12.1 % of cases of female breast cancer by stage

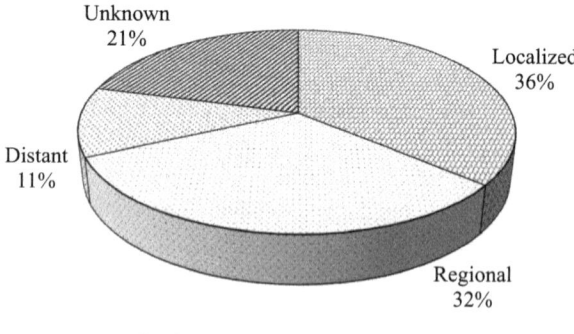

Fig. 12.2 5 year survival of breast cancer by stage

identification of breast cancer. Mammographs are the films the radiologist produces by passing x-rays through breast tissue which the oncologist can further use to suggest appropriate treatment. The diagnosis of breast cancer using mammography may take time due to the unavailability of a specialist in all general hospitals, which may be liable for extending and decreasing the survival rate of the breast cancer inmate.

Over the past few decades, much health-related data have been available due to the tremendous growth of digital technologies in the healthcare sector. This hazardous growth in health-related data has presented significant opportunities for enhancing patient health. As machine learning (ML) approaches aim to develop systems that replicate human intelligence, several machine learning algorithms have been suitably used in the prognosis and diagnosis of disease in recent years [4–8]. Therefore, the early prediction of breast cancer from mammography can be made efficiently using machine learning. Amrane et al. [9] have presented Naïve Bayes (NB) and K-Nearest Neighbor (KNN) for the classification of breast cancer. The empirical results found that KNN obtained the highest accuracy of 97.51%, with a low error rate compared to NB, which received an accuracy of 96.19%.

For categorization of triple-negative and non-triple negative patients who have breast cancer through gene expression data, various ML models such as KNN, NB, Support Vector Machine (SVM), and Decision Tree (DT) have been proposed by Wu et al. [10]. They make use of features selected using distinct threshold values. Further, results reveal that SVM could categorize breast cancer more effectively into two categories with an accuracy of 90% compared to the others. For the prediction of the survival rate of breast cancer patients in Malaysia using breast cancer data collected from the University Malaya Medical Centre, the following techniques—SVM, DT, Random Forest (RF), Logistic regression (LR), Neural Networks (NN) and Extreme Gradient Boosting (EGB) has been presented by Ganggayah et al. [11]. The experimental outcomes indicate that RF attains better accuracy of 82.7% in the prediction of the survival rate of breast cancer patients. Moreover, the study also identified the essential prognostic factors persuading the survival rate of breast cancer patients, which can be used as decision support tools in the healthcare sector.

In recent years, nature-inspired optimization algorithms have significantly solved diverse, complex problems in distinct domains. As nature-inspired optimization algorithms use a stochastic approach for determining the best solution in the ample search space, these algorithms have also been utilized for the efficient prognosis and diagnosis of disease in the healthcare sector and for attaining better results than the conventional methods. Gupta et al. [12] proposed the Optimized Crow Search Algorithm (OSCA) for the early diagnosis of Parkinson's disease. The performance of the OSCA has been evaluated using 20 standard datasets, and the results indicate that the OSCA obtained an accuracy of 100% compared with the standard CCSA (Chaotic Crow Search Algorithm). Moreover, the results also reveal that the OSCA is more stable, reduces the number of features selected and identifies an optimal subset of features. Goel et al. [13] developed MGOA (Modified Grasshopper Optimization Algorithm) for the identification of Autism Spectrum Disorder (ASD) in all stages of life. The efficacy of this system has been assessed using three ASD screening datasets containing data related to distinct age groups. The outcomes reveal that the

MGOA, along with RF, has obtained accuracy, specificity, and sensitivity of 100% at all stages of life compared to the state-of-the-art models.

The popularity of nature-inspired optimization algorithms in diagnosing distinct diseases has also been used to predict and detect breast cancer. Algorithms such as Particle Swarm Optimization (PSO), Ant Colony Optimization (ACO), Bat optimization Algorithm (BA), and Firefly algorithm (FA) have been presented by Anusha and Reddy [14] to diagnose breast cancer in its early stages. Then the performance of these techniques was evaluated using NB, and the outcomes indicate that PSO and FA attained better accuracy of 98%. Moreover, Sharma et al. [15] used PSO, FA, ACO, and Artificial Bee Colony Optimization (ABCO) to enhance breast cancer diagnosis at an initial stage. Then the suitability was evaluated on the UCI Dataset of Wisconsin Diagnostic Breast Cancer using various classifiers such as KNN, RF, DT, and LSVM (Linear SVM). The results show that PSO, along with RF, has obtained 96.45% accuracy compared to others. For segmenting the breast cancer images despite the modality or type of image, another system based on FA has been developed by Kaushal et al. [16]. Then the effectiveness was assessed by comparing the results with K-Means, PSO, DPSO (Darwinian PSO), FEBT (Fuzzy Entropy-Based Thresholding), and FODPSO (Fractional-Order DPSO).

Over the past few years, applying hybrid algorithms has proven to be influential in developing intelligent systems. These various algorithms enhance the searching capability and better handle uncertainty, vagueness, and noisy data [17, 18]. Generally, hybridization of algorithms is obtained by integrating one algorithm with a complementing algorithm. As hybridization of algorithms assists in overcoming the drawbacks of underlying algorithms by considering their merits, these algorithms have also been used in designing intelligent systems in the healthcare domain.

Another hybrid model known as HAW based on ABCO and Whale Optimization Algorithm (WOA) has been developed by Stephan et al. [19] that enhances the accuracy of the breast cancer diagnosis. This suggested system combines the bubble net attacking technique of the WOA with the exploitatory employee bee phase of ABCO. Further, the explorative phase of HAW is used to enhance the weak exploration of the standard ABCO. Then the performance of HAW was evaluated using Levenberg–Marquart (HAW-LM), resilient backpropagation (HAW-RP), and momentum-based gradient descent (HAW-GD) on various datasets of breast cancer, and the results show that HAW-RP attained better performance in terms of accuracy, computational speed and complexity when compared with HAWLM and HAW-GD. Mazen et al. [20] demonstrated the hybridization of the Genetic algorithm (GA) and Firefly Algorithm (FA) to diagnose breast cancer. The biases of the neurons and weights among the layers have been optimized to reduce the fitness function's cost. Then the Wisconsin Breast Cancer Dataset was fed for evaluation, and the empirical outcomes indicate that the GA-based FA attained the lowest MSE (mean squared error) of 0.0014 compared with FA, Biogeography Based Optimization, ACO, and PSO algorithms.

As hybridization of nature-inspired algorithms and machine learning algorithms have been used in the efficient prediction and diagnosis of breast cancer, the present study uses ACO and GA along with the Random Forest (RF) for the early diagnosis of breast cancer. The main contributions of this chapter are summarized below:

- A hybridized evolutionary-based feature selection method and RF classifier are proposed for efficient breast cancer diagnosis.
- The proposed model is segregated into three different modules, namely, Data Preprocessing Component (DPC), Evolutionary Algorithm-based Feature Selection Component (EAFSC), and GACO_RF Component (GRC).
- A hybridization of GA and ACO, termed GACO, is used to select the most relevant features for cancer diagnosis. These chosen attributes are fed to the RF classifier.
- The suggested system is implemented in Python, and the classification accuracy metric analyzes performance.
- The feature selection model is compared with existing evolutionary feature selection methods like Particle Swarm Optimization (PSO), simple GA, and ACO.
- The comparison of the developed algorithm is conducted with some other existing models present in the literature.
- The verification and validation of the proposed system are carried out on the widely used Wisconsin Diagnostic Breast Cancer (WDBC) dataset obtained from the UCI machine learning repository.

12.2 Related Work

Due to the emergence of medical research, several works have been presented for a better diagnosis and prognosis of breast cancer at the initial stage. This section describes such examples carried out on the diagnosis and prognosis of breast cancer using machine learning and nature-inspired optimization algorithms. Al-Quraishi et al. [21] proposed an approach based on a Random Forest (RF) classifier to predict the probability of breast cancer repetition in patients. Then the authors have used the Wisconsin Prognosis Breast Cancer dataset collected from the UCI machine learning repository for computation. Further, they have applied the SMOTE technique to balance the dataset. The experimental results indicate that RF has obtained better accuracy than the deep neural network classifiers in predicting breast cancer recurrence among patients.

Ittannavar and Havaldar [22] proposed a system for the screening and identification of breast cancer. Initially, the suggested method has obtained the mammography images from a digital database and mammographic image analysis society datasets. The quality of the images has been enhanced by using normalization, median filter, and histogram equalization. Then, cancer and non-cancer regions segmentation from the improved pictures was done using a multi-level multi-objective optimization algorithm. Furthermore, Haralick texture features, local directional ternary pattern, and histogram of oriented gradients are used for extracting a feature vector from the segmented regions of enhanced images. Then, appropriate features for breast cancer are selected using infinite feature selection with GA. In addition, the GA benefits from a probabilistic transition rule that assists in investigating the associate neighbor features. Further, simulation outcomes show that the model attains 0.10–7% enhancement in accuracy in comparison with CNN (convolutional neural network), conditional GAN (generative adversarial network), and ELM (extreme learning machine).

For the early detection of breast cancer, an automated disease detection system has been developed by Islam et al. [23]. The system uses five machine learning techniques, such as SVM, RF, KNN, LR, and Artificial neural networks (ANN), to identify breast cancer on Wisconsin Breast Cancer from the UCI machine learning repository. The simulation results showed that ANN attained superior performance of 98.57%, 97.82%, and 98.90% accuracy, precision, and F1 score, respectively, compared to other conventional concepts.

A hybrid feature selection system, known as BOAALO, has been suggested by Thawkar et al. [24]. This model hybridized BOA (Butterfly Optimization Algorithm) and ALO (Ant Lion optimizer) to reduce the dimensionality of feature space. Further, the BOAALO uses three different classifiers, ANN, SVM, and ANFIS (Adaptive Neuro-Fuzzy Inference System), to predict breast cancer as benign or malignant using the optimal subset of features. The evaluation of the BOAALO has been tested using 651 mammogram images, and the results show that BOAALO attained better performance than the standard BOA and ALO approaches. Moreover, BOAALO has been evaluated using a standard dataset against five traditional techniques, and simulation results indicate that BOAALO attained superior performance with a minimal number of features. Table 12.1 illustrates some works on identifying breast cancer using various ML and nature-inspired algorithms.

12.3 Preliminaries

In this section, the working mechanism of the concepts used, such as Data Normalization, Principal Component Analysis (PCA), Genetic Algorithm (GA), Ant Colony Optimization (ACO), and Random Forest (RF), have been described.

12.3.1 Data Normalization

The data normalization procedure scales all the data values of a record in the range of [0, 1]. The normalization is conducted to lessen the influence of high-valued samples on the ability of classifiers [31]. Suppose $D = \begin{pmatrix} x_{11} x_{12} & \cdots & x_{1n} \\ \vdots & \ddots & \vdots \\ x_{m1} x_{m2} & \cdots & x_{mn} \end{pmatrix}$ is a high-dimensional dataset having m rows and n columns. Each point $x_{ij}, \forall i = \{1, \cdots, m\}$ and $j = \{1, \cdots, n\}$ denote an instance. The Min–Max normalization is

Table 12.1 Analysis of other works performed on the identification of breast cancer using ML and nature-inspired algorithms

Author and year	Approach	Dataset	Results	Limitations	Refs.
Macaulay et al. and 2021	Random forest classifier	180 patient's data from the surgical department of Lagos State University Teaching Hospital (LASUTH)	RF obtained an accuracy, sensitivity, specificity, and AUC of 98.33, 100, 96.55, and 98% when Chi-square selected features were included	Limited size dataset	[25]
Resmini et al. and 2021	Genetic algorithm + SVM	UFPE database consists of 60 regular and 38 cancer-detected thermal images	Accuracy = 97.18% and AUC-ROC = 94.79%	Does not consider distinct breast diagnoses	[26]
Habibi et al. and 2020	SVM + PSO	Wisconsin University UCI Machine Learning breast cancer patients database	Classification accuracy = 78.91%	Does not make utilization of a portion of the inertia weight value and the accelerated coefficient value to find the best value	[27]
Saturi et al. and 2021	ACO + PSO	BreakHis dataset	Accuracy = 95.72%	Imbalanced data set	[28]
Fang et al. and 2021	MLP + WOA	MIAS and DDSM dataset	Correct detection rate of MLP + WOA = 93.1%	Shortcomings of optimization algorithms such as premature convergence and being trapped at a local minimal point have not been considered	[29]
Hou et al. and 2020	XGBoost, Deep Neural network, and RF	Dataset consisting of 7127 breast cancer cases and 7127 healthy cases from Breast Cancer Information Management System, West China Hospital of Sichuan University	AUC of XGBoost = 0.742	Important risk factors were excluded from the study	[30]

applied on D that is mathematically illustrated as shown in Eq. (12.1):

$$Norm\_D = \frac{D - D_{min}}{D_{max} - D_{min}} \qquad (12.1)$$

where $Norm\_D$ is the normalized dataset, D_{min}, and D_{max} denotes the minimum and maximum value of the element in D. After scaling the dataset, the PCA technique is applied to the high-dimensional data for dimensionality reduction.

12.3.2 Principal Component Analysis (PCA)

As the resources for visualizing high-dimensional data in graphical form are unavailable, it is hard to identify and express the data's underlying structures (patterns) [32]. Thus, a high-dimensional dataset has been transformed into a low-dimensional one utilizing the PCA technique [32]. This method selects only a few uncorrelated instances from the correlated ones called principal components, which retain a considerable amount of information from the more extensive set. The principal components are sorted in reverse chronological order of their variances and act as a set of new axes for showing the high-dimensional data in lower dimensions.

Initially, the element x_{ij} of a matrix, D is scaled by using Eq. (12.1), producing a normalized matrix $Norm\_D$. After that, PCA is used on the normalized dataset $Norm\_D$. The basic equation of PCA in matrix format is expressed as in Eq. (12.2):

$$Z = W^T R^{-\frac{1}{2}} Norm\_D \qquad (12.2)$$

where $Z = [z_{ij}]$ is the principal component matrix, $R = [r_{ij}]$ is a correlation matrix consisting of the diagonal points of its variance–covariance matrix Q and $W = [w_{1j}, w_{2j}, \ldots, w_{ij}]^T$ is a weight vector.

12.3.3 Genetic Algorithm (GA)

The idea of formulating Darwin's "Survival of the fittest" theory into a Genetic Algorithm (GA) has been first developed by Holland in the year of 1975 [33]. In this process, searching for an optimal solution is done repetitively from an initial set of possible solutions (chromosome). Other methods like chromosome selection, crossover, and mutation operations are also used in GA to achieve the best global solution [33]. In addition, this optimization procedure helps generate a more evolved population, which is more receptive to resolving the problem than its previous counterpart [34].

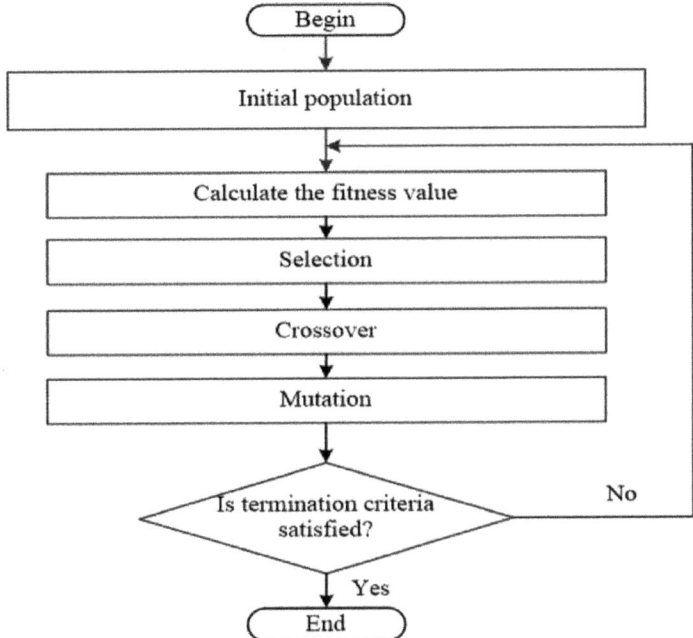

Fig. 12.3 Flowchart of a typical genetic algorithm model

Two crossover techniques, namely, n-point crossover and uniform crossover, are employed to produce offspring by merging any two chosen individuals concerning a crossover rate P_c ranging within [0.6, 1.0] [34]. Three selection methods—roulette-wheel selection, tournament selection, and ranking selection have been applied to pick the chromosomes for crossover operation. Finally, the mutation is used on the generated offspring (solution) with a mutation rate $P_m > 1\%$, so the solution does not get stuck in the local search space. Figure 12.3 depicts the flowchart of a typical GA.

12.3.4 Ant Colony Optimization (ACO)

ACO is based on finding the shortest path between a food source and an ant colony, where a few artificial ants attempt to obtain multiple solutions for a given problem [35]. Each ant searches for the shortest path from other ants to construct solutions through intensification and evaporation processes. The ants follow the pheromone trails to reach the food and communicate with other ants. ACO optimizes a problem by having an updated pheromone trail and moving these ants around in the search space according to simple mathematical formulae over the region's transition probability and total pheromone. ACO generates global ants at each iteration and calculates their fitness to update pheromone. If fitness is improved, then move local ants to better regions and update and evaporate ant pheromone. Figure 12.4 illustrates the working mechanism of ACO.

Let n be the initial ant population and $m_{i,j}^k$ be the movement of the kth ant from state i to state j with a pheromone value δ_{ij} and visibility density γ_{ij}. The probability of an ant movement is presented in Eq. (12.3) as follows:

$$m_{i,j}^k = \frac{(\delta_{i,j})^\alpha \cdot (\gamma_{i,j})^\beta}{\sum_{q \in allowed_i} (\delta_{i,q})^\alpha \cdot (\gamma_{i,q})^\beta} \quad (12.3)$$

where the parameter α is used to regulate the effect of pheromone ($0 \leq \alpha$). Similarly, β defines the significance of visibility ($\beta \geq 1$). $\delta_{i,q}$ and $\gamma_{i,q}$ indicate the pheromone and visibility density when an ant travels from state i to other probable state q, respectively. Upon finding an optimal path, the pheromones are updated as per Eq. (12.4). $\Delta\delta_{i,j}^k$ denotes the quantity of pheromone deposited by the kth ant, and ρ is the evaporation variable ($\rho \in [0, 1]$). The whole procedure will continue till the termination condition is not satisfied. At last, the searching mechanism generates the best traveling path for all ants to follow.

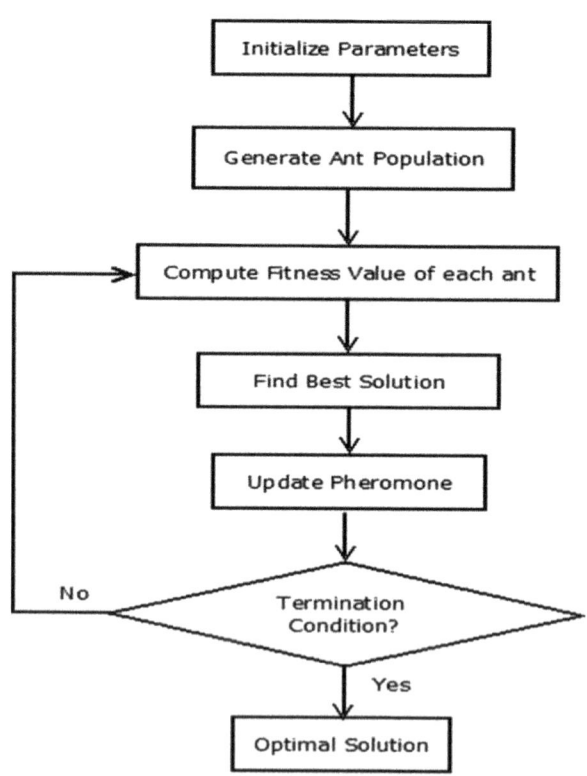

Fig. 12.4 Working mechanism of ant colony optimization algorithm

$$\delta_{i,j} = (1-\rho)\delta_{i,j} + \sum_{k}^{n} \Delta\delta_{i,j}^{k} \qquad (12.4)$$

The ACO algorithm has earlier been used to resolve global search optimization problems as it has shown strong robustness and a suitable dispersed calculative mechanism [36]. However, due to its slow convergence speed, it is highly probable to restrict to the local optimum [36].

12.3.5 Random Forest Algorithm (RF)

The Random Forest (RF) algorithm, an ensemble of decision trees, works on the Bagging principle [37]. Each tree present in the RF has been created independently through bootstrap sampling while considering the randomly selected features from the dataset. The Gini index values of the decision trees are then evaluated, and the final output is dependent on the majority voting. It is to be noted that RF is more tolerant to noise as compared to other decision tree ensembles [38]. Furthermore, RF produces high accuracy and consumes less training time than other ML techniques, making it more desirable to use on a high-dimensional large dataset. Additionally, the RF model's performance is not affected by missing data points, thus making it more robust and reliable. The working mechanism of RF has been presented below.

Suppose a dataset having n features is fed to the RF for model construction. Initially, the RF selects p attributes randomly from those n points where $p \ll n$ and determines a root node using the best split approach. Based on the root node, m decision trees are constructed that produce m opinions. Then a majority voting is done on those responses to get a result. Generally, the Gini Index is used to find a node where the best split can be done [38]. Observe each tree prediction for every incoming sample and allocate the new example to the class with the highest votes.

12.4 Proposed System

Usually, when a machine learning classifier is used on a dataset for classification purposes, its success rate is always dependent on the representation of the features [39]. Thus, selecting the most relevant attributes, known as feature selection, is necessary to improve the efficiency of a classifier [39]. Despite various feature selection techniques, most are plagued by high memory consumption and computational cost [39]. Therefore, in this work, various evolutionary algorithm-based feature selection procedures have been adopted for selecting appropriate features, thus producing a reduced dataset. After that, a supervised classifier is used on the reduced dataset to identify the nature of tumors effectively. The proposed cancer diagnosis model comprises the following three principal components:

12.4.1 Data Preprocessing Component (DPC)

Typically, the cancer database contains high-valued and high-dimensional data. Furthermore, the actual patient records cannot be published due to violating the right to privacy; rather, the researchers anonymize and publish the data for research purposes. Hence, in the current work, one such anonymized real-world breast cancer dataset, known as "Wisconsin Breast Diagnostic Cancer (WDBC)," has been used [27]. The description of the dataset has been presented in Sect. 5.1.

It is to be noted that inaccurate data representation often degrades its quality [40]. Thus, it is vital to smooth the unorganized raw data suitable for analysis. The Data Preprocessing Component (DPC) is incorporated with feature transformation techniques to facilitate the data preprocessing. This module deals with the normalization and dimensionality reduction of all the attributes. Initially, the raw records undergo the data normalization process for converting their values in the [0, 1] range. That is done to ensure that every data point will get equal opportunity rather than the high-valued attributes upon subjecting to a machine learning classifier model. As described in Sect. 3.1, the Min–Max normalization technique has been used to facilitate such a process.

Furthermore, a classifier tends to become overfitted by the high-dimensional dataset since the increase in dimension adversely affects the data space and makes them sparse [41]. The sparse data prevents the classifiers from achieving maximum efficiency by not accurately estimating the training parameters. This phenomenon is referred to as the "curse of dimensionality" problem that a dimensionality reduction technique can overcome. As the name suggests, dimensionality reduction refers to minimizing the number of features (dimension) present in a dataset so that the overfitting issue of classifiers is attenuated [41]. The attribute numbers can be lessened by obtaining a smaller set of features from the original ones (feature selection) or by performing feature extraction (constructing a new attribute set from the old ones).

Furthermore, the newly generated feature set retains all the relevant information from the actual dataset. To decrease the dimension, we used the PCA method described in Sect. 3.2. This technique initially projects the high dimensional data instances in a low dimensional geometric space and later selects the lower dimensional points with higher variance values. Thus, the original dimension is reduced by keeping only the essential features leading to a modified dataset.

12.4.2 Evolutionary Algorithm-Based Feature Selection Component (EAFSC)

The EAFSC module proposes a hybrid of two evolutionary algorithms—Genetic Algorithm (GA) and Ant Colony Optimization (ACO), termed GACO, which is used for selecting the relevant features. The GA is the simplest and vastly used optimization algorithm in feature selection. However, GA needs a longer processing time for large datasets and tends to converge prematurely, affecting achieving the best solution [42]. Similarly, ACO exhibits specific characteristics that may constrict the global search operation to a local one [42]. To deal with this issue, several researchers have developed a hybridization of the Genetic Algorithm (GA) and ACO that has fared well in various application domains like sequence alignment [42] and traveling salesman problem [43, 44]. They have demonstrated the usage of GA for creating feature subsets and ACO to incorporate local search, thereby increasing the performance of both GA and ACO.

The hybridized GACO model follows two steps: (i) employ GA to create solutions for initial ACO pheromones; (ii) continue using ACO till an optimum solution is found. For the more straightforward implementation of the first step, initially, we have encoded the solution space in binary form {0, 1}. It helps in utilizing the total efficiency of GA in generating the initial pheromone population.

Suppose the initial ACO pheromone, and visibility density are δ_{ij} and γ_{ij}, respectively. The relative significance of pheromone is $\alpha(\alpha > 0)$, β defines the importance of visibility ($\beta > 0$). At the same time, ρ signifies the evaporation rate ($\rho \in [0, 1]$). The ant chooses a search route based on the pheromone concentration from a state i to state j. The initial values of δ_{ij} is set as a small random number. The optimal binary-coded individuals generated from the first iteration of GA are given as initial input to γ_{ij}. The movement of kth ant from state i to state j is updated as follows:

$$m_{i,j}^k(0) = \frac{(\delta_{i,j}(0))^\alpha \cdot (\gamma_{i,j}(0))^\beta}{(\delta_{i,j}(0))^\alpha \cdot (\gamma_{i,j}(0))^\beta + (\delta_{i,j}(1))^\alpha \cdot (\gamma_{i,j}(1))^\beta} \quad (12.5)$$

$$m_{i,j}^k(1) = 1 - m_{i,j}^k(0) \quad (12.6)$$

where, $k = (1, 2, \ldots, N)$ ants, $m_{i,j}^k(0)$ $m_{i,j}^k(1)$ are the respective movement probabilities for binary values 0 and 1. $\delta_{i,j}(0)$ and $\gamma_{i,j}(0)$ denotes the pheromone and visibility density for binary 0, respectively. Likewise, $\delta_{i,j}(1)$ and $\gamma_{i,j}(1)$ represents the pheromone and visibility density for binary 1. Similarly, the pheromone values are updated as illustrated in Eqs. (12.7) and (12.8).

$$\delta_{i,j}(0)(t+1) = (1-\rho)\delta_{i,j}(0)(t) + \Delta\delta_{i,j}^{best} \quad (12.7)$$

$$\delta_{i,j}(1)(t+1) = (1-\rho)\delta_{i,j}(1)(t) + \Delta\delta_{i,j}^{best} \quad (12.8)$$

where, $\delta_{i,j}(t+1)$ is the pheromone value at $(t+1)$ iteration and $\Delta\delta_{i,j}^{best} = (1/best\_fit)$, $best\_fit$ is the best fitness value. The accuracy performance metric is used as the fitness function in the proposed GACO-based feature selection technique, while the Support Vector Machine (SVM) algorithm is chosen for calculating the metric. Once the first iteration of GA produces a set of optimal binary-coded populations for ACO to start, the fitness cost is computed using SVM. If the accuracy value of a current individual is higher than that of GA, the ants update their movements as per Eqs. (12.5) and (12.6), while the pheromone values are upgraded as per Eqs. (12.7) and (12.8) respectively.

12.4.3 Proposed GACO_RF Component (GRC)

The proposed GRC module presents a classification method that initially selects the most relevant features from the dataset by employing the hybridized GACO-based evolutionary feature selection method. A test set is obtained from the original preprocessed dataset. Afterward, the Random Forest (RF) classifier is trained and validated by the reduced dataset and applied to the test set for identifying benign and malignant tumors.

12.4.3.1 GACO-Based Feature Selection

It is to be noted that the selection of relevant features is the crux point as it affects the capability of a classifier. The hybrid GACO algorithm has been applied to the dataset to pick out the best attributes that needed further processing. Initially, data preprocessing is applied to the original dataset. After that, the most relevant attributes are chosen by employing the proposed GACO on the processed input data. A wrapper class methodology has been used to estimate the fitness function's cost factors. The SVM classifier has been considered for such a purpose.

The GACO-based evolutionary method produces the optimal feature subset by initially generating some attribute subsets and estimating their feasibility with the help of an objective function, as mentioned in Eq. (12.9).

$$fit(i) = \frac{Accuracy(i)}{1 + \varphi \cdot n(i)} \quad (12.9)$$

where, $fit(i)$ is the fitness value of i th ant. $Accuracy(i)$ signifies the accuracy computed by SVM. $n(i)$ refers to the number of selected attributes, while $\varphi = 0.01$ is a weighting parameter. At last, the model giving the minimal fitness cost value is selected as the optimum, and the corresponding binary encoded attribute list is used as the chosen feature subset. The bits in the reduced feature subset containing binary value one are selected, while the bits with binary value 0 are not chosen.

The suggested GACO-based feature selection algorithm has been presented below. The meaning of notations used are as given follows: $D[m][n]$ is the input preprocessed dataset having size $m \times n$, $iter$ refers to the iteration, population size (pop), , crossover ratio (P_c), mutation ratio (P_m), number of ants (N_A), pheromone rate (α), visibility rate (β), and evaporation rate (ρ).

Algorithm. Proposed GACO-based Feature Selection

Input: $D[m][n]$, $iter = 0$, pop, P_c, P_m, N_A, α, β, ρ

Output: Optimal attribute subset

Method:

Initialize GA parameters: pop, P_c, P_m and construct the initial population

while the algorithm does not reach termination condition:

do

    $iter = iter + 1$

    Compute fitness value using Eq. (9)

    Execute selection, crossover, and mutation operations of GA

    Set the initial pheromone value of ACO as per GA and generate a solution for N_A

    Calculate and update the movement probability of ants using Eq. (5) and Eq. (6)

    Compute the fitness value of each solution generated by ACO and keep the optimal one

    if the solution of ACO is better than GA:

    then

        Replace the current individual

    else:

        The GA individual does not change

    end if

    Update pheromone values using Eq. (7) and Eq. (8)

end while

12.4.3.2 Cancer Detection Using Random Forest

After the reduced feature subset had been obtained from the GACO methodology, the training and validation set were extracted from it by using k-Fold cross-validation method. Several RF models are generated and validated by the train and validation sets. Finally, the structure producing the highest classification accuracy is chosen as the best-performing one. The earlier extracted test set is given to the validated system for identifying the malignant and benign cases.

12.5 Results and Discussions

The proposed system was evaluated on a system with Intel Core i5 CPU@1.60 GHz and 8 GB RAM, running Windows 10 OS. The implementation has been done in Python 3.5 using the Jupyter Notebook. Extensive experiments were carried out on the Wisconsin Diagnostic Breast Cancer (WDBC) labeled dataset to show the efficacy [27].

12.5.1 Dataset Description

The original WDBC dataset has 569 records and 32 features containing information captured from the breast images [27]. The dataset cataloged specific behavioral characteristics of cell nuclei, such as radius, texture, perimeter, symmetry, and many more. Furthermore, these attributes' mean, error, and worst values are also documented, along with the presence of benign or malignant tumors. Out of 32 features, only 30 attributes are real-valued, while one attribute is the label denoting a malignant or benign case and another one is the patient identification number.

12.5.2 Data Preprocessing

The raw dataset is normalized in the range of [0, 1] by using Min–Max normalization as mentioned in Eq. (12.1). For transforming the high-dimensional rows into a low-dimensional ones, the PCA technique has been used on the normalized cancer records (using Eq. (12.2)). After successfully applying the PCA method to them, the GACO model is implemented to extract the most relevant features.

12.5.3 GA Parameters Estimation

Multiple experiments were carried out to determine the optimum values for the following GA parameter—crossover rate (p_c), population size (pop), and mutation rate (p_m). The parameters yielding minimum fitness cost value have been selected as the ideal combination [34]. The cost values obtained during experimentation concerning different combinations of these parameters are given in Table 12.2. The pop values vary in [10, 100] with a step of 10, similarly, p_c ranges [0.6, 1.0] by raising 0.1. Accordingly, a diversified range of p_m have been set [0.02, 0.1] with addition of 0.02 each iteration.

It is observed from the table that GA generates a minimum cost of 9.95e-5 at $pop = 50$, $p_m = 0.02$ and $p_c = 0.8$. In addition, we have also presented the time consumed (in seconds) by the GA fitness function over the iterations ranging from 10 to 100 in Table 12.3. It is evident from the table that the computational time increases proportionally with the number of iterations. Since the GA takes the least computation time at iteration = 10, it has been chosen as the ideal. Following are the optimal parameter values required for efficient working of the GACO module:

- Population Size $pop = 50$
- Crossover Rate $p_c = 0.8$
- Mutation Rate $p_m = 0.02$
- Number of Iteration $= 10$.

12.5.4 GACO Parameter Estimation

In this section, extensive experimentation was carried out to show the performance of the proposed GACO method. After experimentation, we have found the following model parameter values for GA: maximum iteration $(iter) = 10$, population size $pop = 50$, , mutation rate $(P_m) = 0.02$ and crossover rate $(P_c) = 0.8$. It is to be noted that fine-tuning parameter values could yield good results.

Multiple experiments were conducted to determine the optimum values for the GACO parameters—pheromone rate (α) and visibility rate (β). The SVM supervised classifier is the wrapper class for computing the accuracy and the selected attribute list. The tenfold cross-validation is used in the wrapper class for measuring the accuracy. Table 12.4 presents the accuracy values obtained during experimentation concerning different combinations of these parameters. The number of ants (N_A) has been set to 20. The α and β values vary [0.1, 0.9] by step of 0.1. The maximum iteration is set to 40. It is observed from the table that ACO produces the highest accuracy of 98.24% at $\alpha = 0.9$ and $\beta = 0.1$.

Before applying feature selection, the input dataset contained 30 real-valued attributes. After employing the GACO-based feature selection technique, the reduced attribute set contains only 14 features, such as the mean, worst, and error values of tumors' radius, texture, compactness, smoothness, concavity, and perimeter.

Table 12.2 Determination of optimum GA parameters

Population size	Crossover rate (p_c)				
	0.6	0.7	**0.8**	0.9	1.0
(a) $p_m = 0.02$					
10	1.22e-4	9.11e-5	8.73e-5	1.00e-4	7.48e-5
20	2.02e-4	2.88e-4	1.72e-4	2.18e-4	2.57e-4
30	1.73e-4	1.73e-4	1.86e-4	1.66e-4	1.96e-4
40	2.03e-4	1.59e-4	1.99e-4	1.19e-4	1.11e-4
50	1.67e-4	1.52e-4	**9.95e-5**	1.74e-4	3.22e-5
60	2.09e-4	1.77e-4	1.41e-4	1.15e-4	1.69e-4
70	1.14e-4	1.26e-4	1.33e-4	1.37e-4	1.31e-4
80	1.13e-4	1.60e-4	1.45e-4	1.50e-4	1.38e-4
90	1.02e-4	9.80e-5	1.52e-4	1.36e-4	1.16e-4
100	1.42e-4	1.61e-4	1.11e-4	1.17e-4	1.35e-4
(b) $p_m = 0.04$					
10	1.06e-4	1.10e-4	1.47e-4	1.28e-4	1.09e-4
20	2.18e-4	1.92e-4	1.71e-4	1.85e-4	2.10e-4
30	1.33e-4	1.55e-4	1.65e-4	2.13e-4	1.49e-4
40	1.72e-4	1.78e-4	1.26e-4	1.68e-4	1.66e-4
50	1.54e-4	1.28e-4	1.34e-4	1.40e-4	1.72e-4
60	1.39e-4	1.18e-4	1.27e-4	1.62e-4	1.56e-4
70	1.19e-4	1.29e-4	1.11e-4	1.45e-4	1.35e-4
80	9.70e-5	1.33e-4	1.20e-4	1.31e-4	1.15e-4
90	1.62e-4	1.20e-4	1.19e-4	1.55e-4	2.33e-4
100	1.20e-4	1.17e-4	1.14e-4	1.42e-4	1.30e-4
(c) $p_m = 0.06$					
10	1.10e-4	1.13e-4	7.64e-5	9.17e-5	7.08e-5
20	5.51e-4	2.21e-4	2.21e-4	2.13e-4	2.46e-4
30	1.64e-4	2.62e-4	1.96e-4	1.17e-4	2.24e-4
40	1.38e-4	1.04e-4	1.42e-4	1.45e-4	1.88e-4
50	1.29e-4	1.33e-4	1.36e-4	1.27e-4	1.58e-4
60	8.19e-5	1.08e-4	1.55e-4	1.43e-4	1.35e-4
70	1.42e-4	1.31e-4	1.26e-4	1.12e-4	1.37e-4
80	154e-4	1.56e-4	1.09e-4	1.15e-4	1.32e-4
90	1.03e-4	2.01e-4	1.28e-4	1.23e-4	1.28e-4
100	1.37e-4	1.13e-4	1.28e-4	1.24e-4	1.29e-4
(d) $p_m = 0.08$					

(continued)

Table 12.2 (continued)

Population size	Crossover rate (p_c)				
	0.6	0.7	**0.8**	0.9	1.0
10	1.02e-4	9.49e-5	8.27e-5	1.07e-4	8.56e-5
20	1.87e-4	2.22e-4	2.68e-4	1.92e-4	2.43e-4
30	1.60e-4	1.70e-4	1.98e-4	1.63e-4	2.43e-4
40	1.27e-4	3.19e-5	1.23e-4	2.02e-4	2.46e-4
50	1.67e-4	1.28e-4	1.43e-4	1.39e-4	1.33e-4
60	1.38e-4	1.41e-4	1.27e-4	2.04e-4	1.88e-4
70	1.20e-4	1.43e-4	1.27e-4	1.37e-4	1.34e-4
80	1.26e-4	1.41e-4	1.22e-4	1.09e-4	1.52e-4
90	1.21e-4	1.20e-4	1.30e-4	1.34e-4	1.61e-4
100	1.36e-4	2.41e-4	1.21e-4	1.169e-4	1.63e-4
(e) Mutation Rate $p_m = 0.1$					
10	9.52e-5	1.01e-4	7.91e-5	7.47e-5	1.53e-4
20	2.12e-4	2.38e-4	2.19e-4	1.74e-4	2.40e-4
30	1.57e-4	1.56e-4	1.51e-4	1.41e-4	2.29e-4
40	1.69e-4	1.21e-4	2.71e-4	4.46e-5	1.77e-4
50	1.38e-4	1.79e-4	1.43e-4	1.28e-4	3.04e-5
60	1.24e-4	1.31e-4	1.64e-4	3.14e-5	1.63e-4
70	3.60e-5	1.15e-4	1.36e-4	1.25e-4	2.90e-5
80	1.39e-4	1.38e-4	1.75e-4	1.38e-4	3.12e-5
90	1.03e-4	1.30e-4	1.18e-4	1.16e-4	3.73e-5
100	3.33e-5	1.01e-4	9.26e-5	1.69e-4	3.19e-5

Table 12.3 Determination of optimal iteration for GA

Iterations	Computational time (in seconds)	Number of iterations	Computational time (in seconds)
10	**12**	60	38
20	15	70	42
30	20	80	47
40	29	90	51
50	31	100	62

12.5.5 Performance Comparison of Evolutionary Feature Selection Methods

Apart from GA and ACO, another evolutionary algorithm, Particle Swarm Optimization (PSO), is employed for performance comparison. A brief idea of GA has been

Table 12.4 Determination of optimum GACO parameters

α	β	Accuracy	α	β	Accuracy
0.1	0.9	96.31	0.6	0.4	97.37
0.2	0.8	96.92	0.7	0.3	98.22
0.3	0.7	95.25	0.8	0.2	97.37
0.4	0.6	97.37	**0.9**	**0.1**	**98.24**
0.5	0.5	95.61			

illustrated in Sect. 3.3. Likewise, the functionalities of ACO have been presented in Sect. 3.4. The PSO tries to find an optimum solution set by continuously updating the location and velocity of a particle through a fitness function [45]. The current solution swarm estimates an optimal global value once a particle's present velocity and position costs are determined. The following subsection elaborately discusses the proposed GACO algorithm.

This section shows a performance comparison of our proposed GACO model with the three individual evolutionary algorithms GA, ACO, and PSO. The model exhibiting the minimum fitness cost is considered the best [39]. We have set the model parameter values experimentally for GA, ACO, and PSO as follows:

- **GA:** population size $pop = 50$, maximum iteration $= 10$, mutation rate $P_m = 0.02$ and crossover rate $P_c = 0.8$.
- **ACO:** number of ants $= 20$, maximum iteration $= 40$, $\alpha = 1$ and $\beta = 0.2$.
- **PSO:** minimum velocity $= -0.1$, swarm size $= 20$, maximum iteration $= 10$ and maximum velocity $= 0.1$.

Comparative performance analysis of the four feature selection methods is presented in Fig. 12.5. It is visible that the proposed GACO-based feature selection approach generates the minimum cost $= 0.0238$. The GACO technique finds the optimum ant numbers by efficiently utilizing the best GA populated search space.

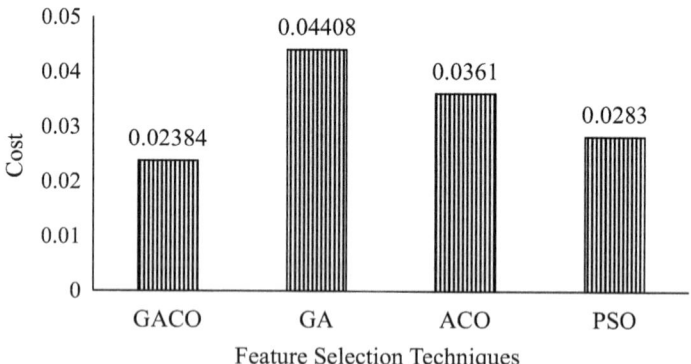

Fig. 12.5 Performance of evolutionary algorithms based feature selection methods

12.5.6 Performance Metric

The performance metric Accuracy measures the ability of the developed work. Accuracy determines the correctness of a classifier. The method producing the highest Accuracy value is considered optimal since it indicates a classifier's efficiency in recognizing a more significant number of inaccurate samples while minimizing false alarms.

$$\text{Accuracy} = \frac{TP + TN}{TP + TN + FP + FN} \quad (12.10)$$

where True Positive (TP) and True Negative (TN) show the correctly classifying samples as positive and negative, respectively. False Positive (FP) and False Negative (FN) depict the Type-I, and Type-II misclassified instances, respectively.

12.5.7 Performance Comparison of Proposed GACO_RF Model

To show the efficacy of our proposed GACO_RF model, we have presented a performance comparison with other evolutionary feature selection-based classifiers. We have employed the RF classifier on the three evolutionary algorithms—GA, PSO, and ACO individually, thus, generating models, namely, GA_RF, PSO_RF, and ACO_RF, respectively. The performance comparison of the proposed GACO_RF model with these models and RF has been provided in Fig. 12.6. It is seen from the figure that the GACO_RF produces the best outcome with a maximum accuracy of 99.122%. The suggested GACO module generates the most relevant features affecting the efficacy of the GACO_RF model. The GA_RF produces the lowest accuracy since the GA can be riddled with early convergence. Meanwhile, the accuracy of only RF and PSO_RF classifiers are almost equivalent as PSO tends to constrict itself in local search space, thus influencing the capability of RF. The ACO_RF produces an accuracy of 96.662%, which is better than the ability of GA_RF, PSO_RF and RF classification models.

Furthermore, a comparative analysis of the proposed GACO_RF model has been presented with four other works present in the literature. Habibi et al. [27] employed the PSO algorithm and SVM to select the essential attributes. Another work suggested using GA-based feature selection to choose relevant data points [46]. They have used ANN with a resilient backpropagation technique to classify the benign breast cells from the malignant ones. Kusuma et al. [47] developed a backpropagated neural network module to detect cancerous breast cells. A PSO-based non-parametric Kernel Density Estimation (KDE) system has been proposed by Sheikhpour et al. [48] for identifying the appropriate cancerous traits. It is evident from Table 12.5 that the GACO_RF model outperforms the other research in terms of accuracy.

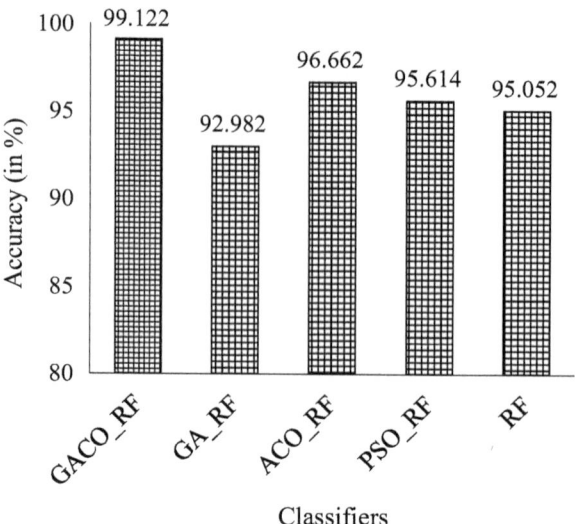

Fig. 12.6 Comparative performance analysis of classifiers

Table 12.5 Performance comparison with other studies

Author—year	Habibi et al., 2020 [27]	Ahmed at el., 2014 [46]	Kusuma et al., 2020 [47]	Sheikhpour et al., 2016 [48]	Proposed GACO_RF
Accuracy (in %)	78.91	98.29	89.80	98.45	99.122

12.6 Conclusion

Correct identification of the nature of the breast tumors with minimal relevant attributes is essential in any patient's and doctor's life. This research proposes a novel approach that uses multiple evolutionary-based optimization algorithms to select features. A hybridized Genetic Algorithm based Ant Colony Optimization (GACO) algorithm has been suggested to choose the most critical features for breast cancer diagnosis. This work further demonstrates the use of the Random Forest (RF) algorithm for accurately classifying breast tumor cells into benign or malignant classes. The effectiveness of the proposed system has been evaluated using the widely available Wisconsin Breast Diagnostic Cancer benchmark dataset. The proposed GACO_RF model has produced 99.12% accuracy, while the GACO module has a minimal cost value of 0.02384.

Moreover, the significance of fusing GA and ACO optimization methods over other optimization algorithms has been demonstrated. Besides, comparative assessment with several other evolutionary algorithm-based classification models reflects the proficiency of the proposed system in effectively distinguishing malignant breast tumors from benign ones. Moreover, an analysis of four other existing studies reflects the supremacy of the developed GACO_RF model. In the future, we aim to develop a multi-objective hybridized GACO system to increase classification accuracy while correctly finding the crucial cancerous traits.

References

1. https://www.who.int/news-room/fact-sheets/detail/breast-cancer. Accessed 14 April 2022
2. https://seer.cancer.gov/statfacts/html/breast.html. Accessed 14 April 2022
3. Lauby-Secretan, B., et al.: Breast-cancer screening—viewpoint of the IARC Working Group. N. Engl. J. Med. **372**(24), 2353–2358 (2015)
4. Ayon, S.I., Islam Md, M., Hossain Md, R.: Coronary artery heart disease prediction: a comparative study of computational intelligence techniques. IETE J. Res. 1–20 (2020)
5. Muhammad, L.J., et al.: Predictive data mining models for novel coronavirus (COVID-19) infected patients' recovery. SN Comput. Sci. **1**(4), 1–7 (2020)
6. Shamrat, F.M.J.M., et al.: Implementation of machine learning algorithms to detect the prognosis rate of kidney disease. In: 2020 IEEE International Conference for Innovation in Technology (INOCON). IEEE (2020)
7. Gogi, V.J., Vijayalakshmi, M.N.: Prognosis of liver disease: using machine learning algorithms. In: 2018 International Conference on Recent Innovations in Electrical, Electronics & Communication Engineering (ICRIEECE). IEEE (2018)
8. Diller, G.-P., et al.: Machine learning algorithms estimating prognosis and guiding therapy in adult congenital heart disease: data from a single tertiary centre including 10 019 patients. Eur. Hear. J. **40**(13), 1069–1077 (2019)
9. Amrane, M., et al.: Breast cancer classification using machine learning. In: 2018 Electric Electronics, Computer Science, Biomedical Engineerings' Meeting (EBBT). IEEE (2018)
10. Wu, J., Hicks, C.: Breast cancer type classification using machine learning. J. Pers. Med. **11**(2), 61 (2021)
11. Ganggayah, M.D., et al.: Predicting factors for survival of breast cancer patients using machine learning techniques. BMC Med. Inform. Decis. Mak. **19**(1), 1–17 (2019)
12. Gupta, D., et al.: Improved diagnosis of Parkinson's disease using optimized crow search algorithm. Comput. Electr. Eng. **68**, 412–424 (2018)
13. Goel, N., et al.: Modified grasshopper optimization algorithm for detection of autism spectrum disorder. Phys. Commun. **41**, 101115 (2020)
14. Derangula, A., Edara, S.R.: Identification of optimized features using nature-inspired meta-heuristics based optimizations in breast cancer detection. Mater. Today: Proc. (2021)
15. Sharma, M., et al.: Bio-inspired algorithms for diagnosis of breast cancer. Int. J. Innov. Comput. Appl. **10**(3–4), 164–174 (2019)
16. Kaushal, C., Kaushal, K., Singla, A.: Firefly optimization-based segmentation technique to analyze medical images of breast cancer. Int. J. Comput. Math. **98**(7), 1293–1308 (2021)
17. Ting, T.O., et al.: Hybrid metaheuristic algorithms: past, present, and future. In: Recent Advances in Swarm Intelligence and Evolutionary Computation, pp. 71–83 (2015)
18. Bouaouda, A., Sayouti, Y.: Hybrid meta-heuristic algorithms for optimal sizing of hybrid renewable energy system: a review of the state-of-the-art. Arch. Comput. Methods Eng. 1–35 (2022)
19. Stephan, P., et al.: A hybrid artificial bee colony with whale optimization algorithm for improved breast cancer diagnosis. Neural Comput. Appl. **33**(20), 13667–13691 (2021)
20. Mazen, F., AbulSeoud, R.A., Gody, A.M.: Genetic algorithm and firefly algorithm in a hybrid approach for breast cancer diagnosis. Int. J. Comput. Trends Technol. (IJCTT) **322**, 62–68 (2016)
21. Al-Quraishi, T., et al.: Breast cancer recurrence prediction using random forest model. In: International Conference on Soft Computing and Data Mining. Springer, Cham (2018)

22. Ittannavar, S.S., Havaldar, R.H.: Detection of breast cancer using the infinite feature selection with genetic algorithm and deep neural network. In: Distributed and Parallel Databases, pp. 1–23 (2021)
23. Islam Md, M., et al.: Breast cancer prediction: a comparative study using machine learning techniques. SN Comput. Sci. **1**(5), 1–14 (2020)
24. Thawkar, S., et al.: Breast cancer prediction using a hybrid method based on butterfly optimization algorithm and ant lion optimizer. Comput. Biol. Med. **139**, 104968 (2021)
25. Macaulay, B.O., et al.: Breast cancer risk prediction in African women using random forest classifier. Cancer Treat. Res. Commun. **28**, 100396 (2021)
26. Resmini, R., et al.: Combining genetic algorithms and SVM for breast cancer diagnosis using infrared thermography. Sensors **21**(14), 4802 (2021)
27. Habibi, R.: SVM performance optimization using PSO for breast cancer classification. Bp. Int. Res. Exact Sci. (BirEx) J. **3**(1), 28–41 (2021)
28. Saturi, R., Premchand, P.: Multi-objective feature selection method by using ACO with PSO algorithm for breast cancer detection. Int. J. Intell. Eng. Syst. **14**(5), 359–368 (2021)
29. Fang, H., et al.: Automatic breast cancer detection based on optimized neural network using whale optimization algorithm. Int. J. Imaging Syst. Technol. **31**(1), 425–438 (2021)
30. Hou, C., et al.: Predicting breast cancer in Chinese women using machine learning techniques: algorithm development. JMIR Med. Inform. **8**(6), e17364 (2020)
31. Tax, D.M., Duin, R.P.: Feature scaling in support vector data descriptions. In: Learning from Imbalanced Datasets, pp. 25–30 (2000)
32. Smith, L.I.: A Tutorial on Principal Components Analysis (2002)
33. Holland, J.H.: Adaptation in Natural and Artificial Systems: An Introductory Analysis with Applications to Biology, Control, and Artificial Intelligence. MIT Press, Cambridge (1992)
34. Bäck, T., Schwefel, H.-P.: An overview of evolutionary algorithms for parameter optimization. Evol. Comput. **1**(1), 1–23 (1993)
35. Dorigo, M., Birattari, M., Stutzle, T.: Ant colony optimization. IEEE Comput. Intell. Mag. **1**(4), 28–39 (2006)
36. Niu, S.H., Ong, S.K., Nee, A.Y.C.: An enhanced ant colony optimizer for multi-attribute partner selection in virtual enterprises. Int. J. Prod. Res. **50**(8), 2286–2303 (2012)
37. Wang, S., et al.: An improved random forest-based rule extraction method for breast cancer diagnosis. Appl. Soft Comput. **86**, 105941 (2020)
38. Chen, Y., et al.: Large group activity security risk assessment and risk early warning based on random forest algorithm. Pattern Recognit. Lett. **144**, 1–5 (2021)
39. Saeys, Y., Inza, I., Larranaga, P.: A review of feature selection techniques in bioinformatics. Bioinformatics **23**(19), 2507–2517 (2007)
40. Kotsiantis, S.B., Kanellopoulos, D., Pintelas, P.E.: Data preprocessing for supervised learning. Int. J. Comput. Sci. **1**(2), 111–117 (2006)
41. Bellman, R., Kalaba, R.: Dynamic programming, invariant imbedding and quasilinearization: comparisons and interconnections. In: Computing Methods in Optimization Problems, pp. 135–145 (1964)
42. Lee, Z.-J., et al.: Genetic algorithm with ant colony optimization (GA-ACO) for multiple sequence alignment. Appl. Soft Comput. **8**(1), 55–78 (2008)
43. Changdar, C., Pal, R.K., Mahapatra, G.S.: A genetic ant colony optimization-based algorithm for solid multiple traveling salesmen problem in fuzzy rough environment. Soft Comput. **21**(16), 4661–4675 (2017)
44. Wan, Y., et al.: A feature selection method based on modified binary-coded ant colony optimization algorithm. Appl. Soft Comput. **49**, 248–258 (2016)
45. Xue, B., Zhang, M., Browne, W.N.: Particle swarm optimization for feature selection in classification: a multi-objective approach. IEEE Trans. Cybern. **43**(6), 1656–1671 (2012)
46. Ahmad, F., Isa, N.A.M., Hussain, Z., Osman, M.K., Sulaiman, N.S.: A GA-based feature selection and parameter optimization of an ANN in diagnosing breast cancer. Pattern Anal. Appl. **18**(4), 861–870 (2015)

47. Kusuma, E.J., Shidik, G.F., Pramunendar, R.A.: Optimization of neural network using Nelder Mead in breast cancer classification. Int. J. Intell. Eng. Syst. **13**, 330–337 (2020)
48. Sheikhpour, R., Sarram, M.A., Sheikhpour, R.: Particle swarm optimization for bandwidth determination and feature selection of kernel density estimation based classifiers in diagnosis of breast cancer. Appl. Soft Comput. **40**, 113–131 (2016)

Milton Keynes UK
Ingram Content Group UK Ltd.
UKHW020606201123
432904UK00002B/26